Medical Emergencies
Diagnosis and Management

Medical Emergencies
Diagnosis and Management

SIXTH EDITION

RICHARD ROBINSON
FRCP
formerly Registrar to the Renal Unit, Guy's Hospital,
London

ROBIN STOTT
MA, FRCP
Consultant Physician, Lewisham Hospital, Lewisham

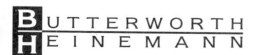

BUTTERWORTH
HEINEMANN

Butterworth-Heinemann Ltd
Linacre House, Jordan Hill, Oxford OX2 8DP

$\mathcal{R}$ A member of the Reed Elsevier group

OXFORD   LONDON   BOSTON
MUNICH   NEW DELHI   SINGAPORE   SYDNEY
TOKYO   TORONTO   WELLINGTON

First published 1970
Second edition 1976
Reprinted with revisions 1977
Reprinted 1979
Third edition 1980
Reprinted 1981
Fourth edition 1983
Reprinted 1985, 1986
Fifth edition 1987
Reprinted 1989 (twice), 1991
Sixth edition 1993

British Library Cataloguing in Publication Data
Robinson, Richard
  Medical Emergencies: Diagnosis and
  Management.—6Rev.ed
  I. Title   II. Stott, Robin
  616.025

ISBN 0 7506 0897 8

Printed and bound in Great Britain

Contents

Foreword

Every well-educated, newly appointed, pre-registration house offi-cer on the way to answer a call to deal with a medical emergency experiences the same anxieties about his ability to discharge his responsibilities when he gets there. One of my own strong memor-ies is set in the casualty room at Johns Hopkins where I was acting as a locum intern: I recall a more senior colleague—long since an eminent professor of medicine—reaching up to take bottles of sterile glucose from the shelf as the comatose (hypoglycaemic) patient was wheeled in on the ambulance trolley. How could one, I wondered, ever match this speedy diagnostic acumen and authori-tative management?

By experience, of course. But also through the knowledge accumulated by those who have faced the situation before and made important contributions by indicating the essential features to enquire about in the history, the signs to seek in the clinical examination, the laboratory measurements to order, and the first steps to take in management.

Emergencies are situations more than any others where one feels the drawbacks of our learning being divided into medical and surgical subjects, and further subdivided now into the organ specialties. House officers have to assemble in a trice knowledge from many sources. In a way, this is the strength of the young pre-registration or post-registration house officer: in this era of fast expanding knowledge he or she is, across the board, most up to date. But it demands a superb memory and a flexibility of thought given to very few of us.

Richard Robinson and Robin Stott realised the need for a pocket manual about the essentials of the current diagnostic, therapeutic and management principles, to deal properly with medical emer-gencies. So they have written this book, to bring together infor-mation widely scattered in textbooks on many subjects. They have set things down on the assumption, correct I believe, that the users will be the graduates of the present era, au fait with current hospital facilities and modern drugs. They have aimed to help them by concise writing. Here and there, the approach may be regarded as didactic, but that hardly matters in the emergency situation. I therefore commend this book to all those young people into whose hands our most seriously ill emergencies first come, with my best wishes to them for quick and accurate diagnosis, and to their patients, for speedy recovery !

W. J. H. Butterfield, OBE, DM, FRCP
Emeritus Regis Professor of Physic,
Addenbrooke's Hospital, Cambridge

Preface

The aim of this book is still to supply a framework of knowledge into which the house physician can fit his or her experience. Some of the facilities mentioned are not available in many hospitals. If, by creating awareness of deficiencies, patient care is improved, this book will be justified.

Since this book was first written we have become acutely aware of another dimension of its subject. The sobering fact is that the bulk of medical emergencies, which attract so much glamour and therefore money, talent and facilities, are preventable. This applies to each of the big four—coronary artery disease, cerebrovascular accidents, acute respiratory failure and overdoses. A moment's thought will show that the causes of each of these lie in the way we respond to our social and economic situation. The increasingly complex technology of medicine has been associated with the increasing isolation of its practitioners. This has led to a pre-empting by doctors of major areas of the patient's involvement with his disease. It is all too easy to treat patients in a life-threatening situation as a physiological preparation, and to over-look the fact that the patient and his family have lived with the roots of his disease, will probably continue to do so, and will have to live with its results.

Effective prevention of these conditions will probably only begin when the responsibility for health care is taken where it belongs—in the community. The effect of this aspect of treatment—which we have almost wholly ignored—will be far greater than the results obtained by the successful management of acute emergencies.

Introduction to the sixth edition

When we look back at the first edition of this book, printed over 20 years ago, we realise the extent to which the factual and technical base of medicine has changed. So also has the whole climate in which we practise medicine. The welcome, and increasing role that patients play in determining the direction of their care, the recognition of the importance of rigorous evaluation of all that we do, and of the impact of thoughtful organisational change on improving the process of care are all features of our present practice. There is also an increasing recognition of the importance of education, housing, economic wellbeing and a healthy environment in the promotion of health. We have only to look at the deteriorating health status of most who live in the third world, as well as those living in poverty in the first world, to understand the importance of all these factors in health. More parochially, there has within hospital practice been a tendency for physicians to become increasingly specialized, a trend which we believe makes the need for care guidelines of the sort contained in this edition more vital than ever.

The emergence of AIDS has altered many aspects of acute medicine beyond recognition. We have therefore included a detailed section on AIDS in this edition. This is the only new chapter, although all the others have been updated and some rewritten. AIDS has also brought into clearer focus the difficult ethical decisions confronting those of us involved in health care work. It is our belief that sharing information honestly and compassionately with our patients (or, where they are incapable, their relatives) is the only basis upon which such decisions can be made. Such sharing demands communication skills which are still sadly lacking—we hope that those reading this book recognise with us that a clear diagnosis and management plan can only be really helpful where it is seen to be the basis for effective communication, and dedicate the book to the furtherance of such communication amongst health care professionals.

Acknowledgements

Cardiovascular	Graham Jackson
Respiratory	Mac Cochrane
Gastrointestinal	Gordon Sladen
Renal	Chisholm Ogg
Endocrine	Stephanie Amiel
Neurology	Richard Hughes
The overdose	Glyn Volans
General/AIDS	Lionel Lewis
Psychiatric and social problems	Derry MacDiarmid
	Judy Delap
Sickle cell anaemia	Mark Dudley

Also Helen Crimlisk, who read and amended the manuscript from the 'user's' point of view.

Cardiovascular

Cardiac arrest[5,10,11,12]

Before you ever have to deal with a cardiac arrest be prepared by:

(1) knowing how to use the defibrillator;
(2) knowing how to inflate the patient with 100% oxygen;
(3) attending a resuscitation programme, or viewing the British Heart Foundation video

DIAGNOSIS

Cardiac arrest can be considered to have occurred if the carotid or femoral pulses are absent. Do not waste time trying to hear the heart. There are three main mechanisms for cardiac arrest.[6, 12]

(i)   Ventricular fibrillation (approx. 80%).
(ii) Asystole (approx. 15%).
(iii) Electromechanical dissociation, where near normal complexes on the ECG are not associated with an output. This is most likely to occur in:

   (a) hypovolaemia;
   (b) tamponade;
   (c) massive pulmonary embolus or tension pneumothorax;
   (d) a huge infarct;
   (e) drug overdose;
   (f) hypothermia;
   (g) electrolyte imbalance;

all of which you should therefore consider and treat as appropriate.

   However initial management of cardiac arrest does not depend on an accurate diagnosis of the cause.

MANAGEMENT

Your aim is to reperfuse both brain and heart by restoring an appropriate heart rhythm. If this is not achieved within 90 s the ultimate prognosis is poor. By far the most important measure is to deliver a 200 J shock to the heart, which should be given immediately a defibrillator is available, and regardless of the cause of the arrest (a shock will not harm those who turn out to have asystole or EMD). If this initial shock is unsuccessful, two further shocks, one of 200 J, the next of 340 J should be tried as necessary. It is both the availability of, and training in the immediate use of defibrillators which is the most important issue in successful resuscitation. In the event of this initial shock regime being unsuccessful, or the defibrillator not being immediately available, you will need to know how to undertake closed cardiopulmonary resuscitation (CPR). If this is started immediately, and carried out efficiently, you will be able to achieve cerebral blood flows greater than 20% of normal—the minimum needed to ensure full neurological recovery. Delay exponentially reduces your chances of achieving this goal.[9] So:

(1) Check the time and thump the sternum firmly. This may restore a reasonable rhythm. If you have immediate access to a defibrillator, as we hope you will have, proceed at once to deliver up to three shocks, the first two using 200 J, the third at 360 J, as necessary (see 11 below). With modern machines which recharge quickly, you should be able to give these three shocks within the crucial 90 s.

(2) Ensure the patient is on a firm surface and start cardiac massage at about 80 compressions per minute. Effective cardiac massage produces a femoral pulse. The forward blood flow is as much dependant on swings in intrathoracic pressure (chest pump mechanism) as direct heart compression (heart pump mechanism)

(3) Get someone to give mouth-to-mouth respiration (the aesthetics of this can be improved by using a laerdal pocket mask, or failing this, laying a handkerchief over the face of the patient). It is essential to tilt the head backwards and displace the mandible forwards to maintain a patent airway while giving mouth-to-mouth respiration. Give 5 compressions to one inflation. Whilst it is not necessary to stop compressing the heart whilst your assistant inflates the chest,[4] it is in practice easier to do so.

(4) Check that the anaesthetist and emergency trolly, ECG, or oscilloscope, and defibrillator have all been sent for.

(5) Get a sucker. The patient will soon vomit if he has not already done so.

(6) Establish intravenous access by whichever method you feel most adept at.

(7) Endotracheal drug administration.[7] If you cannot establish i.v. access, two and a half times the i.v. dose of adrenaline, lignocaine and atropine can be given via the endotracheal tube, in 10–20 ml of saline. You should disperse the drug by the use of positive pressure ventilation with a few hyperinflations.

(8) If the anaesthetist is not forthcoming insert the cuffed endotracheal tube yourself—size 7–8 for an average sized female and 8–9 for a male. Re-acquaint yourself with this technique by practising after each unsuccessful cardiac arrest. The patient must not become hypoxic. If you have difficulty intubating, stop every 30 s and re-inflate as in (3) above for 1–2 min before attempting to intubate again.

(9) Check that the tube is in the trachea by pressing the chest and getting a puff back up the tube, by looking for equal movement of the chest wall, and by auscultating to ensure that you can hear breath sounds over the apex and base of both lungs. Anchor the tube to the face by taping or strapping.

(10) Attach the patient to your source of oxygen supply and inflate once every 5 s or after every fifth compression.

(11) **Ventricular fibrillation**. Deliver a 200 J shock with the defibrillator as soon as it arrives. In cardiac arrest due to ventricular fibrillation (VF) this is by far the most important treatment. Delay, in order to establish the nature of the cardiac arrhythmia, lessens the chances of successfully provoking a return to sinus rhythm. Delivering a shock will do the patient no harm if the heart is in asystole or electromechanical dissociation. Points to remember are:

    (i) Straddle the electrodes across the heart—preferably one on the anterior chest wall and one just outside the cardiac apex.

    (ii) You will probably be using defibrillator pads, but if not, do not get electrode jelly smeared across the skin between the electrodes—it will conduct current. (caution—KY jelly does not contain electrolytes and is less efficient).

    (iii) Do not stand in puddles of blood or saline.

    (iv) If you are not using defibrillator pads, ensure that the electrodes are smeared with fresh jelly at each attempt.

    (v) Ensure that no one else is touching the patient or the bed.

(12) Attach the patient to an ECG or an oscilloscope as soon as possible. Machines in which the defibrillator paddles also act as ECG electrodes are now the norm.

(13) If VF persists after three attempts at DC conversion (the last using 360 J)

    (i)   Give adrenaline 1 mg (1 ml of 1:1000 solution) (the UK resuscitation council now recommend giving adrenaline before lignocaine, in the hope that it will improve the cerebral and coronary circulation). Then give 10 sequences of CPR, following the normal routine of five compressions to one breath.

    (ii)   Now try and defibrillate again, using three shocks of 360 J as necessary.

    (iii) If you are not successful, repeat the cycle of adrenaline and CPR and defibrillation, as outlined in 13 (i) and (ii) above, three times.

    (iv) If, after these three cycles your patient is still in VF, the situation is now desperate, and recovery unlikely. Try giving lignocaine 100 mg.

    (v)   If, after a further three cycles of adrenaline and CPR and defibrillation, you are still unsuccessful, one or more of the following drugs are worth trying intravenously:

        (a) Bretylium tosylate 5 mg/kg i.v. (followed by 100 mg i.m. hourly to a maximum of 2.0 g). Should you successfully control VF, maintain a lignocaine infusion 2–4 mg/min for 24 hours.

        (b) Magnesium sulphate 5–10 mmol of a 20% solution (6–12 ml)

    Bad prognostic signs are:

    (i)   Steadily decreasing amplitude of fibrillation. The amplitude may be increased by giving further doses of adrenaline.

    (ii)   A tendency for DC shock to cause asystole.

(14) **Aystole**. Once that it has become clear that the heart is in asystole try to restart a normal rhythm or at least provoke VF, which you can then treat as outlined above.

    (i)   Give:

        (a) 10 ml of 1:10 000 adrenaline (or 1 ml of 1:1000 adrenaline) i.v., which now has precedence over atropine, followed by 10 sequences of CPR, following the normal routine of 5 compressions to one breath

(b) then atropine 3 mg i.v., which you should give once only. This relieves the cholinergic depression of the sinus and a.v. nodes. Its use is associated with increased survival from asystolic arrest.[3]

(ii) If you have provoked fibrillation, proceed as for the treatment of VF.

(iii) If you have not provoked fibrillation repeat the dose of adrenaline as in (i a) above.

(iv) We, in common with the UK Resuscitation Council, no longer recommend the use of intracardiac adrenaline.

(v) If, after the return of the heart rhythm, your patient remains persistently bradycardic, pacing may be required.

(15) Remember that recovery from aystole is uncommon. Unless aystole is associated with hypothermia, it is unwise to persist with resuscitation for more than about 15 min.

(16) **Electro-mechanical dissociation (EMD).** Here, the correction of any of the provoking causes should get first priority (see under diagnosis). If this is not effective, give adrenaline as you would in VF.

Whilst all the above is going on, 10–15 min will have elapsed. By this time the patient should be reasonably pink. If he is not, consider the following:

(i) Efforts at ventilation are insufficient. The usual tendency is to under-estimate the rate and depth of ventilation needed and it is sometimes salutary to measure the blood gases during a cardiac arrest.

(ii) The patient has inhaled masses of vomit. Suck this out through the endotracheal tube. If your resuscitation is subsequently successful remember to give high doses of corticosteroids as a prophylaxis to vomit induced 'shock lung' (see p. 97).

(iii) The patient has had a massive pulmonary embolus. The lungs will resist inflation.

(iv) The oxygen supply has run out. You don't know when this occurred so carry on.

(v) The patient has a pneumothorax (see p. 85).

(17) Sodium bicarbonate—for a long time we have been aware that infusion of $NaHCO_3$ may give rise to a paradoxical increase in intracellular acidosis. For this reason its routine use is not now recommended. However, if during a prolonged arrest the arterial pH is less than 7.1, as measured on blood gas analysis, we suggest giving 50 ml of 8.4% $NaHCO_3$ (50 mmol).

(18) Calcium chloride 5–10 ml of a 10% solution i.v. the use of this is now contentious—we only give it for specific indications, such as a recent blood transfusion, or in patients known to be on calcium channel blockers or to have hyperkalaemia or hypocalcaemia.

(19) Other points to bear in mind are:

    (i) The cause of the arrest: acute hypoxia, fits, upper airways obstruction, electrolyte disturbances such as hypo- or hyperkalaemia, and digoxin poisoning, are potentially reversible. Severe brain injury, massive pulmonary emboli and ruptured aortic anaeurysms are not.

    (ii) Full recovery has been recorded after the pupils have been fully dilated. This sign is not in itself a sufficient reason for stopping.

    (iii) Do not forget cardiac tamponade (p. 65). If due to a tense effusion it may be necessary to aspirate the pericardial space or if due to blood clot an emergency thoracotomy (at the bedside) is indicated. So call those who have appropriate experience. The heart may then be defibrillated directly using internal paddles. A thoracotomy may also have to be performed if you are not obtaining an adequate circulation for some other reason, e.g. regurgitant heart valves.

    (iv) Finally—and more rapidly acquired with experience than you might think—try and keep a detached attitude. When the situation is under control, e.g. the drip is up, the patient is being inflated and the ECG or oscilloscope is running, get someone else to do the cardiac massage, step back and decide what you are going to do next and for how long you are going to continue.

(20) There is increasing interest in measures which might help reduce the effects of cerebral ischaemia which occur as a consequence of the reduced cerebral circulation during cardiopulmonary resuscitation. There is preliminary evidence that

calcium channel blockers may help. Other measures used to reduce intracranial pressure (see p. 220) have also been tried, without obvious benefit. We, in common with others, do not think these therapies are justified at present.[11]

(21) Although open heart massage has become unfashionable, it is important to remember that it is a much more efficient way of generating blood flow than is closed massage.[9] The situations where this is the process of choice, are indicated below:

(i) Where treatable intrathoracic pathology has caused the cardiac arrest, e.g. uncontrolled haemorrhage.

(ii) When you cannot produce a carotid pulse by sternal compression.

(iii) As a last step in treating intractable VF. This may particularly occur in hypothermia (see p. 291).

Technique

(a) This should only be undertaken by those who have the necessary surgical training. Cut through skin and muscle overlying the 4th or 5th intercostal space. Pierce other intercostal structures with a blunt instrument, and spread open the intercostal space with your fingers or a rib spreader.

(b) Compress the heart by placing your right hand behind it, with the thenar eminence and a thumb in front of it.

(c) All drugs, except for HCO_3, may safely be given via the intracardiac route.

(d) Defibrillation. Use insulated paddle electrodes with saline soaked paddles. Place one behind the left ventricle, the other in front of the heart. Use 0.5 J / kg body weight initially, increasing the energy as necessary.

(22) The cause of the arrest, the age of the patient and the response to treatment are all factors to take into account when deciding to abandon resuscitation. However, a large survey found no survivors among patients in whom resuscitation attempts had lasted more than 30 min.[2]

(23) After successful resuscitation from the arrest, check the arterial blood gases, ECG, electrolytes and a chest x-ray, to identify any residual abnormalities which may require treatment, and transfer your patient to a coronary care unit for monitoring. It is probably safe to use fibrinolytics (see p. 12)

if the evidence for a myocardial infarct as the cause of the arrest is clear-cut.

References

1   Aitkenhead A. (1986) Cerebral protection. *Br. J. Hosp. Med.* **35**: 290.

2   Bedell S. E. *et al.* (1983) Survival after cardiopulmonary resuscitation in the hospital. *N. Engl. J. Med.* **809**: 569.

3   Camm A. J. (1986) Asystole and electromechanical dissociation. *Br. Med. J.* **292**: 1123.

4   Chandras N., Rudiboff M., Weisfeldt M. I. (1980) Simultaneous chest compression and ventilation at high airway pressure during cardiopulmonary resuscitation. *Lancet* **i**: 175.

5   Chamberlain D. A. (1989) Advanced life support. *Br. Med. J.* **299**: 446.

6   Chamberlain D. A. (1986) Ventricular fibrillation. *Br. Med. J.* **292**: 106.

7   Leader (1988) Intratracheal drugs. *Lancet* **i**: 743.

8   Sabin H. I. *et al.* (1983) Accuracy of intracardiac injections determined by post-mortem study. *Lancet* **ii**: 1054.

9   Safar P. (1984) Recent advances in cardiopulmonary–cerebral resuscitation: a review. *Ann. Emerg. Med.* **13**: 856.

10 Skinner D. (1989) Monitoring resuscitation. *Br. Med. J.* **298**: 1597.

11 Yatsu F. M. (1986) Cardiopulmonary–cerebral resuscitation. *N. Engl. J. Med.* **314**: 446.

12 Guidelines for advanced life support—A statement by the advanced life support working party of the European resuscitation council (1992) *Resuscitation* **24**: 111.

Myocardial infarction

DIAGNOSIS

(1) Myocardial infarction usually presents with a history of severe crushing retrosternal chest pain, often radiating to the neck and arms. The patient often perspires and is nauseated. Those with previous angina fail to obtain the usual relief from nitrates.

(2) However, it may present in a number of indirect ways, particularly in the elderly, for example:

  (i)   Acute left ventricular failure.
  (ii) Unexplained hypotension (particularly postoperatively).
  (iii) A peripheral embolus.
  (iv) Fainting, giddy turns, palpitations or collapse.
  (v)   A stroke.

Remember that pain may be felt in the traditional referral sites only.

(3) Now that the early benefits of the thrombolytic therapy are clear, early diagnosis of infarction is very important.[23] Unfortunately, it is sometimes difficult to be certain if infarction has occurred. Serial ECGs and cardiac enzymes usually resolve the dilemma, but not before the thrombolytic window of opportunity has passed, as the creatinine phosphokinase (CPK) rise does not occur until between 6 and 10 h of the infarct, at which time ECG changes are almost always present. A good history, coupled with ST elevation, are the criteria we use before giving thrombolytics. A proportion of patients with ischaemic chest pain, transient ST segment depression and normal CPK may have the pre-infarction syndrome (see p. 23). Only if these changes fail to resolve within 2 h of treatment would we assume infarction has taken place, and give thrombolytics, as this group have not yet been shown to benefit from thrombolytic therapy.

Cardiac Troponin T, a unique myocardial antigen, is released into the circulation earlier than CPK, and is more specific. It may well have a role in helping the early diagnosis of infarction.[14]

MANAGEMENT

You must establish intravenous access as soon as possible. Drugs must be given i.v. both for speed and because absorption from other routes is less certain when perfusion is diminished. Then:

(1) Control pain.

  (i) Diamorphine 5 mg i.v. or morphine 5–10 mg i.v. (each with prochlorperazine 12.5 mg i.m.—we are wary of cyclizine, as it has a cardiodepressant effect)[22]—are still the drugs of choice.

  (ii) Isosorbide dinitrate, given in a starting dose of 2 mg/h, and increasing to 10 mg/h as necessary, may be used to relieve pain which persists despite opiates. Until the i.v. infusion is under way give sublingual glyceryl trinitrate 0.5 mg. Nitrates may have other benefits (see (3) below).

  (iii) Under no circumstances withhold these drugs from patients suffering from myocardial pain. If you are worried by the possibility of respiratory depression, monitor the blood gases and treat appropriately. (p. 73). Where necessary, respiratory and circulatory depression due to narcotics can be counteracted by:

   (a) Naloxone 0.4–1.2 mg i.v. in divided doses over 3 min.
   (b) Doxapram, by continuous infusion, 1.5 mg/min to a maximum of 2.5 mg/min.

(2) Arrhythmias must be treated (see p. 26).

(3) Therapy directed at reducing infarct size and thus minimizing the risk of sudden death, and maximizing the long-term outlook, should be started as soon as possible.

  (i) Give aspirin—150 mg orally initially, then 75 mg orally each day.[10, 11]

  (ii) Fibrinolytics. Streptokinase, the cheapest and most readily available of these is as good as any, and should be given as soon as possible. [10, 11] Give 1.5 million units in 100 ml of normal saline i.v. over 30 min. In patients who have recently received streptokinase (5 days to 12 months), the presence of antibodies is likely to make a subsequent dose of the drug ineffective. They should therefore be given an alternative thrombolytic, such as tissue plasminogen activator (t–PA) 0.5–0.75 mg/kg body weight, i.v. over 90 min.[15, 25]

Absolute contraindications to fibrinolytics are active bleeding or a bleeding diathesis, aortic dissection, proliferative diabetic retinopathy and pregnancy. Relative contraindications are severe hypertension—(systolic >200 mmHg, diastolic >115 mmHg, active peptic ulceration, recent stroke or GI bleed (within the past 2 months), and recent trauma or surgery (within the past 10 days). If you observe these contraindications, the incidence of side effects is small.[18]

Fibrinolytics are maximally effective if given within 4 h, but a small benefit persists up to 12–24 h.

(iii) There is increasing evidence that i.v. heparin as an initial bolus of 5000 IU and then 1000 IU/h for at least 24 h adjusted to keep the PTT about twice normal, further reduces infarct size and reocclusion.

(iv) Nitrates. Pooling of all the presently available trial data suggests that i.v. nitrates, given as for pain relief, may reduce infarct size and hospital mortality.[26] We do not presently give nitrates to all our infarcts, but do use it freely.

(v) Beta-Blockers. When given intravenously within 12 h of the onset of pain, these prevent early cardiac rupture. They seem to have a synergistic effect with thrombolytics. Most clinicians now give 5–10 mg of atenolol i.v. as soon as possible, and 50 mg orally each day thereafter.[5] Clearly, nobody with contraindications to beta-blockers (av dissociation, pulmonary oedema, systolic blood pressure <100 mmHg, pulse rate <60/min or concurrent administration of any other antiarrhythmic) should be given this therapy.

(vi) The angiotensin converting enzyme inhibitor captopril, initially 25 mg twice daily provided that there has been no adverse response to a 6.25 mg test dose, has been shown in one trial to improve ventricular function post infarct.[20] We do not use it as yet.

(vii) Neither percutaneous coronary angioplasty (PTCA) nor bypass grafting confers any benefit in those patients given thrombolytics, and has no place in uncomplicated acute infarcts.[8, 21] The role of PTCA in cardiogenic shock, and in those patients in whom fibrinolytics are contraindicated, is being evaluated.

(4) Heart failure.

    (i)   May be aggravated by pain or arrhythmias, which should be treated appropriately. Otherwise impaired ventricular function results from either loss of functioning muscle, (the common early cause) or from mechanical disruption of the ventricular wall (VSD or tamponade), or valves (mitral incompetence). Mechanical problems usually occur between the second and tenth day.

    (ii)   Invasive haemodynamic studies in normals show that cardiac output is between 2.2 and 4.3 l/m²/min. If the measured output falls below 2.2 l/m²/min, clinical symptoms of poor perfusion (cool peripheries, hypotension, oliguria, urinary output <20 ml/h and a tendency towards mental confusion) appear. This clinical state is best called pump failure.[7]

        Normal subjects have a pulmonary capillary wedge pressure (PCWP a measure of left ventricular end diastolic pressure, and an indirect measure of left atrial pressure) of <18 mmHg. If the PCWP >25 mmHg, the

Table 1

Group	Clinical features	Haemodynamic characteristics	Average mortality
a	No pulmonary oedema	Normal PCWP <18 mmHg	1%
	Good perfusion	Normal cardiac output >2.2 l m⁻² min⁻¹	
b	Pulmonary oedema	Raised PCWP >25 mmHg	10%
	Good perfusion	Normal cardiac output >2.2 l m⁻² min⁻¹	
c1	No pulmonary oedema Poor perfusion	PCWP <18 mmHg Low cardiac output <2.2 l m⁻² min⁻¹	20%
c2	As above, but with a high central venous pressure—see text		
d	Pulmonary oedema Poor perfusion	PCWP >25mm/Hg Low cardiac output	60%

signs of pulmonary oedema develop—dyspnoea, late inspiratory crackles at the lung bases, added heart sounds, engorgement of the upper lobe pulmonary veins on the CXR, which may also show radiological evidence of oedema. This clinical state is best designated pulmonary oedema due to left ventricular failure.

(iii) Haemodynamic studies in patients with myocardial infarction, measuring cardiac output and wedge pressures, have shown there to be four groups of patients (a–d below). These invasive studies correlate well with the clinical picture, and so we use the following clinical classification on which to build a rational approach to therapy (see Table 1).

TREATMENT

All these groups require treatment as outlined in (1)–(3) above.

Group a

No further treatment.

Group b

(1) Nitrates (see p. 13), and a diuretic such as frusemide 20–40 mg i.v., are the best means of reducing the elevated wedge pressure, and thus relieving pulmonary oedema.

(2) You should monitor the dose in accordance with your patient's response. Clinical improvement often precedes both radiological improvement and the disappearance of physical signs. Excessive diuresis can cause hypovolaemia, so be aware of the discordance between symptoms and signs when adjusting the diuretic dose.

(3) It is probable that captopril, in an initial dose of 6.25 mg b.d., will be useful here, but this is as yet unproven.

(4) If you are not controlling the failure with these measures, further treatment should be as for group d.

Groups c and d

These two constitute the entity sometimes called 'cardiogenic shock'.[4] Before embarking on therapy it is invaluable to have a

Swan–Ganz catheter in place to measure both cardiac output and PCWP. You should also measure central venous pressure. This will distinguish between those patients in group c who have hypovolaemia, where the CVP will be low, and those with predominantly right-sided ventricular damage, in whom the CVP will be high.[2]

Group c

(1) Both hypovolaemia and predominantly right-sided failure can cause the combination of a low cardiac output and a low or normal PCWP. The central venous pressure, low in hypovolaemia, is raised in right-sided failure, and will therefore separate these two categories.

Hypovolaemia after an infarct is more common than generally appreciated,[4] in part related to the anorexia, sweating and vomiting that accompany infarction, and needs urgent treatment. Proceed as follows:

   (i)   Give i.v. Haemocel, plasma or albumin, until the PCWP approaches 18 mmHg or the CVP approaches the upper range of normal (see p. 14) without the development of tachypnoea.

(2) If the initial CVP was high, or the PCWP and cardiac output do not respond to the above treatment, you are dealing with right ventricular failure.[2] Assuming this is due to an infarct (remember that pulmonary embolism and cardiac tamponade cause a similar haemodynamic picture), proceed as follows.

   (i)   These patients require volume expansion and thus a high right-sided filling pressure before they will improve. So stop any diuretics and vasodilators, and be sparing with opiates, as all these reduce right-sided pressures.
   (ii) Give fluids as for hypovolaemia. Give the fluid in boluses of 200 ml. You may require up to a litre.
   (iii) If this fails to improve cardiac output, give inotropic agents—dobutamine is probably the best.

(3) For persistent pump failure in these group c patients who have not responded to an adequate volume replacement and heart rate, proceed as for group d.

Group d

(1) Many of these patients will die, but treatment may occasionally be gratifyingly successful. Rational treatment is based on the idea that the ischaemic myocardium will function best given an optimal supply of oxygen and a minimum amount of work to do. We cannot often improve oxygen supply, so the above aim is best achieved using vasodilators. These come in two guises:

    (i)   venodilators, which act primarily to reduce the pulmonary capillary wedge pressure and thus the pre-load on the left ventricle;

    (ii)   arteriodilators, which reduce peripheral resistance, and thus the after load on the left ventricle.

(2) Therefore use:

    (i)   Sodium nitroprusside 0.5–10 μg/kg/min.[17] Nitroprusside which, because it has a roughly equal effect on veins and arteries, is called a balanced vasodilator, has a half-life of 2–5 min. It may cause profound hypotension (though, paradoxically this is less likely to happen with iller patients). Careful titration of the dose using intra-arterial monitoring is therefore mandatory. If you cannot use nitroprusside for lack of intra-arterial monitoring, use:

    (ii)   Salbutamol, 3–20 μg/min. This acts primarily as a vasodilator and may be managed using routine reading of CVP and BP.

(3) The persistence of unacceptably poor perfusion is indicated by:

    (i)   An hourly urine output of less than 0.5 ml/kg/h.

    (ii)   A core peripheral (rectal/toe) temperature gap of $>5°$ C.

(4) In these circumstances, there is little alternative but to resort to inotropic agents, with the possible dangers of increasing the oxygen demand of the myocardium more than supply to it. The choices are:

    (i)   Dopamine and/or dobutamine 2–5 μg/kg/min. In this dose range dopamine has little overall effect on systemic resistance; however, the preferential increase in renal flow makes it the catecholamine of choice. If a dopamine infusion of 5 μg/kg/min has not restored perfusion, it is wise to add dobutamine, starting at a dose of 2.5 μg/kg/min, and increasing to 10 μg/kg/min as necessary. Dobutamine is a more potent inotrope than dopamine, but does not have the renal vasodilator effect. Thus using the two together optimizes the benefits of both, and also makes good pharmacological sense.

(ii) If neither of these is available, use isoprenaline, 0.5–10 μg/min.

(5) Digitalization is a form of inotropic support which seems to have little theoretical advantage over the catecholamines. However, some clinicians feel unhappy if their patients are not digitalized in these circumstances. Give digoxin in an initial dose of 1.0 mg i.v., and then 0.5 mg 6-hourly to a maximum of 2.0 mg.

(6) Infuse 500 ml of 20% glucose, containing 39 mmol KCl and 20 units of soluble insulin (GIK) over 6 h. This is said to improve myocardial contractility, but its use is controversial. This same regime may also be helpful in the 'sick cell syndrome'. Here the sodium pump, which is responsible for the extrusion of sodium from cells, falters. The intracellular sodium rises as the extracellular sodium falls, and the altered ionic milieu causes widespread, and often disastrous, metabolic consequences. The sick cell syndrome often occurs as a terminal event in many serious illnesses, and so the above regime is only occasionally helpful.

(7) Emergency percutanous transluminal coronary angioplasty (PTCA) may be of avail in this group of patients—you should discuss the possibilities with your local cardiologists.

Further points to consider are:

(1) Anxiety. Many patients are already aware of their diagnosis, and it provides for them a most potent intimation of mortality. Reassurance is of paramount importance, if necessary supported by diazepam 5–10 mg i.v. or 2–5 mg t.d.s. orally. Lorazepam 1–4 mg i.v. or 1–2 mg t.d.s. orally is another excellent sedative.

(2) Give oxygen (40%) via an MC mask as even patients with minor infarcts may have a low Pao_2.

(3) Anticoagulants. Heparin 5000 units s.c. 8 hourly started within 8 h of the infarction, prevents thrombo-embolism as effectively as conventional full anticoagulation.[24] In addition,

hypertension and peptic ulceration are not contraindications to this regime. Full anticoagulation should probably be used in patients with a full-thickness anterior infarct, as this group is particularly prone to form intraventricular clots (which are best detected by echocardiography),[9] with the associated risk of stroke.[13] To achieve this, i.v. heparin should be given by continuous infusion using a suitable pump. Check baseline partial thromboplastin time (PTT) and prothrombin time (PT). Start with a loading dose of 5000 units i.v. over 5 min, and then give 1400 units hourly. Check the partial thromboplastin time after 6 h, and daily thereafter, and alter the infusion rate as detailed below to keep the PTT between 1.5 and 2.5 times normal.

PTT ratio	Change in heparin infusion rate
>7	Discontinue the infusion, and measure PTT again in 2 h
5.1–7.0	Reduce to 900 units/h
4.1–5.0	Reduce to 1100 units/h
3.1–4.0	Reduce to 1300 units/h
2.6–3.0	Reduce to 1350 units/h
1.5–2.5	No change
1.3–2.4	Increase to 1600 units/h
<1.2	Increase to 1800 units/h

Continue the heparin for 5 days. In the evening of the last 3 days give warfarin 9 mg orally. On the sixth day, switch to warfarin exclusively, with the dosage monitored by the prothrombin time.[6] Remember that heparin is inactivated by dextrose; only infuse it in normal saline. Heparin should also be used for 24 hours after streptokinase (see p. 12).

(4) Check the blood sugar—many patients with an infarct get stress-induced hyperglycaemia, and raised sugar may predispose towards arrhythmias.[3] Persistent hyperglycaemia should be treated in the acute situation, with an i.v. insulin infusion (see p. 163) commencing at a dose of 2 unit/h. Subsequent doses should be given as indicated below:

Blood glucose (mmol/l)	>4	4–	8–	12–	22+
Insulin (U/h)	0	0.5	1	2	4

There is some evidence that careful control of the blood sugar after infarction improves the prognosis, probably by reducing the incidence of cardiac arrhythmias.

(6) Pericarditis. Pericarditis and minor pericardial effusions are common after a myocardial infarct.[12]

    (i)   Pericardial pain is quickly relieved with a non-steroidal anti-inflammatory drug.

    (ii)   The presence of pericarditis should not influence your decision about anticoagulants. Contrary to what you might expect, these can be safely used in patients with pericarditis.[12]

(7) Routine lignocaine prophylaxis.[16] The concept of warning arrhythmias has proved to be unhelpful, and VF occurs both with and without warning after myocardial infarction. The incidence decreases exponentially with time, and, as a primary electrical problem, is rare after 24 h. Some would therefore advocate routine lignocaine prophylaxis after all infarcts. Although this prevents VF, it predisposes to asystole, and so should not be used routinely. We reserve its use for those who have had an episode of VF. In this group, give a bolus of 100 mg i.v. and then give a continuous infusion of 4 mg/min for 1 h. Reduce the dose to 2.0 mg/min, and then stop the infusion after 24 h. In people over the age of 65, or with hepatic dysfunction, reduce the above dose by one-third.

(8) Magnesium. Recent evidence suggests that 50 mmol of magnesium (as $MgCl_2$) infused in 1000 ml of isotonic glucose over the 24 h after admission, and a further 16 mmol in the next 24 h, reduces the mortality of patients with an acute myocardial infarction. The initial enthusiasm for this has been tempered by experience, but pending definite evidence that it does harm, we still use it.[19]

REFERENCES

General

Bradley R. A. (1977) *Studies in acute heart failure*. London: Edward Arnold.

Specific

1   Breckenbridge A. (1982) Vasodilators in heart failure. *Br. Med. J.* **284:** 763.

2   Caplin J. (1989) Acute right ventricular infarction. *Br. Med. J.* **299:** 69.

3   Clark R., English M. (1985) Effects of intravenous infusion of insulin in diabetics with acute myocardial infarction. *Br. Med. J.* **291**: 303.

4   de Bono D. (1988) Cardiogenic shock. *Hospital Update*, January, p. 1083.

5   Drug and Therapeutic Bulletin (1990) β-blockade after acute myocardial infarction. **28**: 45.

6   Fennerty A. (1988) Anticoagulants in venous thrombo-embolism. *Br. Med. J.* **297**: 1285.

7   Forrester J. S., Diamond G., Chaterjee K. *et al.* (1976) Medical therapy of acute myocardial infarction by application of haemodynamic subsets. *N. Engl. J. Med.* **295**: 1356. (See also (1977) **296**: 971, 1034, 1093.)

8   Guerci A. (1989) TIMI II and the role of angioplasty in acute myocardial infarction. *N. Engl. J. Med.* **320**: 663.

9   Hoffman T. *et al.* (1990) Echocardiographic evaluation of patients with clinically suspected arterial emboli. *Lancet* **336**: 1421.

10   ISIS Collaborative Group (1988) Randomized trial of i.v. streptokinase, oral aspirin, both, or neither among 17,187 cases of suspected acute myocardial infarction:isis II. *Lancet* **ii**: 349.

11   Julian D. (1988) A milestone for myocardial infarction. *Br. Med. J.* **297**: 497.

12   Leader (1986) Pericardial effusion after acute myocardial infarction. *Lancet* **i**: 1015.

13   Leader (1991) Left ventricular thrombosis and stroke following myocardial infarction. *Lancet* **i**: 759.

14   Leader (1991) Troponin T and myocardial damage. *Lancet* **338**: 23.

15   Loscalzo J. (1988) Tissue plasminogen activator *N. Engl. J. Med.* **319**: 925.

16   Lown B. (1985) Lignocaine to prevent ventricular fibrillation —easy does it. *N. Engl. J. Med.* **313**: 1154.

17   Passamani E. R. (1982) Nitroprusside in myocardial infarction. *N. Engl. J. Med.* **306**: 1168.

18   Petch M. (1990) Dangers of thrombolysis. *Br. Med. J.* **300**: 483.

19   Rasmussen H. *et al.* (1986) Intravenous magnesium in acute myocardial infarct. *Lancet* **i**. 234.

20   Sharpe N. *et al.* (1991) Early prevention of left ventricular

dysfunction after myocardial infarction with angiotensin converting enzyme inhibition. *Lancet* **337:** 872.

21   SWIFT (1991) Should we intervene following thrombolysis? *Br. Med. J.* **302:** 555.

22   Tan L. (1988) Detrimental haemodynamic effects of cyclizine in heart failure. *Lancet* **i:** 560.

23   Timmis A. (1990) Early diagnosis of acute myocardial infarction. *Br. Med. J.* **301:** 941.

24   Warlow C., Terry G., Kenmore A. C., *et al.* (1973) Double blind trial of low doses of subcutaneous heparin in the prevention of deep vein thrombosis after myocardial infarction. *Lancet* **2:** 934.

25   White H. (1991) Thrombolytic treatment for recurrent myocardial infarction. *Br. Med. J.* **302:** 429.

26   Yusuf S. (1988) Effect of intravenous nitrates on mortality in acute myocardial infarction: an overview of the randomized trials. *Lancet* **i:** 1088.

Preinfarction syndrome (unstable angina)[3]

DIAGNOSIS

The preinfarction syndrome consists of the following.

(1) Recurrent angina at rest.
(2) Increasing angina not rapidly relieved by glyceryl trinitrate.
(3) Variable and transient ECG changes—e.g. a 2 mm or more depression of the ST segment, or inversion of T waves.
(4) Normal cardiac enzyme levels.

It is that part of the spectrum of ischaemic heart disease which lies between stable effort angina and myocardial infarction. Not infrequently, we find difficulty in knowing at which precise point in the spectrum an individual patient is; when there is this dilemma, we prefer to err on the side of assuming a myocardial infarct has taken place, with the implication that we can then give fibrinolytic agents in the knowledge that they will help.

One in seven of patients with unstable angina will progress to an infarct if left untreated.

Most patients with unstable angina have eccentrically placed, fissured, atheromatous plaques upon which either platelet emboli or thrombus form. Vasoconstrictive substances released from platelets are also important in this process. These together cause the reduction in blood supply underlying the condition.[2,5] The main therapeutic endeavour is to increase perfusion with vasodilators and anti-thrombus and anti-platelet agents. In addition, the role of substances which block the platelet-induced vasoconstrictors, such as the 5 HT_2 receptor antagonist ketanserin, is now being actively explored.[5]

MANAGEMENT

(1) Anxiety and pain are managed as in a myocardial infarction (see p. 18).
(2) Aspirin should be given for its antiplatelet effect as soon as

possible.[6,7] The dose is controversial. We use 150 mg each day.

(3) Nitrates. Give glyceryl trinitrate 0.5 mg sublingually, and set up an infusion of isosorbide dinitrate, initially at 2 mg/h. This can be increased to a maximum of 10 mg/h. You should use the lowest dose which will achieve pain relief while not dropping the systolic arterial pressure below 90 mmHg. After your patient has been pain-free for 6 h, start oral nitrates and tail off the i.v. infusion.

(4) Beta-blockers. The reason for the efficacy of these in unstable angina is by no means clear, but several studies have reported benefit from their use.[8] We use atenolol 50 mg/day, and start this at the same time as the nitrates, provided there are no contraindications, e.g. a history of asthma or heart failure, a systolic blood pressure below 100 mmHg or a pulse rate below 50/min.

(5) If despite these measures your patient is still getting pain 24 h later, add nifedipine 10–20 mg t.d.s. However, calcium channel blockers should not be used for unstable angina unless your patient is on beta-blockers, as when used alone they do not help.[4]

(6) Heparin. This should be used early and by the i.v. route. Start an i.v. infusion of heparin, with an initial bolus of 5000 units and then 1400 units each hour adjusted to keep the PTT around twice normal, (see p. 19) as soon as possible, and continue the infusion for at least 3 days.

(7) Fibrinolytics. As we have intimated above, in the section on diagnosis, the role of fibrinolytics in unstable angina, as distinct from established myocardial infarction, is not yet defined. We anticipate that trials now in progress will rectify this problem: until then we err on the side of not giving them.

(8) Coronary angiography. Patients who are not pain-free within 48 h despite the above therapy, should be considered for angiography, with a view to either angioplasty or coronary artery surgery.[1,3]

REFERENCES

1   De Feyter P. J. *et al.* (1985) Emergency coronary angioplasty in refractory unstable angina. *N. Engl. J. Med.* **313:** 342.

2 Fuster V., Cheesebro J. (1986) Mechanisms of unstable angina *N. Engl. J. Med.* **315:** 1023.

3 Hargreaves A., Boon N. (1991) Management of unstable angina. *Hospital Update*, February, p. 98.

4 Held P. *et al.* (1989) Calcium channel blockers in acute myocardial infarction and unstable angina: an overview. *Br. Med. J.* **299:** 1187.

5 Hillis L., Lange R. (1991) Serotonin and acute ischaemic heart disease. *N. Engl. J. Med.* **324:** 688.

6 RISC Group (1990) Risk of myocardial infarction and death during treatment with low dose aspirin and intravenous heparin in men with unstable coronary disease. *Lancet* (1990) **336:** 827.

7 Theroux P. *et al.* (1988) Aspirin, heparin or both to treat acute unstable angina. *N. Engl. J. Med.* **319:** 1105.

8 Yusuf S. *et al.* (1983) Reduction in infarct size, arrhythmias and chest pain by early intravenous beta blockade in suspected acute myocardial infarction. *Circulation* **67** (Suppl. 1): 32.

Cardiac arrhythmias

These may be supraventricular arising from the atria (atrial) or from around the A-V node (junctional) or ventricular (arising below the A-V node). They cause too rapid a heart action (tachycardia), occasional irregularities in rhythm (extrasystoles) or too slow a heart action (bradycardia). Also included in this section are arrhythmias where there is an abnormal relationship between atrial and ventricular contraction (conduction defects).

Arrhythmias are encountered commonly after myocardial infarction. They may occur terminally after a period of hypotension and congestive cardiac failure in which case they are usually resistant to treatment (so-called secondary arrhythmias). However, they may also occur as a temporary disturbance in a heart capable of maintaining an adequate circulation. It is in this group, the primary arrhythmias, that treatment may be life-saving.

Arrhythmias may be potentiated or even caused by the following.

(1) Pain and anxiety—always ask your patient specifically about the presence of pain; he or she may be stoical.
(2) Hypoxia (which is often impossible to detect clinically).
(3) Acidosis.
(4) Hypo- or hyperkalaemia.
(5) Hypo- or hypercalcaemia.
(6) Hypomagnasaemia.

Correction of these abnormalities may stop the arrhythmia and will certainly make it more amenable to treatment.

Arrhythmias cause their adverse effects in one or more of the following ways:

(1) Loss of atrial transport, which may cause a 25% reduction in the cardiac output.
(2) Increase in myocardial oxygen requirement, coupled with decreased supply. Tachycardias (>100 beats/min), while causing a rate-dependent increase in consumption, also cause decreased perfusion because of the invariable shortening of diastole. Bradycardias (<40 beats/min), while lengthening diastole, diminish perfusion by reducing cardiac output.
(3) Loss of synchronous, or organised ventricular contraction,

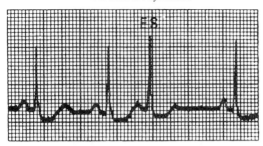

Fig. 1 Supraventricular extrasystole. The small pointed P wave can be seen deforming the preceding T wave. (ES = extrasystole.)

leading to reduced output. Ventricular fibrillation is the most extreme form of this.

SUPRAVENTRICULAR ARRHYTHMIAS

Atrial ectopics (Fig. 1)

These may be caused by digoxin and catecholamines. They may occur in otherwise normal hearts, especially during pregnancy. They may occur after myocardial infarction when they are usually benign, but may occasionally herald atrial tachycardia or fibrillation. In none of these situations is any treatment required, other than reassurance.

Supraventricular tachycardia

(1) *Sinus tachycardia* comes on gradually. Its rate is affected by posture, exercise, atropine and is usually below 150 beats/min. There is always an underlying cause such as left ventricular failure (LVF), anxiety, fever or hypoxia, which should be looked for and treated as necessary. It needs to be differentiated from:

(2) *Paroxysmal tachycardia* (Fig. 2) which comes on abruptly. Its rate (usually > 150 beats/min) is unaffected by any of the above but may be terminated by vagal stimulation. If your patient is not on digoxin, you can:

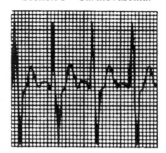

Fig. 2 Supraventricular tachycardia. The P wave can clearly be seen preceding each QRS complex.

(i)   Do nothing, if there is no evidence of failure, and the patient tells you that the attacks are short-lived.

(ii)   Induce vagal stimulation. The Valsalva manoeuvre while supine is the best way of effecting this.[8]

(iii) The treatment of choice in patients whose circulation is compromised is synchronised DC reversion, which should be undertaken with your patient anaesthetised. Give the shock observing the usual precautions (see p. 6) starting at 100 J and increasing the stimulus by 50 J until 400 J are reached. In the rare circumstances that this is ineffective, try placing one 'paddle' on the patient's back behind the heart and one in front. If DC reversion has been unsuccessful, you should try it again after giving one of the drugs mentioned below.

(iv)   If DC reversion is either not available or not considered necessary, the following drugs may be useful.

(a)   Adenosine, which has a very short half life (10–30 s), is not negatively inotropic, and is highly effective in blocking A-V nodal conduction and is the drug of choice. Give an initial dose of 6 mg i.v., and increase to 12 mg, and then 18 mg as necessary.[3]

(b)   Verapamil, a depressor of A-V nodal function, 5 mg i.v. repeated at 5 min intervals to a maximum of 20 mg is usually effective. This should not be used if any other anti-arrhythmic drugs have been given before it, or if the patient is suspected of having

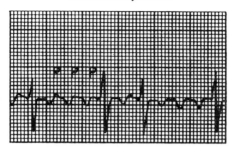

Fig. 3 Atrial Flutter. The first three flutter waves are marked 'P'. The ventricles respond at a varying 1:2–1:3 ratio.

poor ventricular function, as it is negatively inotropic, and irreversible asystole may occur.

(c) Beta-blockers. These are still used in some places as first line therapy. Atenolol, given in 5 mg aliquots i.v. at 5 min intervals to a maximum of 20 mg is a reasonable choice.

(d) Assuming your patient is not already on digoxin, digoxin may be used (see p. 18).

(e) Try the Valsalva manoeuvre again if your drug treatment has been unsuccessful.

(f) Amiodarine 5 mg/kg infused over 20 min through a long intracath may be tried.[7] If this is successful it may be continued as a continuous infusion—600–1200 mg over 24 h.

Atrial flutter (Fig. 3)

This may occur after myocardial infarction and with cardiomyopathies, ASD and systemic infections. It is not, unlike atrial fibrillation, associated with mitral stenosis or thyrotoxicosis. The atrium flutters at an average rate of 300 beats/min. As the ventricles cannot respond at this rate there is always some degree of 'block' which may vary (Fig. 3).

(1) The treatment of choice for the patient whose circulation is compromised is DC reversion, to which flutter is very sensitive. Therefore start with a 40 J shock, and increase as necessary.

(2) If this either fails or is not deemed necessary, digitalise the

patient. This may cause a reversion to sinus rhythm, or progression to atrial fibrillation.

(3) Adenosine, verapamil or atenolol may be given as for atrial tachycardia. These drugs do not revert the flutter to sinus rhythm, but merely reduce the ventricular rate.

Atrial fibrillation and flutter fibrillation[12] (Figs 4 and 5)

(1) For practical purposes these are the same thing.

(2) The most common cause is acute or chronic ischaemic heart disease, but it also occurs in hypertensives, in ethanolic heart disease, in association with mitral valve disease, thyrotoxicosis, sub-acute bacterial endocarditis, atrial septal defect, pericarditis and after thoracotomy.

(3) If the ventricular rate is sufficiently fast to cause cardiac failure the treatment of choice is digitalisation—combined if necessary with diuretics and oxygen (see pp. 15 and 18 respectively). Continue that dose of digoxin which maintains the ventricular rate between 70 and 80 beats/min.

(4) If digoxin fails, use either:

   (i) amiodarone—see above;
   (ii) flecanide, an agent which slows intra-atrial conduction, as well as producing A-V block, in a dose of 2 mg/kg i.v. infused over 10 min. It is said to terminate about 70% of cases of atrial fibrillation, and is safe to use in this situation, although you should remember that it is negatively inotropic.

(5) Remember that resistant atrial fibrillation may be a complication of pericarditis. If you are having trouble controlling atrial fibrillation, make sure you have either excluded pericarditis, or treated it with a non-steroidal.

(6) DC reversion can be used if drug therapy has failed.

Sinus bradycardia

Sinus bradycardia may occur with vasovagal attacks, intracranial hypertension, myxoedema (see p. 188) and in athletes in training. It is occasionally caused by beta-adrenergic blocking agents, and by digoxin itself.

Bradycardia may also cause all the signs of severe cardiovascular collapse when it occurs after inferior myocardial infarction. In this

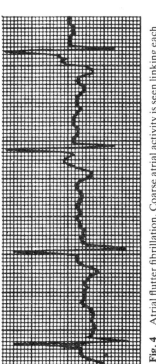

Fig. 4   Atrial flutter fibrillation. Coarse atrial activity is seen linking each QRS complex.

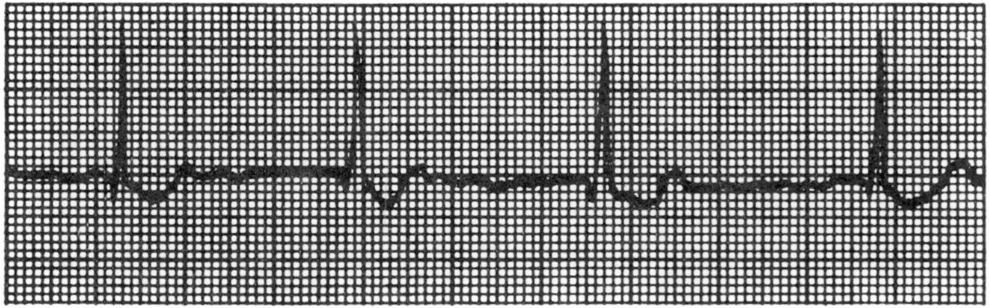

Fig. 5   Atrial fibrillation. Small-amplitude atrial activity links each QRS complex.

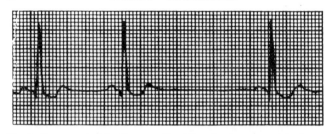

Fig. 6 Sinus arrest. After the second beat there is a temporary delay in sinus activity before the third beat is initiated.

situation give atropine 0.6 mg i.v. Repeat this dose if there is no effect within 5 min. Response is usually prompt and gratifying. Atropine may provoke ventricular fibrillation, urinary retention and glaucoma, and it is unwise to give more than 2.4 mg.

Isoprenaline (see p. 18) may be used if atropine fails. Rarely, pacing may be necessary.

Sinus arrest[5] (Fig. 6)

Sinus arrest may be caused by many of the anti-arrhythmic drugs, hyperkalaemia, autonomic instability (as in the Guillain-Barré syndrome), and myocardial infarction. Short periods of sinus inactivity may progress to permanent sinus arrest and if they occur a transvenous intracardiac pacemaker should be passed urgently. Prior to this sinus rhythm may be restored by a sharp precordial blow or by atropine 0.6–2.4 mg i.v.

JUNCTIONAL ARRHYTHMIAS (Figs 7, 8, 9)

Junctional rhythms represent the action of a natural pacemaker at variable sites in the bundle of His which takes over as a result of sinus node dysfunction—the commonest causes of which are digoxin toxicity, myocardial infarction and myocarditis. If the rate is sufficiently slow to cause cardiac failure, atropine 0.6–2.4 mg i.v. may provoke the sinus node to return at the normal rate. Failing this, isoprenaline (see p. 18) may encourage acceleration of the junctional rhythms. Junctional tachycardias are treated as for their atrial counterparts.

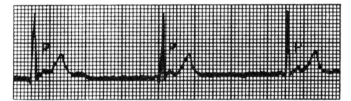

Fig. 7 Junctional rhythm. The P wave of each beat is clearly seen deforming the ST segment.

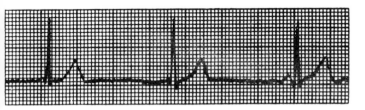

Fig. 8 Junctional rhythm. The P wave is seen immediately preceding each QRS complex.

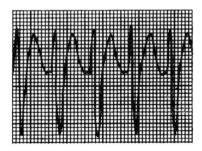

Fig. 9 Junctional tachycardia. A small P wave is seen immediately preceding each wide QRS complex.

VENTRICULAR ARRHYTHMIAS

Ventricular ectopics (Fig. 10)

Ventricular ectopics occur in myocardial infarction and in cardio-myopathies or as a result of digoxin toxicity.

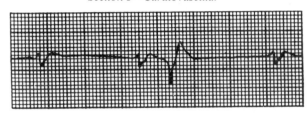

Fig. 10   Ventricular ectopic beat.

(1) They may herald ventricular tachycardia or fibrillation (death, although sudden, is not always unannounced) if:

   (i)   they interrupt the T wave or ST segment of the preceding complex (in technical terms, if their coupling intervals is short);

   (ii) they are of multifocal origin;

   (iii) they are frequent (more than 10/min);

   (iv) more than two occur in succession.

However, the relevance of these warning arrhythmias has certainly been overstated, and anyway, no specific drug treatment has been proved to be of benefit.[1]

(2) They may be provoked by pain, hypoxia or hypokalaemia, all of which should be corrected. Enthusiasm for treating persistent ectopics is waning, as there is no good evidence that treatment forestalls progression to more serious arrhythmias. We do not usually treat them. If treatment is deemed necessary give lignocaine 100 mg over 2–3 min i.v. as a bolus followed by an infusion at 4 mg/min. Reduce the infusion dose as soon as possible, usually within 1 h, to 2 mg/min.

(3) If this fails, use the following.

   (i)   Disopyramide 2 mg/kg i.v. over 10 min, as a loading dose, and then up to 1 g/day i.v. or orally.

   (ii) Procaine amide. Give 100 mgm i.v. diluted in 5% dextrose, at a rate not exceeding 25–50 mg/min. This dose can be repeated at 5–10 min intervals until the arrhythmia is controlled, adverse reactions occur or the maximum of 1.0 g has been given. To maintain therapeutic levels, give 2–6 mg/min by continuous infusion.

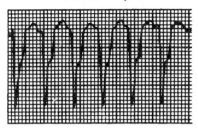

Fig. 11 There is no easily discernible P wave in this recording and it is impossible to tell whether this is a supraventricular tachycardia with bundle branch block or ventricular tachycardia.

    (iii) Amiodarone 5–10 mg/kg i.v. over 20 min then 600–1200 mg via a continuous infusion over 24 h.

    (iv) Bretylium tosylate (see p. 6).

After myocardial infarction a few ventricular ectopics are very common. Suppression of these, at least with flecanide, may, paradoxically, increase the death rate,[10] and we do not use a specific drug treatment.

Ventricular tachycardia (Fig. 11)

(1) Both ventricular tachycardias and supraventricular tachycardia with bundle branch block give rise to broad complex tachycardias.[2] The two may be difficult to distinguish, because:

    (i) The clinical signs which frequently occur in ventricular tachycardia, namely

        (a) occasional cannon waves,

        (b) varying intensity of first heart sound, are not always present and can occur in SVT with bundle branch block.

    (ii) The ECG features commonly associated with ventricular tachycardia, namely

        (a) P waves in varying relationship to QRS complexes,

        (b) slight irregularity of the QRS complex and rate, may occur in either condition.

    (iii) The wider the complex and the more unlike it is to conventional bundle branch block, the more likely it is to be ventricular in origin. Accomplished electrocardiographists can tell the difference on a 12 lead tracing, and if you are lucky enough either to be one of this rare breed, or you know that the same broad complex is present in both sinus rhythm and the tachycardia, then you can be confident in your diagnosis. However, treating ventricular tachycardias as supraventricular ones is often disastrous,[9] so, if in doubt, always assume you are dealing with a ventricular tachycardia.

Electrophysiological studies, the ultimate arbiter of a tachycardia's origin, show that eight out of ten wide complex tachycardias are indeed ventricular in origin. Adenosine (see p. 28 above) can also be used to distinguish between the two, as it reverses most SVTs and does not compromise the VTs.

(2) DC reversion, the treatment of choice, is almost always effective. If it is not, check that the patient is not hypoxic, anxious or in pain or electrolytically unbalanced. If you do not have the equipment, or DC reversion is unsuccessful, use drugs as for ventricular ectopics. If the situation is deteriorating, contact a specialist unit for advice. They may be able to offer either paired or coupled pacing.

(3) If you have to use a drug in circumstances in which you are not sure of the origin of the arrhythmia, use amiodarone (see above).

(4) Digoxin should never be used in patients with ventricular arrhythmias.

(5) If there has been no recent myocardial infarct, we do not give lignocaine following the correction of a ventricular arrhythmia, as there is no conclusive evidence that it is helpful in preventing further arrhythmias.

Ventricular fibrillation (Fig. 12)

This is, of course, one of the causes of cardiac arrest (see p. 5).

HEART BLOCK

This can take one of the following forms.

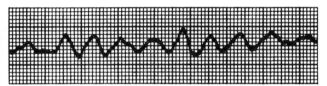

Fig. 12 Ventricular fibrillation.

(1) *First degree* which is defined as a P–R interval prolonged for more than 0.22 s (Fig. 13). This occurs in digoxin overdosage, coronary artery disease, myocarditis and excessive vagal tone. It is of little significance and is not treated unless:

   (i)   it lengthens and/or
   (ii) dropped beats start to occur.

Either may herald complete heart block and if (i) or (ii) occurs following a myocardial infarct, insertion of a temporary transvenous pacemaker should be considered.

(2) *Second degree.* Here the ventricles do not always respond to atrial contraction. There are two types of second degree block, first clearly distinguished by Mobitz and designated Mobitz type I and type II.

   (i)   Mobitz type I—in this type of block, there is a progressively lengthening P–R interval culminating in a dropped beat (the Wenckebach phenomenon) (Fig. 14) or the conducted beat has a prolonged P–R interval (Fig. 15a). The prognosis of Mobitz type I block may not be as good as we used to think. Normal conduction may often be

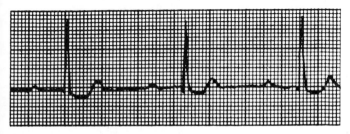

Fig. 13 First degree heart block. The P–R interval is greatly prolonged to 0.36 s.

restored with atropine 0.6–2.4 mg i.v. or, failing this, dopamine (see p. 17). If these fail, or the patient's cardiac output is compromised or the degree of block progresses a pacemaker should be inserted.

(ii)   Mobitz type II—here the conducted beat has a constant P–R interval (Fig. 15b). The ratio between non-conducted atrial contractions may be as great as 5:1. Since Mobitz type II block often progresses to complete heart block, a transvenous pacemaker should be inserted as soon as possible. Sympathomimetic agents should be used with care in this type of block, as an increase in atrial rate may increase the ratio of atrial to ventricular beats, causing the ventricular rate to slow. Use atropine while getting ready to pace your patient.

(3) *Complete heart block* (Fig. 16). Here the ventricular activity bears no temporal relationship to atrial activity. It is usually due to fibrous replacement of the conducting system, but may occur after myocardial infarction. It may rarely be caused by digoxin toxicity, or trauma to the bundle of His (e.g. after cardiac surgery). Complete heart block may

  (i)   cause congestive cardiac failure;
  (ii) cause hypotension and poor tissue perfusion;
  (iii) be punctuated by attacks of ventricular asystole, tachycardia or VF (Stokes–Adams attacks).

Treatment of complete heart block

(1) When complete heart block occurs following myocardial infarction, a temporary transvenous pacemaker should be inserted immediately, under fluoroscopic control.[11] Sinus rhythm usually returns within one week of infarction, but may take up to three. If it does not, permanent pacing will be required.

(2) In other circumstances, if the low heart rate is causing symptoms, a permanent pacemaker should be inserted, if necessary preceded by a temporary wire as in (1) above. If pacing is not available, or while things are being organised, either give i.v. dopamine (see p. 17) or alternatively 5 mg isoprenaline in 500 ml of dextrose infused at a rate of 10 μg (1 ml)/min, until the ventricular rate is above 60 beats/min.

(3) Complete heart block may be presaged by the following.

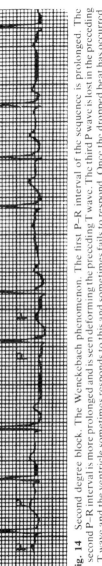

Fig. 14 Second degree block. The Wenckebach phenomenon. The first P–R interval of the sequence is prolonged. The second P–R interval is more prolonged and is seen deforming the preceding T wave. The third P wave is lost in the preceding T wave and the ventricle sometimes responds to this and sometimes fails to respond. Once the dropped beat has occurred the sequence is then repeated (Mobitz type I block).

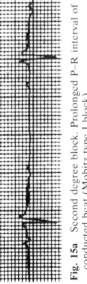

Fig. 15a Second degree block. Prolonged P–R interval of conducted beat (Mobitz type I block).

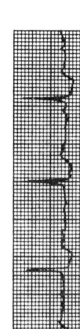

Fig. 15b Second degree block. Normal P–R interval of conducted beat (Mobitz type II block).

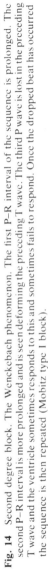

Fig. 16 Complete heart block. The first three P waves are marked. They can be seen to be beating quite independently of the QRS complex.

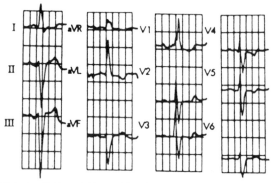

Fig. 17   Right bundle branch block with left axis deviation. (Reproduced
with permission from, Stock J. P. P. and Williams, D. O. (1974) *Diagnosis
and Treatment of Cardiac arrhythmias*. London: Butterworths.)

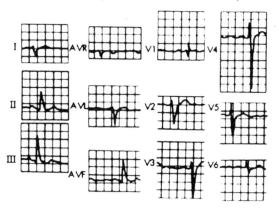

Fig. 18   Right bundle branch block with right axis deviation. (Reproduced
with permission from, Stock J. P. P. and Williams, D. O. (1974) *Diagnosis
and Treatment of Cardiac arrhythmias*. London: Butterworths.)

    (i)   A lesser degree of block (see p. 37).

    (ii)   A combination of left axis deviation (signifying left
           anterior hemi-block) and right bundle branch block (Fig.
           17), or right axis deviation (signifying left posterior hemi-
           block) and right bundle branch block (Fig. 18). Both of

these configurations imply that at least two out of three of the conducting bundles are damaged, some of these patients progressing to complete block, as may patients developing left bundle branch block following myocardial infarction.

(iii) The ECG configurations in (i) and (ii) above, or the development of left bundle branch block, are an indication for pacing if:

(a) they develop after an anterior wall myocardial infarction;

(b) they are associated with symptoms attributable to Stokes–Adams attacks.[6]

REFERENCES

General

Aronson J. K. (1985) Cardiac arrhythmias; theory and practice. *Br. Med. J.* **290:** 487.

Hart G. *et al.* (1985) Physiology of cardiac conduction: *Br. J. Hosp. Med.* **32:** 128.

Specific

1   Campbell R. W. (1983) Treatment and prophylaxis of ventricular arrhythmias in acute myocardial infarction. *Am. J. Cardiol.* **52:** 55c.

2   Griffiths M. J., Camm J. (1989) Broad QRS complex tachycardia. *Hospital Update* July, p. 531.

3   Griffiths M. J. *et al.* (1988) Adenosine in the diagnosis of broad complex tachycardias. *Lancet* **i:** 672.

4   Koch-Weser J. (1979) Disopyramide. *N. Engl. J. Med.* **300:** 95.

5   Leader (1977) Sick sinus syndrome. *Br. Med. J.* **i:** 4.

6   McAnulty J. *et al.* (1982) Natural history of 'high risk' bundle branch block. *N. Engl. J. Med.* **307:** 137.

7   Mason J. W. (1987) Amiodarone. *N. Engl. J. Med.* **316:** 455.

8   Mehta D. *et al.* (1988) Relative efficacy of various physical manoeuvres in the termination of junctional tachycardias. *Lancet* **i:** 1181.

9   Rankin C. A. *et al.* (1987) Misuse of intravenous verapamil in patients with ventricular tachycardia. *Lancet* **ii:** 472.

10   Ruskin J. (1989) The cardiac arrhythmia suppression trial. *N. Engl. J. Med.* **321:** 386.

11   Sclarovsky S. *et al.* (1984) Advanced early and late atrioventricular block in acute inferior wall myocardial infarction. *Am. Heart J.* **108:** 19.

12   Selzer A. S. (1982) Atrial fibrillation revisited. *N. Engl. J. Med.* **306:** 1044.

Acute pulmonary oedema

DIAGNOSIS

(1) Acute pulmonary oedema is usually caused by a rise in pulmonary capillary pressure overcoming the osmotic pressure of plasma proteins. The rise in pulmonary capillary pressure is usually caused by left ventricular failure, in which case:

   (i) There is usually a history of increasing dyspnoea, fatigue, anorexia and orthopnoea, which may be accompanied by a dry cough and possibly attacks of paroxysmal nocturnal dyspnoea with production of pink frothy sputum.

   (ii) Examination reveals a frightened, gasping patient who is pale and cyanosed with cold peripheries and who is pouring with sweat. The arterial pressure may be high with a narrow pulse pressure, and in addition pulsus alternans may be present. A third heart sound and loud P2 may be present but are usually difficult to hear because of lung sounds—there are widespread loud crackles and wheezes over the lung fields. The sputum is pink and frothy.

   (iii) The chest x-ray is usually characteristic with semi-confluent mottling spreading from the hila, and enlarged upper lobe pulmonary veins. In addition there may be left ventricular enlargement, Kerley 'B' lines and pleural effusions. The left ventricular end diastolic pressure will be raised—see (iv) and (v) below. There may also be evidence of an obvious cause.

   (iv) The pulmonary capillary pressure (PCP) at which pulmonary oedema secondary to left ventricular failure occurs depends on the serum albumin level. At a normal serum albumin level of 32 g/l, pulmonary oedema due to heart failure will only occur when the PCP is above 25 mmHg. At lower albumin concentrations, pulmonary oedema will occur when the PCP is less than 18 mmHg. A simple formula (serum albumin (g/l) x 0.57 expressed as mmHg) gives an approximation to this critical pressure (but see p. 337).

(v)   The pulmonary capillary pressure is essentially the same as the left atrial pressure (which in its turn reflects the left ventricular end diastolic pressure). The left atrial pressure is usually measured indirectly using a Swan–Ganz catheter with its tip wedged in a small pulmonary artery (see p. 387).

(2) Pulmonary oedema can also occur in patients who are severely ill for other reasons (e.g. septicaemia, acute renal failure) and who do not have a raised left atrial pressure. Here the likely cause is transudation of fluid from damaged capillaries. The appearance and management of these patients differs from those in left ventricular failure (see section on shock lung, p. 97).

(3) Acute pulmonary oedema has to be distinguished from:

(i)   Asthma (see p. 80), for in both conditions the patient prefers sitting up, tachycardia is present and both may have inverted T waves on the ECG. In asthma there is more high-pitched wheeze and fewer crackles than in acute pulmonary oedema. The patient is not grey and sweaty unless in extremis, when parts of the lung fields are virtually silent; there is a quick inspiratory snatch and a prolonged expiratory phase; pulsus paradoxus may be present, the sputum is white and very sticky; the chest x-ray is usually normal or shows hyperinflation of the lungs. When, as sometimes happens, the main clinical evidence for pulmonary oedema is wheezing, the clinical situation and chest x-ray help distinguish it from asthma.

(ii) Pulmonary embolus (see p. 52).

(iii) Acute or chronic respiratory failure may mimic acute pulmonary oedema and be preceded by a history of orthopnoea. $Paco_2$ before morphine and oxygen are given may help distinguish between the two, and must be measured if there is any doubt. Unfortunately, patients who have no pre-existing lung disease may sometimes have a raised $Paco_2$ when in LVF.[1]

(iv) Other causes of acute shortness of breath (see p. 71) which are less easily confused.

(4) The causes of pulmonary oedema must be considered, especially the following treatable conditions.

(i)   Myocardial infarction (see p. 11).
(ii)   Severe hypertension (see p. 48).
(iii)   Mitral stenosis and regurgitation, aortic valve disease and left ventricular aneurysms.
(iv)   Sub-acute bacterial endocarditis.
(v)   Cardiac arrhythmias (see p. 26).
(vi)   Water and salt overload, especially in an anuric patient (see p. 157).
(vii)   Pulmonary embolus. This may so compromise oxygen supply to the heart that left ventricular failure develops.
(viii) Cardiac tamponade (see p. 65).
(ix)   Cardiomyopathy.
(x)   Left atrial myxoma or ball valve thrombus (seen once in a lifetime).

MANAGEMENT

Management involves reducing the pulmonary oedema as follows.

(1) Sit the patient up if he has not already done so himself, either in a cardiac bed or with the legs over the side of the bed.
(2) Give the following.

(i)   *Oxygen* by either MC mask or nasal catheter 4–6 l/min. If the patient has chronic respiratory failure give 28% O_2 initially by a Ventimask. If the Pao_2 is less than 5.3 kPa (40 mmHg), increase the percentage of oxygen while monitoring the $Paco_2$ (see p. 44).
(ii)   *Morphine* 5–10 mg and an antiemetic such as prochlorperazine 12.5 mg i.v. If the patient has chronic respiratory failure there is no safe sedation. If he is very distressed, probably the best thing to do is to give a small dose of morphine together with doxapram (1 mg/kg i.v.) and treat respiratory depression as necessary, while monitoring the blood gases.
(iii)   *Frusemide* 40–80 mg i.v.
(iv)   *Nitrates.* These venodilators reduce pre-load, and hence left ventricular end diastolic pressure. Glyceryl trinitrate, 0.5 mg sublingually or isosorbide dinitrate from 2 to 10 mg/hour i.v. are important adjuncts to therapy.
(v)   *Aminophylline* helps to reduce bronchospasm and in addition may lower the pulmonary venous pressure. A

loading dose of 5 mg/kg slowly over 30 min followed by an infusion at 0.5 mg/kg/h attains adequate blood levels safely, but may occasionally cause headaches and nausea. The dose may need modifying in old or very ill patients (see p. 82).

(vi) A *cardiac glycoside*. If the patient has not had a cardiac glycoside within the past five days, give digoxin (see p. 18).

(3) Having given (ii)–(vi) above, reassure the patient and then leave the nurse to make observations. Do not hover looking anxious. This will increase the patient's anxiety.

(4) If, three-quarters of an hour later, the patient is

　(i)　the same:

　　　(a) repeat the dose of frusemide and
　　　(b) give a further 5 mg of morphine, both intravenously;

　(ii)　worse:

　　　(a) let one pint of blood—this is best done with an ordinary blood donor's set.
　　　(b) cuffing the limbs is now known to be ineffective in LVF.[2]

(5) If, despite these measures, the patient continues to deteriorate, consider using continuous positive airways pressure (CPAP), or if this fails to improve matters putting him on a ventilator. Positive pressure ventilation will reduce the venous return, lower the arterial pressure, and force the oedema back out of the alveoli. This may hold the situation until the other measures have taken effect.

INVESTIGATION AND TREATMENT OF THE CAUSE

(1) A chest x-ray and ECG should be taken as soon as possible.

(2) If an arrhythmia is thought to be the cause, the ECG should be continuously displayed on a cardiac monitor. The arrhythmia is treated in the usual way (see p. 26). In particular, atrial fibrillation may be an important contributory cause in an already jeopardised myocardium.

(3) Many patients with acute pulmonary oedema have a transiently elevated arterial pressure. However, if there is evi-

dence of previous hypertension (hypertensive retinopathy, left ventricular hypertrophy and the diastolic pressure is maintained at >110 mmHg) steps should be taken to lower it (see p. 49).

(4) Acute pulmonary oedema will require the following treatments in special circumstances:

    (i)   *Mitral stenosis*—is an indication for an emergency valvotomy if the patient is already on adequate medical treatment.

    (ii)   *Anuria*—is an absolute indication for dialysis.

    (iii) *Papillary muscle* and *ventricular septa* can rupture following myocardial infarction and may be amenable to surgical repair. These two problems are best diagnosed by echocardiography.

    (iv) *Cardiac tamponade*—is an indication for paracentesis of the effusion without delay.

    (v)   A *cardiac aneurysm*—intractable cardiac failure may be controlled by resection of the redundant muscle.

    (vi) *Atrial myxoma* or ball valve thrombus—can be relieved, it is said, by re-positioning the patient, head down.

REFERENCES

1   Leader (1972) Blood gas tensions in acute pulmonary oedema. *Lancet* **i:** 1106.

2   Leader (1975) rotating tourniquets for left ventricular failure. *Lancet* **i:** 154.

Hypertensive emergencies[2,3]

DIAGNOSIS

(1) Hypertension may be regarded as critical and requiring urgent treatment when:

  (i) It is causing hypertensive encephalopathy.[6] This causes periodic attacks of severe headache, accompanied by vomiting, convulsions, confusion, deterioration of vision, possibly focal neurological signs and eventually coma. On examination the systolic and diastolic arterial pressures are usually more than 200 mmHg and 140 mmHg respectively. The fundus shows florid hypertensive changes and the urine contains protein.

  (ii) It occurs in association with dissection of an aortic aneurysm (see p. 63).

  (iii) It occurs in association with acute or chronic renal failure (see p. 149).

  (iv) It occurs in the eclampsia and pre-eclampsia of pregnancy.

  (v) It occurs in association with the use of 'recreational' drugs—commonly cocaine hydrochloride, but also with sympathomimetic drugs such as amphetamine and lysergic acid diethylamide.

  (vi) It occurs in a patient on monoamine oxidase inhibitors who has eaten tyramine-containing foods.

  (vii) It occurs in accelerated or malignant hypertension. Here there are retinal haemorrhages and proteinurea, and the diastolic arterial pressure is usually above 120 mmHg.

  (viii) It is causing left ventricular failure (see p. 46).

(2) Because of the improvement in the treatment of hypertension, emergencies are now uncommon—less than 1% of hypertensives will ever have a crisis.

(3) Target organ damage resulting from high arterial pressure can be seen directly in the fundus and can be inferred from clinical and ECG evidence, namely:

(i)   deepest S wave in right ventricular leads plus tallest R wave in left ventricular leads add up to more than 36 mm;

(ii)   ST depression plus T wave inversion in left ventricular leads, indicative of left ventricular strain.

(4) Remember that there are dangers in lowering blood pressure acutely,[2,7] particularly in

(i)   the elderly, where too rapid reduction may compromise cerebral renal or myocardial blood flow;

(ii)   patients with cerebral infarction, intracerebral or subarachnoid haemorrhage, in whom hypotensive therapy should be withheld unless the hypertension is extreme (diastolic greater than 130 mmHg). In these circumstances the blood pressure should be reduced by 20% over 24 h.

(5) We therefore use i.v. therapy sparingly. Only in categories (i)–(vi) in section (1) above do we recommend i.v. therapy. In other circumstances, we use oral therapy.

MANAGEMENT

Reduction of diastolic arterial pressure to 100 mmHg is all that should be attempted (but see section (4, ii) above). Further reduction may reduce cerebral blood flow to such an extent that neurological symptoms occur. Special care is needed in treating patients who have cerebral infarction with associated severe hypertension (see (4) above). The arterial pressure may be lowered rapidly with any one of the following drugs.

(1) Sodium nitroprusside.[10] This is the drug of choice. If your pharmacy has no access to the ready-made solutions, make up a fresh solution of 50 mg sodium nitroprusside in 500 ml of 5% dextrose (0.01% solutions). Sodium nitroprusside has an immediate effect, a duration of action of only 3 min, and is given continuously i.v. An incremental infusion rate in the dose range 0.3–10.0 μg/kg/min may be required for short periods of time. It is mandatory to measure thiocyanate and cyanide levels with exceptionally high doses, but at doses of under 10 μg/kg/min no adverse side effects have been noted. Cyanide poisoning can be reversed by giving hydroxy

cyanocobalmin 1000 μg i.v. or, in severe cases, the specific antidote to cyanide poisoning, dicobalt EDTA in a dose of 300 mg i.v.

(2) Hydralazine.[5] This is still the drug of choice in the hypertensive emergencies of pregnancy. Give 10 mg i.v. or i.m. It takes about 20 min to have an effect, and lasts from 3 to 6 h. The dose may be repeated every 30 min as necessary. Common toxic effects are tachycardia, headaches, nausea and vomiting. Occasional dizziness, flushing and sweating, dyspnoea, angina, paraesthesia and urticaria may occur.

(3) Diazoxide (Eudomid).[4] Give 5 mg/kg rapidly i.v. The onset of action is between 1 and 5 min and the duration 6–12 hours. The dose may be repeated as necessary to a total dose of 600 mg. Side effects are the development of hyperglycaemia and sodium and water retention.

Hydralazine and diazoxide both increase cardiac stroke volume and cardiac work; thus in patients with dissecting aneuryrsm or with pulmonary oedema, sodium nitroprusside is preferable. In patients with dissection, the nitroprusside should be preceded by a drug which has a negative inotropic effect—propranolol 2 mg i.v. is a suitable choice.

(4) Labetalol. Give an i.v. bolus 20–80 mg every 5–10 min, up to 300 mg. It acts within 5–10 min, and lasts 3–6 h. Labetalol is particularly useful in hypertensive crisis associated with catecholamine excess—(v) and (vi) in section (1), p. 48—as is phentolamine (see below). Labetalol can also be used in pregnancy, and in acute dissection.

(5) Oral therapy.

    (i) Nifedipine. Given by the sublingual or buccal route, the onset of action is between 5 and 10 mins, the duration 3–6 hours. Start with a dose of 10 mg, with a further 10 mg dose in 20 min if there is no initial response.[11,9]

    (ii) Captopril. A 25 mg sublingual dose produces a fall in pressure within 5 min, and a useful hypotensive action for hours.[8]

Although the sublingual route has been vigorously promoted, it may have been overplayed; swallowing the tablets may be just as effective.[9] An alternative is a combination of a beta-blocker, such as atenolol 100 mg, and a diuretic (bendrofluazide 5–10 mg) which produces a smooth fall in arterial pressure over 12–24 h and is often all that is required (see (4) on p. 49).

(5) If you do use i.v. therapy, treatment with diuretics, in doses adequate to maintain urinary output, and oral hypotensives should start at the same time.

(6) Hypertensive crisis in phaeochromocytoma must be treated with an alpha-adrenergic blocking drug. Give phentolamine 5.0–10 mg i.v. at 5 min intervals until the arterial pressure is controlled and thereafter at 2–4 h intervals, or as needed to keep the arterial pressure under control. Phentolamine, which acts within 1–2 min, and has a duration of action of 3–10 min, may also be given as a continuous infusion at a rate of 0.2–0.5 mg/mm. Labetalol or sodium nitroprusside may also be used in this situation.

REFERENCES

1   Bertel O. *et al.* (1983) Nifedipine in hypertensive emergencies. *Br. Med. J.* **286:** 19.
2   Calhoun D. A., Oparil S. (1990) Treatment of hypertensive crisis. *N. Engl. J. Med.* **323:** 1177.
3   Gifford, R. (1991) Management of hypertensive crisis. *JAMA* **266:** 829.
4   Koch-Weser J. (1976) Diazoxide. *N. Engl. J. Med.* **294:** 1271.
5   Koch-Weser J. (1976) Hydralazine. *N. Engl. J. Med.* **295:** 320.
6   Leader (1979) Hypertensive encephalopathy. *Br. Med. J.* **2:** 1387.
7   Leader (1989) Severe symptomless hypertension. *Lancet* **2:** 1369.
8   Leader (1991) Hypertensive emergencies. *Lancet* **338:** 220.
9   Messerli F. *et al.* (1991) Sublingual nifedipine for hypertensive emergencies. *Lancet* **338:** 881.
10 Palmer R. F., Lasseter K. C. (1975) Sodium nitroprusside. *N. Engl. J. Med.* **292:** 294.

Pulmonary embolus[12,17]

DIAGNOSIS

(1) Pulmonary embolus, depending on its size, may present as one of four clinical pictures, the last three of which may overlap to some extent.

    Group A   Sudden death. The diagnosis is established at post mortem.

    Group B   circulatory failure. Syncope or collapse occur in 80%, acute dyspnoea in 70% and central chest pain in 35% of this group. This group of patients needs to be distinguished from those with myocardial infarction (see below).

    Group C   Pleuritic pain and haemoptysis, unaccompanied by signs of circulatory failure. This needs to be distinguished from pneumonia (see below).

    Group D   Shortness of breath alone. This characteristically insidious onset of multiple pulmonary emboli should always be considered in a patient with a history of slowly progressive dyspnoea.

(2) The signs on examination will again vary according to the size of the embolus.

    (i)   The signs of pulmonary hypertension may be present if approximately two-thirds of the area of the pulmonary arterial bed is obstructed. These signs, which occur in a major pulmonary embolus (group B above), include:

        (a) a giant 'a' wave in the jugular venous pulse;
        (b) a powerful para-sternal heave;
        (c) a right atrial gallop (triple heart sounds heard loudest in the pulmonary area);
        (d) accentuation of the pulmonary second sound;
        (e) tachypnoea, tachycardia, cyanosis and hypotension are also frequently present.

    (ii)   The signs of pulmonary infarction. This does not invariably follow pulmonary embolus but is usually present if pleuritic pain occurs—characteristically group C. A pleural friction rub is heard and if the infarct is large this is followed in about 48 h by dullness, decreased breath sounds and crackles over the site of the infarct.

(3) The legs should always be examined for signs of deep vein thrombosis (DVT).[6,14,15] These thrombi, of course, are the source of the embolus. There may be pain in the calf. The signs are:

(i) delayed cooling of the exposed leg;
(ii) increased size of the calf, the careful measurement of which should be compared with the other leg. These are two of the most reliable signs of deep vein thrombosis. In addition there may be:
(i) accentuation of the venous pattern and oedema of the ankle and foot;
(ii) tenderness on palpation of the calf muscles or Hunter's canal.

(4) The presence of thrombi in the veins above the knee (the usual source of emboli) can be confirmed simply by ultrasound and impedence plethysmography.[6,15] Remember, though, that the absence of DVT does not exclude a pulmonary embolus— all the clot may have travelled to the lung by the time of your investigations. Remember also that Homan's sign is falsely positive or falsely negative too often to be of any value, and that 70% of DVTs give rise to neither signs nor symptoms.

(5) Investigations include the following.

(i) Chest x-ray. Frequently there may be no evidence of large pulmonary emboli on an ordinary chest x-ray. Collapse of part of a lung may be inferred from an elevated diaphragm (the first sign to develop) and increased translucency of one lobe or lung. As the infarct becomes haemorrhagic the characteristic wedge shaped shadow appears. In addition, the pulmonary artery diameter may be enlarged (more than 17 mm in a man and more than 16 mm in a woman) or the pulmonary artery may even be seen to terminate abruptly—'pulmonary cut off'.

(ii) ECG. The ECG may be initially normal, but may change rapidly in the early phases of the illness. Characteristic patterns of change are:

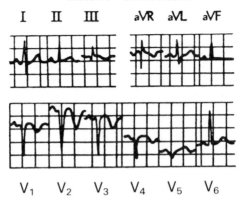

Fig. 19 ECG in pulmonary embolism. (Reproduced with permission from, Oram S. (1984) *Clinical Heart Disease*, 2nd edn. (London: Heinemann Medical.)

(a) an attempt to develop right axis deviation—an S wave in I—a Q wave in III with a raised ST segment and inverted T wave (but not also in II as in inferior myocardial infarction) and inverted T waves across the right ventricular chest leads with clock-wise rotation (Fig. 19);

(b) development of right bundle branch block (RBBB);

(c) any of the conventional ischaemic patterns, presumably provoked by low coronary artery blood flow. In fact sinus tachycardia, supraventricular tachycardias and atrial fibrillation are commoner than RBBB or S wave in lead 1, Q wave in lead 3 and T wave inversion in lead 3.

(iii) A perfusion scan of the lungs may reveal areas of diminished flow at a time when the chest x-ray is normal, and a normal perfusion scan effectively excludes pulmonary embolus. It is helpful to combine the perfusion scan with a ventilation scan. A gross mismatch, showing a segmental or larger area of underperfusion of normally ventilated lung, is characteristic of pulmonary embolism, but you need to be aware that smaller matched defects can occur in pulmonary emboli[16,17]. Thus scans allow you to make confident therapeutic decisions in two groups—

those patients with a high probability of emboli usually prove to have them on a pulmonary angiogram, and patients with normal scans in whom the diagnosis is virtually excluded. This leaves an intermediary group (around 40% of scans) where the scan does not help to solve the clinical dilemma, because in this group the overall rate of angiographically defined pulmonary emboli is 40%.[11] It is in this group that the other diagnostic aids, particularly the definition of venous thrombosis, are most useful.

(iv) Arterial blood gases. The Pao_2 is usually below 8.0 kPa (60 mmHg) in substantial embolization.

(v) Pulmonary angiography is the only certain way of diagnosing pulmonary embolus. It may demonstrate absent or incomplete filling of the pulmonary vasculature. The indications for this investigation—which is quick and is of minimal inconvenience to the patient if the specialised equipment and experience are available—are discussed below. Retrograde venography undertaken at the same time may show the source of the embolus in the pelvic or leg veins.[2]

(vi) Bilirubin, LDH and ALT levels are seldom diagnostically helpful.

MANAGEMENT

Group A is fatal by definition. Group B is frequently fatal. Group C should always be treated urgently because some 30% of patients who survive one embolus have a second which is fatal in about 20%. Patients in group D also require urgent treatment but are not, unlike groups B and C, in mortal danger. Management involves:

(1) Establishing the diagnosis. As indicated above, physical examination of the acute case may be helpful, but is seldom conclusive. Additional information is needed from the chest x-ray, arterial blood gases and ECG which should all be obtained as soon as possible. Pulmonary angiography, being the only certain diagnostic measure, should be undertaken in any patient in whom there is clinical suspicion of a major pulmonary embolus.

(2) Restoring the systemic circulation. This is the first consideration in group B and is most effectively achieved by moving the embolus. How to do this is controversial, but:

(i)   If the heart has stopped cardiac massage may not only restart it, but may also break up and disperse the embolus.

(ii) If the patient is in shock or deteriorating rapidly with signs of progressive right heart failure, and is not responding to, or not able to have fibrinolytics, pulmonary embolectomy should be undertaken. This will only be required in 2–6% of patients with major pulmonary embolus.[9] Heparin should then be used postoperatively.

(iii) Thrombolytics (fibrinolytics) may be infused into the pulmonary arteries through the catheter with which the angiogram has been done.[10] These agents are plasminogen activators; the plasmin so generated is a proteolytic enzyme. By digesting fibrin, it dissolves clots. Absolute contraindications to the use of fibrinolytics are active bleeding or a bleeding diathesis, aortic dissection, proliferative diabetic retinopathy and pregnancy. Relative contraindications include recent trauma or surgery (within the preceding ten days), recent stroke or GI bleed (within the past two months), active peptic ulceration and severe hypertension (systolic arterial pressure of >200 mmHg, or diastolic arterial pressure of >115 mmHg). Give one of the following.

(a) Streptokinase (which is cheap, but is allergenic). Give an initial dose of 250 000 units in 30 min and then infuse 100 000 units/h for 24 h.

(b) If for any reason you cannot use streptokinase, tissue plasminogen activator (tPA) in a dose of 100 mg infused through a peripheral vein over 2 h is an effective alternative.[3]

(c) Urokinase (which is expensive but not allergenic) is used occasionally. Give 4400 IU/kg over 10 min, and then 4400 IU kg/h for 24 h. If the initial response is unsatisfactory continue the infusion at the same rate to a total of 700 000 units.

These fibrinolytics are potentially hazardous, in that severe bleeding may occur during the infusion. To minimize the chances of bleeding, you should:

      minimise the physical handling of the patient;

      discontinue parenteral medicine wherever possible, and substitute appropriate oral therapy;

      minimise all invasive procedures;

      apply compression bandages at the site of vessel punctures;

      avoid concurrent anticoagulation, or treatment with anti-platelet drugs.

If bleeding does occur, stop the fibrinolytic agent (the half-life of which is usually only ½ h), and give fresh whole blood. Failing this, give fresh frozen plasma and cryoprecipitate to replace the fibrinogen and other coagulation factors. Epsilon amino caproic acid, in a dose of 5 g, can be given in the rare event of the above measures being unsuccessful.

(iv) Monitoring fibrinolytic therapy. The best way to do this is the whole blood euglobin lysis time, the next best is the thrombin time. These are not generally available, and the partial thromboplastin time is a reasonable alternative. Take a preinfusion control value, and repeat 4 h after the infusion has started. If the PTT is increased, you can assume that systemic lysis has been achieved.

(v) After completing the thrombolytic therapy, a continuous infusion of heparin should be started as soon as the PTT falls to less than twice the control value.[5]

(vi) While definitive measures are being initiated, you may have to support the circulation. To this end, it is important to keep the right atrial pressure (and thus the right ventricular filling pressure) high. A pressure of 12 mmHg above the sternal angle appears to be optimal for maximising right-sided stroke work in this situation. The right atrial pressure tends to be high anyway in major pulmonary emboli but if less than 12 mmHg infuse Haemaccel or dextran 70 under CVP control. You will probably only need a few hundred ml, so be wary. If raising the right ventricular filling pressure is to no avail, use inotropic agents.

(3) Reversing hypoxia. This is always present because intrapulmonary shunting, alveolar hypoventilation and impaired perfusion occur.[4] Oxygen via an MC mask is partly effective in relieving this hypoxia.

(4) Relieving pain. Give diamorphine, 5 mg i.v. preceded by prochlorperazine 12.5 mg i.m.

(5) In groups C and D the systemic circulation is not jeopardised and none of the measures (i)–(iii) under (2) above is required. However, in all groups, whatever the initial treatment, you can minimize the chance of further thrombi forming, and therefore of further embolization, by anticoagulating your patient. This should be undertaken as indicated on p. 18.

(6) Removal or exclusion of any remaining deep vein thrombi. These have first to be identified either by retrograde phlebography at the same time as the pulmonary arteriogram, or by bilateral ascending femoral phlebography. After identification either direct surgical removal or proximal ligation of the affected vein can be undertaken, depending on the site of the thrombus. An alternative is to infuse fibrinolytic agents locally or systemically, in the doses given above.[8,10] In practice, it is only rarely that you will need to do any more than give systemic thrombolytics.

(7) Pregnancy. In the particular circumstances of pulmonary embolism in pregnancy, anticoagulation should be commenced with heparin, as advocated on p. 18. Warfarin is best not used since it is teratogenic and is also associated with an increased incidence of ante-partum haemorrhage.[7]

(8) Remember that the prevention of venous thrombosis is the key to the prevention of pulmonary embolism.[1]

(9) Vena caval filters. In patients who have recurrent pulmonary emboli, despite all the above treatments, you may need to consider the insertion of a vena caval filter.[11]

REFERENCES

1   Collins R. *et al.* (1988) Reduction in fatal pulmonary embolism and venous thrombosis by perioperative administration of subcutaneous heparin. *N. Engl. J. Med.* **318:** 1162.

2   Dow J. D. (1973) Retrograde phlebography in major PE. *Lancet* **2:** 407.

3   Goldhaber S. Z. *et al.* (1988) Randomized controlled trial of recombinant tissue plasminogen activator versus urokinase in the treatment of acute pulmonary embolism. *Lancet* **ii:** 293.

4   Hayes S. P., Bone R. C. (1983) Pulmonary emboli with respiratory failure. *Med. Clin. North Am.* **67:** 1179.

5   Hull R. (1986) Continuous intravenous heparin compared with intermittent subcutaneous heparin in the initial treatment of proximal vein thrombosis. *N. Engl. J. Med.* **315:** 1109.

6   Leader (1989) Diagnosis of deep vein thrombosis. *Lancet* **ii:** 23.

7   Leader (1979) Thrombo-embolism in pregnancy. *Br. Med. J.* **1:** 1661.

8   Leader (1981) Streptokinase and deep venous thrombosis. *Lancet* **i:** 1035.

9   Leader (1989) Surgery for pulmonary embolus? *Lancet* **i:** 198.

10   Marder V. (1988) Thrombolytic therapy: current status. *N. Engl. J. Med.* **318:** 1512.

11   McCullom C. (1987) Vena caval filters: keeping the big clots down. *BMJ* **294:** 1566.

12   Oakley C. M. (1970) Diagnosis of pulmonary embolism. *Br. Med. J.* **2:** 773.

14   Sandler D. A. *et al.* (1984) Diagnosis of deep venous thrombosis: comparison of clinical evaluation, ultrasound, plethysmograph, and venoscan with x-ray venogram. *Lancet* **ii:** 716.

15   Salzman, E. W. (1986) Venous thrombosis made easy. *N. Engl. J. Med.* **314:** 847.

16   Spies W. B. *et al.* (1986) Ventilation/perfusion scintigraphy in suspected pulmonary embolus, correlation with pulmonary angiography and refinement of criteria of interpretation. *Radiology* **159:** 383.

17   Windebank W. (1987) Diagnosing pulmonary embolism. *Br. Med. J.* **294:** 1369.

Peripheral embolus[1,3-5]

DIAGNOSIS

(1) Obstruction of blood supply to an organ usually causes a sudden onset of severe pain, numbness and loss of function. The basis for obstruction is usually either embolus or thrombosis superimposed on local atheromatous disease. It may be impossible to decide between the two. Where there is clinical doubt, arteriography should be undertaken, as the treatment may differ.

(2) The diagnosis should be considered in anyone in whom the above mentioned symptoms occur, especially when there is an obvious source of embolus, e.g. recent myocardial infarction, atrial fibrillation, mitral stenosis.

(3) Thus:

    (i) *In the limbs*: look for the six Ps—pain, pallor, pulselessness, paraesthesia, paralysis, and perishing cold. The diagnosis is usually fairly clear. However it may be mimicked by a deep vein thrombosis which occurs in a leg with pre-existing obstructive arterial disease. Here also the leg is painful, pale and pulseless, but may be differentiated from infarction by the development of oedema, which occurs only late in infarction. In addition, an arterial embolus is experienced first as pain which passes into numbness.

    (ii) *In the gut*: causes abdominal pain with vomiting and possibly the passage of blood per rectum. There may be signs of peritonitis and impending intestinal obstruction. The patient rapidly deteriorates if infarction of the bowel has occurred. Diagnosis is made at laparotomy.

    (iii) *In the kidney*: the patient complains of acute loin pain and haematuria symptoms which may also be caused by a stone. An IVP and renogram should distinguish between the two, and an arterial occlusion can be confirmed by selective renal arteriography.

    (iv) *In the carotid circulation*: causes the onset of neurological signs, e.g. hemiplegia. If this occurs in a setting where an embolus is likely, early arteriography, preferably a DVI, should be undertaken to determine the site of the block.

(4) Emboli are not infrequently multiple. All the peripheral pulses should be carefully palpated.

MANAGEMENT

(1) Control of pain with i.v. morphine (see p. 12).
(2) Conservation of the ischaemic area. This is only really possible in the limbs, which, pending definitive therapy, should be:

(i) exposed in a dependent position;
(ii) cooled, using a portable fan.

(3) Minimising further thrombus formation. This is only practical in acute limb ischaemia, where you should give i.v. heparin (see p. 19), irrespective of whether you deem surgery likely or not.[1] Anticoagulants may also prevent further emboli (see (5) below).
(4) Removal or dissolution of the obstruction.[1] As a general principle this should be undertaken whenever possible. Thus:

(i) *In the limbs*: if the diagnois of embolus is clear, surgery should be undertaken without delay, if necessary under local anaesthetic. Otherwise, first perform an arteriogram; if there is a thrombosis, low dose streptokinase (5000 units/h) should be infused through the arterial catheter until patency is restored,[2] or there is no improvement between successive 12-hourly arteriograms. This regime is accompanied by 67% reperfusion rates. In neither case is a 'wait-and-see' policy justified. If the above treatments are either unsuccessful or impossible, the following regime may be helpful. Give alternate bottles of 20 ml 95% alcohol in 500 ml of saline with 500 ml dextran 70 in 5% dextrose 6-hourly.
(ii) *In the gut*: if at all possible, embolectomy and revascularisation of the bowel should be undertaken immediately. If infarction has occurred survival without operation is extremely rare.
(iii) *In the kidney*: operation should be considered, at which

either the embolus or the kidney is removed depending on the viability of the latter.

(iv) *In the extracranial carotid arteries*: immediate embolectomy under local anaesthetic may be considered, but enthusiasm for this approach is waning (see p. 92).

(v) *In the intracranial carotid artery*: anticoagulants should be started after you have shown on CT scan that the infarct is not haemorrhagic.

(5) Prevention of further occlusion. After the primary therapy has been undertaken a course of anticoagulants should be started (see p. 19) as they probably reduce the incidence of further embolism or thrombi.

(6) Atrial fibrillation, which is often present, should be controlled as necessary.

(7) These patients often have significant atherosclerotic disease, and it is prudent to give them aspirin 75 mg/day.

REFERENCES

1 Campbell W. B. (1989) Managing acute limb ischaemia. *Br. Med. J.* **299:** 526.

2 Earnshaw J. (1987) Management of acute lower limb arterial ischaemia. *Hospital Update* January, p. 15.

3 Sewell I. A. (1985) Sudden arterial occlusion. *Hospital Update* June, p. 363.

4 Sewell, I. A. (1985) Management of sudden arterial occlusion. *Hospital Update* June, p. 449.

5 Thompson J. E. (1980) Peripheral arterial surgery. *N. Engl. J. Med.* **302:** 491.

Dissections of the thoracic aorta[1,2,3]

DIAGNOSIS

(1) The process of dissection may be intensely painful. Pain which, in contrast to myocardial infarction is usually maximal at the onset of the problem, may be experienced in the chest, the back, the abdomen or the legs, depending upon the origin of the aneurysm. It may spread from one site to another depending on the direction and extent of the dissection. In almost half the cases, however, pain is slight and the diagnosis is made from a chance finding on chest x-ray, from a sudden drop in the arterial pressure, or from the signs of ischaemia (see p. 60).

(2) The signs include the following.

    (i)   Shock (see p. 334) which may be due to severe pain or to loss of blood.

    (ii)   Signs of ischaemia in the:

        (a) myocardium—myocardial infarction;
        (b) limbs—apart from gross signs (see p. 60) a difference of 20 mmHg between the systolic arterial pressures of opposite limbs indicates arterial obstruction in the limb with the lower pressure;
        (c) brain—a hemi- or quadriplegia;
        (d) kidneys—if both kidneys are involved, as is usually the case, there is severe oliguria with a few red cells or complete anuria;
        (e) gut (see p. 60);
        (f) spinal cord—paraplegia.

    (iii)   Aortic regurgitation.
    (iv)   Haemopericardium.
    (v)   Left pleural effusion.

(3) Investigations include:

    (i)   Chest x-ray. In 80% of patients with dissection, there is widening of the mediastinum, often accompanied by a left pleural effusion. When you are in doubt, repeat the x-ray every 24 h in order to detect changes in the contour of the aorta.

(ii) Echocardiography. This may show widening and the characteristic double lumen of the aorta. If transoesophageal recordings are made the sensitivity and specificity of this procedure are over 90%.[2]

(iii) Both CT and MRI imaging can identify dissection, and are being used more frequently for this purpose.[1]

(iv) Aortography. This is the definitive investigation for a dissecting aortic aneurysm and most surgeons will want it undertaken if operative treatment is considered.

MANAGEMENT

The priorities of medical management, which should be undertaken in close collaboration with surgical colleagues, are as follows.

(1) Relief of pain. Any one of the following combinations may be given and repeated as often as necessary provided the patient is not dangerously hypotensive.

    (i) Heroin 5–10 mg i.v. plus prochlorperazine 12.5 mg i.v.
    (ii) Morphine 10 mg i.v. plus prochlorperazine 12.5 mg i.v.

(2) Lowering the blood pressure if raised (see p. 49).
(3) Relief of cardiac tamponade (see p. 67).

Further management should be discussed with a cardiovascular surgeon who should be consulted as soon as the diagnosis has been considered.

REFERENCES

1   Desanctis R. *et al*. (1987) Aortic dissection. *N. Engl. J. Med.* **317**: 1060.

2   Erbel R. *et al*. (1989) Echocardiography in diagnosis of aortic dissection. *Lancet* **i**: 457.

3   Leader (1988) Acute aortic dissection. *Lancet* **ii**: 827.

Cardiac tamponade[1,3]

This term implies restriction of cardiac function by mechanical constriction of the heart. This is usually caused by a tense pericardial effusion, or by a haemopericardium (which may follow a dissecting aneurysm, a chest injury or a myocardial infarction). It may also be caused by blood clots surrounding the heart even when the pericardium has been left widely open, as after thoracic surgery.

DIAGNOSIS

(1) There may be a preceding history of precordial pain followed by increasing dyspnoea.

(2) The signs are those of:

    (i) Decreased cardiac output. Despite a tachycardia, the patient is hypotensive, the pulse pressure is small and the peripheries are poorly perfused. In addition pulsus paradoxus is usually present. This may be demonstrated by measuring the systolic arterial pressure in expiration and inspiration. If there is a fall of >10 mmHg on inspiration then constriction is present.

    (ii) Increased pressure in the systemic and pulmonary veins. The jugular venous pressure is raised, and either does not descend or goes up further on inspiration (Kussmaul's sign). Similarly the respiratory rate is raised and the patient is occasionally orthopnoeic, with wheezes and possibly crackles in the chest.

    (iii) The effusion itself. It may be possible to demonstrate an increased area of dullness around the precordium, or at the back, mimicking a pleural effusion. In addition, the apex beat is impalpable and the heart sounds are muffled. However, a third heart sound can usually be heard. Thus, the diagnosis should always be considered in a patient with severe left ventricular failure and/or hypotension.

    (iv) The above signs develop sequentially, over a variable time course. The progression seen serves as a useful guide to grading the severity of the effusion, as outlined below.

    (a) *Grade 1*. JVP and heart rate are both increased, but cardiac output is normal.

    (b) *Grade 2*. As above, with the addition of pulsus paradoxus and mild hypotension.

    (c) *Grade 3*. As above, with in addition a poor cardiac output and muffling of the heart sounds.

(3) Chest x-ray shows a globular heart (the water-bottle heart), which is relatively immobile on screening. The extent of the effusion is best estimated by echocardiography, which has the great advantage of being non-invasive.

(4) The ECG may be of low voltage and there may be widespread inversion of T waves.

(5) If cardiac tamponade needs to be relieved urgently, the signs are usually gross (i.e. Grade 3)—the pulse almost disappearing on inspiration. The degree of severity may be caused by a surprisingly small effusion.

(6) Tamponade needs to be differentiated from other causes of a poor cardiac output with a raised JVP, importantly:

    (i)   severe congestive cardiac failure;

    (ii) pulmonary embolus (see p. 53);

    (iii) right ventricular myocardial infarction (see p. 11);

    (iv) superior vena-caval obstruction—the immobility of the neck veins and suffusion of the face should help you here.

the distinction between these various categories is sometimes very difficult on clinical grounds. If you do not have echocardiogram facilities to help you, assume a pericardial effusion is present, and treat accordingly.

MANAGEMENT

(1) The heart must be decompressed:

    (i)   if the patient is distressed;

    (ii) if the systolic arterial pressure is <90 mmHg and/or the jugular venous pressure is more than 10 cm.

(2) If trauma is the cause of the tamponade, the treatment is urgent thoracotomy. Pericardiocentesis is, in this circumstance, at best a holding manoeuvre, and should not delay surgery.

(3) Manage non-traumatic tamponade as follows.

(i) If the patient is in extremis, insert a wide bore needle in the 4th intercostal space over the precordium and advance until fluid is obtained. This may release enough fluid—often surprisingly little—to relieve the heart.

(ii) Otherwise the site of choice is the xiphisternal angle.[4] Sit the patient up at 45°, insert the needle 3 cm below the xiphisternum at an angle of between 30° and 45° to the skin. Apply suction to the needle, and push it slowly upwards and backwards towards the left shoulder until fluid is obtained, and then aspirate as much fluid as you can. The heart may be difficult to feel, but usually produces ectopic beats when scratched. If you have your needle connected to an ECG machine, as you should, you will get an appropriate recording (Fig. 20).

(iii) If the effusion is haemorrhagic, you may wonder if you have unwittingly entered a cardiac chamber. Place a few ml of the fluid in a glass tube—intracardiac blood will clot, haemorrhagic effusion will not.

(iv) To minimise the chances of your entering a cardiac chamber, it is helpful to attach your aspiration needle to the 'V' lead terminal on the ECG cable. This can be done by means of an insulated wire with a clip on each end—failing this, just attach the wire with Sellotape. Figure 20 shows the electrocardiograms obtained when the needle tip is advanced to three different sites.

(v) Both volume expansion and vasodilators have been advocated. There is good evidence that both are ineffective.[2]

REFERENCES

1   Callahan M. L. (1984) Pericardiocentesis in traumatic and non-traumatic cardiac tamponade. *Ann. Emerg. Med.* **13:** 924.

2   Kerber R. E. *et al.* (1982) Haemodynamic effects of volume

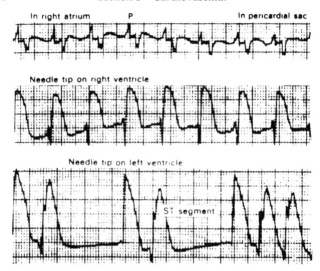

Fig. 20 Electrocardiogram obtained from the needle tip at three sites. (Reproduced with permission from Dr A. Hollman and the editors of *Medicine*.)

expansion and nitroprusside compared with pericardiocentesis in patients with acute cardiac tamponade. *N. Engl. J. Med.* **307:** 929.

3   Leader (1980) Cardiac tamponade. *Br. Med. J.* 505.
4   Lindsay D. (1988) Cardiac tamponade. *Cardiology in Practice* September, p. 34.

Respiratory

Respiratory failure[1]

DIAGNOSIS

(1) This is defined in terms of altered blood gases—an arterial oxygen tension (Pao_2) of less than 8 kPa (60 mmHg) with or without an arterial CO_2 tension ($Paco_2$) of above 6.7 kPa (50 mmHg).

(2) Both hypoxia (low Pao_2) and hypercarbia (raised $Paco_2$) are difficult to pick up clinically, for the following reasons.

(i) The classical signs of hypoxia[2] are either non-specific (disturbances of consciousness, ranging from mild confusion to coma), or difficult to assess (cyanosis).

(ii) Hypercarbia[7] may give rise to a spectrum of mental changes similar to those of hypoxia. It may also cause a flapping tremor, peripheral vasodilatation, papilloedema and early morning headaches, which again are not specific for a rising $Paco_2$.

Hence arterial blood gas measurements are mandatory if the diagnosis is suspected.

There are three patterns of respiratory failure.

(1) *Pure ventilatory failure* which gives rise to a raised $Paco_2$ and a low Pao_2. Examples of this are:

(i) depression of the respiratory centre by drugs;

(ii) neurological conditions such as poliomyelitis, myasthenia gravis, Guillain-Barré syndrome;

(iii) primary alveolar hypoventilation (Pickwickian syndrome).

(2) *Hypoxaemic failure* due to local disturbances of the ventilation–perfusion relationship. This gives rise to a low Pao_2, with a low or normal $Paco_2$.[2] Examples of this are:

(i) 'pure' emphysema;

(ii) asthma in the initial stages of an attack (see Fig. 21, p. 81);

(iii) pneumonia (see p. 104);

(iv) left ventricular failure (but see p. 44);

    (v)   fibrosing alveolitis;

    (vi)   adult respiratory distress syndrome–shock lung (see p. 97).

(3) *A mixture of ventilatory and hypoxaemic failure.*

    (i)   This combination of alveolar hypoventilation and deranged ventilation–perfusion relationships produces a low Pao_2, with a raised Pco_2. The example of this type of failure is chronic bronchitis with emphysema, and in late severe asthma.

    (ii)   Such patients frequently have a permanently low Pao_2 and may have a permanently high $Paco_2$ (and therefore a high serum HCO_3). However, if, with a raised $Paco_2$, the serum HCO_3 is relatively normal (below 30 mmol/l), and the pH is therefore low, the implications are that renal compensation has not occurred, and the respiratory failure has come on over a short time. This further implies that there are reversible elements, such as an acute infection with associated sputum retention, increasing airways obstruction and often heart failure.

    (iii) This is the commonest clinical setting for respiratory failure.

ACUTE OR CHRONIC BRONCHITIS PRECIPITATING RESPIRATORY FAILURE

Diagnosis

(1) The patient often has a history of increasing breathlessness, increasing volumes of purulent sputum and, occasionally, pleuritic pain. All this in the setting of chronic obstructive airways disease.

(2) Examination reveals a breathless, often pyrexial patient, who may be confused, cyanosed and have a tachycardia.

(3) There may be evidence of hypercarbia (see above).

(4) There will be a prolonged expiratory phase, with variable crackles and wheezes.

(5) The signs of collapse, consolidation, effusion or pneumothorax must also be sought as any of these can exacerbate the situation.

(6) Signs of right-sided heart failure (raised neck veins, oedema and a palpable liver) are often present.

Management[3]

Initial investigations, in order of priority, are as follows.

(1) Arterial blood gases and pH.
(2) PEFR measurement.
(3) Chest x-ray, most importantly to exclude a pneumothorax.
(4) Culture of sputum and blood.
(5) Knowledge of haemoglobin, electrolytes and urea, whereas not immediately useful, will be required.

The aim of management is to increase intracellular O_2. Experience with tissue oxygen electrodes is limited and as yet this is measured indirectly by the Pao_2. The Pao_2 should be increased to at least 6.7–7.3 kPa (50–55 mmHg), achieved preferably with a fall, or at least without a substantial rise in $Paco_2$.

Each of the factors, enumerated above, which contribute to the combination of ventilatory and hypoxaemic failure must be tackled.

(1) Infection.

    (i) The commonest infecting organisms are *Streptococcus pneumoniae* and *Haemophilus influenzae*. Both are usually sensitive to amoxycillin 250 mg 8-hourly (parenterally or orally), tetracycline 500 mg 6-hourly (i.m. or orally, not i.v.) or cotrimoxazole tabs. ii b.d. In some parts of the UK there are significant numbers of *H. influenzae* resistant to amoxycillin—consult your microbiologist to get information about your setting, and be guided in your antibiotic therapy accordingly.

    (ii) If the infection has been contracted in hospital, or if for other reasons you suspect that the infection may be caused by resistant staphylococci, add i.v. or i.m. flucloxacillin 500 mg 6-hourly.

    (iii) If the sputum purulence has not decreased after 48 h, consider changing the antibiotic, but consult your bacteriologist first. Remember that sputum culture and sensitivity tests may be misleading, so do not change antibiotics exclusively on the basis of information from these.

(2) Sputum retention.

    (i)   A patient's outlook may be transformed if energetic and regular physiotherapy 'raises the sputum'.

    (ii)   Initially physiotherapy must be given 2-hourly throughout the 24 h, and if necessary you must teach both day and night nurses how to give appropriate physiotherapy.

    (iii)   The sputum should be loosened by clapping the chest for 3–4 min, after which the patient should take a few quick deep breaths and then cough. Ideally this should be done in appropriate bronchial drainage positions. This is rarely feasible, but at least place the patient first on one side and then on the other. If the patient is too confused to cooperate, give physiotherapy after nikethamide or doxapram. The sputum may be sticky, and intermittent humidification through a Wright's nebuliser can aid expectoration (4 ml of warm saline is as effective as anything and is certainly cheapest). If despite these measures the patient still cannot bring up sputum, it must be sucked up by one of the following means.

    (iv)   Nasotracheal suction. Sit the patient up and with a gloved hand pass a soft catheter with a round end (off suction lest the pharynx and trachea be traumatised) through a nostril and into the pharynx. A convenient arrangement for this is to attach the catheter to one limb of a Y connector, which is itself attached to a sucker. Suction is then applied by occluding the other limb. To be of maximum benefit, the catheter must pass between the cords. Encourage the patient to cough, and, as s/he exhales, advance the catheter and then suck. If the patient cannot phonate, you are probably through the cords. Advance the catheter into each main bronchus in turn. This is a potent stimulus to coughing and you should leave the catheter down until more sputum is forthcoming. If laryngospasm occurs, attempts to pass the catheter into the trachea should not be repeated.

    (v)   Bronchoscopy. This should be undertaken if, despite nasotracheal suction, the patient continues to deteriorate, especially if the sputum retention produces lobar collapse. Flexible bronchoscopes have made this a much less traumatic event than previously and, given the

circumstances, the patient's memory for the event is hazy.
(vi) Tracheal toilet through an endotracheal tube.

(3) Airways obstruction. The reversible component may be due to:

(i) sputum retention;
(ii) mucosal inflammation;
(iii) bronchospasm.

Treatments of (i) and (ii) have been discussed. Bronchospasm must be assumed to be present and must be treated, as follows.

(a) Give nebulised salbutamol (5 ml of salbutamol mixed with 3 ml of saline) over 3 min four times each day.
(b) The addition of ipratropium has not been found to confer additional benefit in patients with COAD, and we do not use it.[5,6]
(c) Aminophylline i.v. 5 mg/kg initially and then 0.5 mg/kg per hour thereafter. As well as being a bronchodilator, aminophylline may increase the force of diaphragmatic contraction. The dose may need adjusting in old or very ill patients and, of course, in those who have been on oral theophylline. You should measure the levels at 8 and 24 h (see p. 82).
(d) Steroids may also be given. Even if your patient does not benefit from steroids when well, they are useful in reversing the additional bronchial obstruction present in acute exacerbations. So give hydrocortisone 100 mg 8-hourly.

(4) Oxygen therapy.[8] Oxygen should be given in sufficient concentration to raise the Pao_2 to at least 6.0 kPa (45 mmHg) and preferably 7.3 kPa (55 mmHg). To aim higher than this is unnecessary and in view of the potential danger of oxygen therapy in this type of ventilatory failure, undesirable. The danger of oxygen therapy arises because patients with a chronically raised $Paco_2$ rely not only on a rise in $Paco_2$, as normal, but on a fall in Pao_2 to stimulate respiration—the so-called 'hypoxic drive'.[4] A sudden rise in Pao_2 may reduce this hypoxic drive, and thus depress ventilation.

This causes a further rise in $Paco_2$, and may precipitate CO_2

narcosis. So after you have measured arterial blood gases, start with the 28% oxygen mask. Measure the arterial gases again after one hour. If:

(i) The Pao_2 is above 7.3 kPa (55 mmHg) and $Paco_2$ has not gone up by more than 1.3 kPa (10 mmHg), continue using 28%.

(ii) The Pao_2 is below 7.3 kPa (55 mmHg) and the $Paco_2$ has not gone up more than 1.3 kPa (10 mmHg), progress to 35% O_2 by Ventimask (8 l/min). Measure the $Paco_2$ again in a further hour and if situation (ii) still obtains, you may progress to stronger concentrations of oxygen.

(iii) The $Paco_2$ has risen more than 1.3 kPa (10 mmHg). You are in grave danger of inducing CO_2 narcosis. Do not increase (or lower) O_2 concentration but intensify all other aspects of treatment, particularly the conjunction of physiotherapy and respiratory stimulants. If the $Paco_2$ goes on rising, despite this, you will have to decide if intermittent positive pressure respiration (IPPR) should be used. This can be a difficult decision, and depends particularly on the usual respiratory status of your patient. If he is a respiratory cripple, then IPPR is unlikely to be of lasting benefit and you may have difficulty weaning him off the ventilator.

(iv) Occasionally, patients are given high oxygen concentration by mistake, or in ignorance. This may lead to the rapid development of CO_2 narcosis. It is always best to assume that deterioration in the condition of a patient with ventilatory and hypoxaemic failure is due to CO_2 narcosis. Faced with this deteriorating situation:

(a) do not immediately increase the inspired O_2 concentration;

(b) prevent anybody else from doing so;

(c) measure the blood gases;

(d) if the chest signs have changed, repeat the chest x-ray to exclude pneumothorax or massive pulmonary collapse;

(e) intensify physiotherapy;

(f) if the Pao_2 is above 7.3 kPa (55 mmHg) and the $Paco_2$ either above 12 kPa (90 mmHg), or has risen by more than 1.3 kPa (10 mmHg) from your initial

reading, reduce the O_2 to 28% by Ventimask, and use a respiratory stimulant;
(g) if the Pao_2 is below 4.7 kPa (35 mmHg) as well as $Paco_2$ being high, give a respiratory stimulant without altering the oxygen concentration until the $Paco_2$ has improved;
(h) keep measuring the blood gases. You may have to consider IPPR if things go on deteriorating.

(5) Respiratory stimulants. These are used to:

(i)   wake up the patient and help him to co-operate;
(ii) counteract CO_2 narcosis (as above);
(iii) counteract respiratory depression.

Remember in this context, that you must not sedate patients in respiratory failure. In fact, always write **NO NIGHT SEDATION** on their charts, so that no one else sedates them either! The best drug to use is doxapram, in a dose of 1.5 mg/min, increasing by 0.5 mg/min at ½-hourly intervals if there has been no improvement to a maximum of 3.0 mg/min. Ethamivan 5% 2.5 ml i.v. may also be used, as may nikethamide 2–5 ml (0.5–1.25 mg) i.v. repeated ½ hourly as necessary. If respiratory depression is due to opiates, naloxone, which is a specific opiate antagonist, can be used in doses of 0.4 mg given i.v. over 3 min. This may be repeated to a total dose of 1.2 mg. As it has a shorter duration of action than the opiates, it may need to be repeated.

(6) Heart failure. The measures outlined above result in a substantial diuresis. However, in the presence of gross or persistent CCF:

(i)   Give diuretics.
(ii) Give digoxin, particularly if the patient has uncontrolled atrial fibrillation. Patients in respiratory failure have an enhanced sensitivity to digoxin. This is therefore best not used unless there is atrial fibrillation.
(iii) Do not forget that weight is a useful indicator of fluid balance—so weigh your patient daily.
(iv) In polycythaemic patients diuresis may cause increased sludging of blood, and precipitate thrombosis. This may be prevented by venesection of 3 units of blood over 3 days and replacement with an equal amount of Haemaccel or dextran 70. This in itself may be sufficient to

improve renal blood flow and initiate a diuresis; we consider this mode of therapy to be desirable in men with a PCV >54 and >50 in women.

PURE VENTILATORY FAILURE

(1) There are occasions when the underlying problem is rapidly reversible, i.e. administration of naloxone to persons with opiate-induced respiratory depression (see above).

(2) If no such specific therapy is available, the initial decision is when to institute artificial respiration.

(3) To make a decision you have to make appropriate measurements:

    (i)   Minute volume (measured with a Wright spirometer). If this is over 4 1/min the patient is very unlikely to require artificial ventilation.

    (ii) Vital capacity (measured with a portable, bedside vital-ograph). If the vital capacity remains above 1.5 l, artificial ventilation will probably be unnecessary. The vital capacity should be measured at least daily in patients with progressive neurological lesions.

    (iii) The blood gases should be measured if there is any doubt about the patient's respiratory status. If the Paco$_2$ is raised, artificial ventilation should be instituted.

(4) Physiotherapy should be given routinely to help prevent sputum retention and infection.

(5) In unconscious patients without a gag reflex, or patients whose disease affects swallowing as well as breathing, inhalation of secretion or vomit must be prevented, by passing an endotracheal tube.

(6) All this should be done in conjunction with the anaesthetists.

HYPOXAEMIC FAILURE

Treatment of the underlying disease should of course be initiated.

(1) Oxygen may be given by an MC mask (which delivers a concentration of 50–60% to the mouth, if the flow rate is 6 1/min) as there is no risk of CO$_2$ narcosis. However, be sure not

to raise the Pao$_2$ too high, above 13.3 kPa (100 mmHg) because high oxygen concentration can be damaging to lung tissue.

(2) Artificial ventilation should be resorted to if the Pao$_2$ cannot be maintained above about 6.7 kPa (50 mmHg), or if the effort of breathing is becoming intolerable.

REFERENCES

1   Clark T. J. H. (1972) Respiratory failure. *Br. J. Hosp. Med.* **7:** 692.

2   Flenley D. C. (1978) Clinical hypoxia—causes, consequences and correction. *Lancet* **i:** 542.

3   Howard P. (1983) Drugs or oxygen for hypoxic corpulmonale? *Br. Med. J.* **287:** 1159.

4   Leitch A. G. (1981) The hypoxic drive to breathing in man. *Lancet* **i:** 428.

5   O'Driscoll B. R. *et al.* (1989) Nebulized salbutamol with and without ipratropium bromide in acute airflow obstruction. *Lancet* **i:** 1418.

6   Rebuck A. (1987) Nebulized anticholinergic and sympathomimetic treatment of asthma and COAD in the emergency room. *Am. J. Med.* **82:** 58.

7   Weinberger S. *et al.* (1989) Hypercapnia. *N. Engl. J. Med.* **321:** 1223.

8   Woo S. W., Hedley Whyte J. (1973) Oxygen therapy—the titration of a potentially dangerous drug. *Br. J. Hosp. Med.* **9:** 487.

Severe attacks of asthma[3,7]

DIAGNOSIS

(1) Recurrent reversible attacks of wheezing are the hallmarks of asthma and if despite treatment such an attack lasts for more than 6 h, this is a serious situation with a real risk of unexpected death.[1]

(2) Pulmonary oedema may cause wheezing and mimic asthma quite closely (see p. 44) but other causes of dyspnoea (see p. 375) are usually easily differentiated from asthma.

(3) An attack is usually precipitated by a combination of factors, which include infection, allergy and emotion.

(4) Severe attacks are characterised by:

    (i)   A patient who is too breathless to speak.

    (ii)   A persistent tachycardia of more than 110 beats/min.

    (iii) Pulsus paradoxus.[8] In acute asthmatic attacks paradox is usually, but not invariably present. When it is present the degree of paradox reflects the degree of airways obstruction. In a severe attack the fall in systolic arterial pressure between expiration and inspiration may be as much as 13.3 kPa (100 mmHg), the normal difference being not more than 0.7 kPa (5 mmHg).

    (iv) A 'silent' chest. There is insufficient air being moved to cause a wheeze.

    (v)   A respiratory rate above 25 breaths/min.

    (vi) A peak expiratory flow rate (PEFR) <40% of the predicted normal, or of the best obtainable result if this is known (<200 l/min if the best result is not known.).

    (vii) Hypercapnia. Fig. 21 demonstrates that in most cases of asthma the Pa_{CO_2} is low; a patient with a high Pa_{CO_2} is mortally ill. Some authorities suggest that any asthmatic who has a Pa_{CO_2} above 6.7 kPa (50 mmHg) when first seen should be ventilated forthwith, but in most circumstances it is reasonable to undertake management as outlined below.

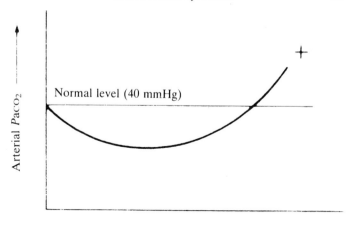

Fig. 21 Relationship between the $Paco_2$ and the severity of the asthmatic attack. (40 mmHg = 5.3 kPa.)

MANAGEMENT

Measurements of pulse rate, respiratory rate, degree of paradox and arterial blood gases are mandatory. So is an initial chest x-ray, as a pneumothorax (see p. 85) or massive pulmonary collapse (see p. 90) may complicate an asthmatic attack, and require treatment in its own right. Peak expiratory flow rate (PEFR) and, if you have a spirometer, forced expiratory volume in one second (FEV_1) are essential base line measurements, changes of which provide a simple way of assessing progress. Put up a drip and then treat the following aspects.

(1) The wheezing.

    (i)   Hydrocortisone 4 mg/kg i.v. stat. and 3–4 mg/kg i.v. 6-hourly thereafter until the patient is better. Oral prednisone 40 mg/day should be started at the same time, as corticosteroids may take 6–8 h to take effect.

    (ii)   Salbutamol. Give nebulised salbutamol (5 ml of salbutamol mixed with 3 ml of saline) on two occasions about

1 h apart. If, on the basis of PEFR, there is no improvement, you should try one of the other bronchodilators mentioned below, as well as continuing salbutamol 4–hourly.

If your patient is not improving with the nebulised treatment, switch to i.v. salbutamol. Give 12.5 μg/min by continuous infusion, a regime which has been shown to be more effective than the use of nebulisers.[4]

(iii) Ipratropium bromide,[6] an inhaled atropine-like compound, causes bronchodilatation by blocking vagal reflexes, and has an additive effect with salbutamol. Give 250–500 μg in 4 ml of saline solution by nebulisers on two occasions, 1 h apart.

(iv) It makes good pharmacological sense to alternate nebulised salbutamol and ipratropium bromide, giving one or other initially at hourly, and then at 2–hourly intervals. This may pose logistic problems, but is an ideal to strive towards.

(v) Remember that the use of nebulisers has been associated with paradoxical bronchial constriction, a risk which can be avoided if you use isotonic and preservative-free nebuliser solutions.[7]

(vi) Aminophylline. This should be considered if the above measures are not improving things. It should be given at a loading dose of 5 mg/kg infused over 30 min, and 0.5 mg/kg each hour thereafter, aiming to obtain a serum level between 8 and 20 mg/l. (45–110 μmol/l). Plasma levels should be checked after 8 and 24 h, and if your patient has CCF, liver disease or is taking oral theophylline, cimetidine, ciprofloxacin or erythromycin the above recommended doses should be halved. In smokers the maintenance dose should be increased to 0.9 mg/kg/h. Your patient should be on a cardiac monitor if theophylline is used.

(vii) Adrenaline should be avoided unless you can be certain that your patient has not been using an aerosol, in which case give adrenaline 1:1000 0.5 ml subcutaneously.

(2) Hypoxia. Use the highest concentration of oxygen available, and set a high flow rate. Retention of CO_2 is not aggravated by treatment with oxygen in patients with acute asthma. Your aim is to raise the Pao_2 to 10.7 kPa (80 mmHg).

(3) Distress. A severe asthmatic attack is alarming for all. However, you must not resort to sedation to allay the anxiety of your patient; rely on massive and repeated verbal reassurance. Try to exude confidence (which you will be far from feeling). Your patient's distress is entirely justified. He will be relieved as soon as he begins to get better; if he deteriorates, hypnotics only make matters worse.

(4) Acidosis. Correction with appropriate amounts of $NaHCO_3$ as calculated from the base deficit (see p. 342) can give rise to a considerable improvement.

(5) Potassium. Hypokalaemia often occurs in acute asthma, and may be aggravated by salbutamol. Potassium supplements should be added to the i.v. solutions as necessary. The maximum safe infusion rate is 30 mmol KCl/h, and lower rates are often adequate.

(6) Inspissated plugs of sputum. These are present in the airways of most severe asthmatics. Physiotherapy is not likely to shift them, and is both impracticable and undesirable in the acute attack. As mentioned in (9) below, hydration is helpful in shifting these plugs.

(7) Intensive care. Most patients with asthma can be looked after on a general medical ward. However, patients with the following features require intensive care.

    (i)   Hypoxia (Pao_2 <8 kPa) despite receiving 60% inspired oxygen.

    (ii) Hypercapnia ($Paco_2$ <6 kPa).

    (iii) Onset of exhaustion.

    (iv) Confusion or drowsiness.

    (v) Unconsciousness.

    (vi) Respiratory arrest.

A few of these patients may require ventilation (0.3% of patients with acute asthma), and you will need to discuss this possibility with your anaesthetic colleagues. Many intensivists will now use continuous positive airways pressure (CPAP) developed by a face mask; this may further reduce the need for ventilation.

(8) Infection. Recent trials have questioned the routine use of antibiotics in acute asthma.[5] However, we feel their use is usually justified, so give either amoxycillin (250 mg orally or i.v. 6-hourly) or oral tetracycline (500 mg g.d.s.) or cotrimaxazole (tabs ii b.d.). Remember, though, that yellow sputum

in asthmatics may be due to eosinophils induced by allergy as well as neutrophils induced by infection.

(9) Dehydration. Should be assumed to be present and should be corrected with adequate i.v. fluid (1.5 l of 5% dextrose and 500 ml of 0.9 N saline in the first 24 h is a reasonable amount, although up to 6 l of fluid may be needed). Correction of dehydration helps make the sputum less tenacious.

(10) Allergy. Removing the patient to hospital often removes her from the allergen. Clearly she must be prevented from coming into contact with any allergens to which she has a known sensitivity.

REFERENCES

1 Benatar S. R. (1986) Fatal asthma. *N. Engl. J. Med.* **314:** 423.

2 Brodie M. J. *et al.* (1988) Therapeutic monitoring of theophylline. *Hospital Update* February, 1208.

3 British Thoracic Society (1990) Guidelines for the management of asthma in adults—acute severe asthma. *Br. Med. J.* **301:** 797.

4 Cheong B. *et al.* (1988) Intravenous B agonists in severe acute asthma. *Br. Med. J.* **297:** 448.

5 Graham V. A. L. *et al.* (1982) Routine antibiotics in hospital management of acute asthma. *Lancet* **i:** 418.

6 Gross N. J. (1988) Ipratropium bromide. *N. Engl. J. Med.* **319:** 486.

7 Leader (1988) Nebulisers and paradoxical bronchoconstriction. *Lancet* **ii:** 202.

8 McGregor M. (1979) Pulsus paradoxus. *N. Engl. J. Med.* **301** (9): 478.

Pneumothorax

This is often due to the rupture of a subpleural bleb in an otherwise fit person, usually a young adult male. It may also complicate other respiratory conditions, such as asthma, chronic bronchitis or emphysema.

DIAGNOSIS

(1) In a fit person:

   (i) Symptoms may be confined to mild breathlessness or pleural pain, even when one lung is wholly collapsed.

   (ii) The signs are in combination diagnostic:

   (a) decreased movement on the affected side (not always present);

   (b) displacement of the trachea and apex beat away from the affected side (indicating mediastinal shift) may be present or absent, depending on the pressure in the pneumothorax;

   (c) increased resonance on the affected side (not always easy to detect);

   (d) distant breath sounds on the affected side (a good sign);

   (e) sometimes additional and often bizarre sounds may be heard—clicks or rubs.

(2) However, the history, symptoms and signs may be absent or be thought to have an alternative explanation in patients who have other lung disease, such as emphysema or asthma. These patients may already be familiar from their previous episodes of infection or reversible airways obstruction—which look exactly similar. Their breath sounds may be difficult to hear at the best of times and a small pneumothorax may be impossible to detect. As they have no respiratory reserve and a missed diagnosis may be disastrous, they must always have a chest x-ray at each presentation.

(3) A pneumothorax is easier to see on a chest x-ray taken in expiration.
(4) Tension pneumothorax—this should always be considered if your patient is getting worse and developing mediastinal shift, in which case you should aspirate the air with a cannula immediately without waiting for an x-ray.

MANAGEMENT

If the patient is not breathless, has no associated lung disease and has a shallow pneumothorax (<30% reduction in lung volume on x-ray—in effect, if the edge of the lung is less than one inch away from the edge of the rib cage), it is reasonable to allow the air to resorb spontaneously. Otherwise, mechanical removal of the air is required. Traditionally, we have used a chest drain with an underwater seal to effect the removal of air. Recently, simple aspiration with a cannula has been used, and seems to be effective, less painful, associated with a shorter hospital stay and with fewer complications. We describe both methods below.

Simple aspiration

We believe this to be the method of choice in patients with unilateral pneumothorax and without associated lung disease.

(1) Infiltrate the skin in the mid axilla with local anaesthetic and insert a 16 gauge i.v. cannula. Withdraw the needle, and connect the remaining plastic cannula through a three-way tap to a 60 ml syringe. The third outlet of your tap should be connected to a length of tubing, the other end of which is placed in a jug of sterile water.
(2) Aspirate the air gently, 60 ml at a time, and expel it through the water.
(3) When you feel resistance on the aspirating syringe (probably due to re-expanded lung impinging against your cannula), or you have aspirated 2 l of air, stop your aspiration, and take a check x-ray.
(4) If the lung is re-expanded, or you are left with a shallow (>30% volume) pneumothorax, merely observe your patient for 24 h and take an x-ray after this. If the situation is unchanged or improving, no further intervention is required.

(5) If on either of the occasions outlined in (4) above, there is a persisting large pneumothorax, the implication is that there is a persistent leak, and you should insert an intercostal drain.

(6) A simple way of predicting whether there is a continuing leak or not is to measure the presence of a marker gas in your aspirated air. Minute, and therefore ecologically legitimate, doses of inhaled CFC detected in the aspirate indicate that there is a continuing leak, and that formal drainage will be necessary.[4]

Intercostal drain

(1) An intercostal drainage tube should therefore be inserted:

   (i)   if simple aspiration fails;
   (ii) in any patient who has co-existent lung disease;
   (iii) in the presence of, or history of, pneumothorax on the other side.

(2) The management of the intercostal drainage tube. The site of choice for insertion of the intercostal tube is in the midaxillary line in the 4th or 5th intercostal space. The midclavicular line in the 2nd intercostal space is a poor alternative because sucking chest wounds have been known to occur after withdrawal of the tube and it leaves an unsightly scar. To enable a problem-free insertion we recommend blunt dissection of the chest wall,[3] preferring this to macho heavies leaning all their weight on the tube, and risking spearing the patient to the bed! The tube is attached to an underwater seal, e.g. a thoracotomy drainage bottle with 100 ml of sterile water in it, the tip being directed up to the apex. Check the position on chest x-ray. Make the patient cough a few times every hour to allow the air to escape from the chest. If the level in the underwater tube stops swinging, either:

   (i)   The lung has re-expanded and is blocking off the end of the tube. In this case clip off the tube, re-x-ray 24 h later and if the lung has not gone down, remove the tube. If the lung has gone down again continue to drain until the lung re-expands, then clip off and take another x-ray etc.
   (ii) The holes in the tube may be occluded by chest wall or partially re-expanded lung. Withdraw slightly and rotate.
   (iii) The tube is blocked and it needs 'milking'. If this does

not unblock the tube try to suck the tube free with a 50 ml syringe. If this does not work flush the tube out by introducing 50 ml of sterile water into the chest. Finally, change the tube.

(iv) If the lung does not expand even though the tube is patent, attach the outlet tube of the thoracotomy bottle to gentle suction (5–10 cmH$_2$O). Obviously the level will stop swinging. Take the tube off suction every hour to check that the tube is not blocked. If despite insertion of an intercostal tube and application of suction the lung still does not expand, consider bronchoscopy. This may clear the main airways of sputum and allow air to enter while the lung re-expands.

(v) If an air leak either persists or recurs:

    (a) check the connection of the intercostal tube to the drainage bottle;

    (b) seal the entry site of the intercostal tube in the chest by packing it with Tulle-gras to form an airtight dressing;

    (c) increase the suction pressure to 10–15 cmH$_2$O if the leak is very free. If the air leak continues there is probably a patent bleb on the lung surface. This will probably seal off in 36–48 h. Keep the tube on suction until the leak stops. Suck for a further 12 h, take off suction and watch the level in the underwater tube. If the chest maintains a negative pressure, i.e. the fluid level in the tube remains above the fluid level in the bottle, all is well. Clip off and x-ray again in 24 h. If the lung is still expanded take the tube out. If the two levels approximate and air begins to escape again, recommence suction and seek the advice of a thoracic surgical unit.

(3) Do not allow the thoracotomy bottle to be moved off the floor. If it is put on the bed locker, the contents will pass from the bottle into the chest. Keep two Spencer Wells clips handy, and clip the tube off whenever you want to move the bottle or the patient.

(4) Physiotherapy should be routine for all patients with pneumothorax in an attempt to prevent sputum retention occurring. Remember to give any necessary pain relief prior to physiotherapy.

(5) Pain control. Both the illness and its treatment are painful. Give opiate analgesia as necessary, measuring arterial gases if there is any possibility of CO_2 retention (see p. 73).

(6) If the diagnosis of the pneumothorax has been delayed (>5 days), try simple aspiration first, as brisk re-expansion carries the risk of inducing unilateral pulmonary oedema.[1]

(7) Some 20–50% of primary spontaneous pneumothoraces recur. A Danish study suggests that instilling talc in 250 ml of saline into the pleural space, stopping drainage for 2 h thereafter, and encouraging the patient to move around during this time, significantly reduces relapse. We think that talc pleurodesis should therefore be used with pleural intubation,[2] but do remember that this is painful, and give appropriate analgesia.

REFERENCES

Henderson A. F. *et al.* (1986) Re-expansion pulmonary oedema: a potentially serious complication of delayed diagnosis of pneumothorax. *Br. Med. J.* **291**: 593.

2 Leader (1989) Spontaneous pneumothorax. *Lancet* **ii:** 843.

3 Parmar J. R. (1989) How to insert a chest drain. *Br. J. Hosp. Med.* **42:** 231.

4 Seaton D. *et al.* (1991) spontaneous pneumothorax: marker gas technique for predicting outcome of manual aspiration. *Br. Med. J.* **302:** 262.

Massive pulmonary collapse

This is the term used to describe the complete collapse of a lobe or a lung. It may occur, of course, due to a spontaneous pneumothorax or following a chest injury with a sucking chest wound. The following remarks are confined to the absorption collapse which follows occlusion of one of the main airways.

DIAGNOSIS

(1) It may present itself as:

    (i)   sudden shortness of breath, with or without chest pain;

    (ii)   sudden worsening of an episode of acute infective bronchitis or asthma;

    (iii) fever, tachypnoea and tachycardia in an already ill patient, e.g. after major surgery;

    (iv) mental confusion.

(2) The signs are usually obvious. There is diminished movement on the affected side. The mediastinum is displaced towards the side of collapse, as demonstrated by shifting of the trachea and apex beat. There is dullness to percussion. If the major bronchi are obstructed, the breath sounds are diminished and there are usually no crackles. However, if the major bronchi remain patent but the peripheral bronchi are obstructed, the signs are those of consolidation, i.e. bronchial breathing, crackles and increased conduction of the spoken and whispered voice. It is most commonly caused by:

    (i)   a tenacious plug of sputum;

    (ii)   the endotracheal tube, at intubation performed for any reason, being inserted into one of the main bronchi, thus causing collapse of the other lung;

    (iii) a foreign body which may be radio-opaque, e.g. classically a fragment of tooth after dental anaesthesia;

    (iv) a carcinoma obstructing one of the main airways;

    (v)   extrinsic pressure on the bronchus, e.g. hilar glands, aortic aneurysm.

MANAGEMENT

(1) If the diagnosis is suspected, a chest x-ray and the appropriate lateral film should be taken. This will demonstrate the volume of lung collapsed, possibly also a foreign body in the trachea or bronchi, or malposition of an endotracheal tube.

(2) Management is directed towards removal of obstruction and obviously depends on the cause (see above). The following are the two most common causes.

    (i)   *Sputum*. If the patient is severely hypoxaemic or comatose, as, for example, after an operation, bronchoscopy should be undertaken immediately. Apart from this contingency there should be time to measure the arterial blood gases, and to assess the effects of vigorous physiotherapy with chest percussion and coughing. If this fails to produce an improvement within a few hours (as judged by a second chest x-ray), bronchoscopy should be undertaken. The timing will depend on the clinical state and the blood gases.

    (ii)   *Foreign body*. Removal through a bronchoscope (usually a rigid one) should be undertaken without delay.

Other causes are less common and, as they are not usually amenable to urgent treatment, are outside the scope of this book.

Acute laryngeal obstruction

Acute laryngeal obstruction is a life-threatening emergency and if it is total and unrelieved, the patient will die in 3 min. Partial obstruction with stridor, cyanosis and a hoarse voice is dangerous and, if progressive, urgent treatment is necessary to prevent death. In total obstruction, speech is impossible. The diagnosis is usually clear from the history. The cause is also fairly obvious.

(1) Trauma: strangulation, laceration, inhaled foreign bodies which, in adult practice, are usually a piece of food inhaled while the victim is eating, burns, irritant gases.
(2) Inflammatory: acute epiglottitis (see p. 298)[1] laryngotracheobronchitis.
(3) Angioneurotic oedema.
(4) Tumours: laryngeal obstruction may occur as a primary presentation, or during radiotherapy to already diagnosed tumours.
(5) Diphtheria—now very rarely and only in a non-immunised person.

It should not be confused with the obstruction caused by the tongue flopping back into the pharynx. This is, of course, easily relieved by lifting the jaw forward and inserting a pharyngeal airway.

MANAGEMENT

(1) Establish a better airway. Intubation may be difficult and occasionally impossible in these patients. So, once diagnosed, an experienced anaesthetist should be called urgently together with a surgeon proficient in tracheostomies.
(2) While awaiting their arrival, administer O_2 and obtain a tracheostomy set. Heliox (79% helium, 21% oxygen) mixture, if available, is more effective as the helium makes the mixture less dense. It therefore effectively, albeit only temporarily, reduces stridor.
(3) If the patient continues to deteriorate with deepening cyanosis (despite vigorous respiratory efforts) and increasing pulse

rate, and the anaesthetist has not yet arrived, an emergency tracheostomy should be performed. This is a simple operation.

(i)   Place the patient on his back with the neck extended.
(ii) Ask an assistant to hold the arms.
(iii) Steady the trachea between thumb and finger and slide a sharp knife between, preferably, the third and fourth tracheal rings.
(iv) Rotate the blade through 90° to maintain an airway and insert tracheal dilators.

(4) In angioneurotic oedema or post-radiotherapy oedema, hydrocortisone i.v. 200 mg plus 0.5–1.0 ml 1:000 adrenaline i.m. may reduce the obstruction sufficiently to avoid intubation.

(5) Patients with tumours and those undergoing a course of radiotherapy should be referred to the ENT surgeons immediately.

(6) The Heimlich manoeuvre. [2,3] If you are confronted with the problem of acute laryngeal obstruction from inhalation outside of the hospital environment (the café coronary syndrome), use of Heimlich's manoeuvre may be life-saving. The principle here is that a rapid upward thrust from below the xiphisternum pushes the diaphragm up, and forcefully expels air from the mouth. Any obstructing object is likewise forcefully and dramatically expelled. The technique can be carried out in people sitting, standing or lying.

(i)   *Victim sitting or standing*   The rescuer either stands or kneels behind the victim, encircling the victim's waist with one of his arms. With one hand, he makes a fist, and places his thumb slightly above the navel, and well below the tip of the xiphoid process, then covers the fist with his free hand, and presses into the victim's abdomen with a quick upward thrust. It may be necessary to repeat this thrust up to six times, although 60% of people are relieved of their obstruction after only two thrusts. The obstructing object may be expelled with such force as to hit a wall 3.7 m away, and should be identified whenever possible.

(ii) *Victim lying*   The victim is placed on his back, with his face looking directly forward. Facing the victim, the rescuer kneels astride him. He puts the palm of one hand between the navel and xiphisternum, places the other on top of it, and pushes upwards and inwards.

REFERENCES

1 Baker A. J. (1986) Adult epiglottitis. *N. Engl. J. Med.* **314:** 1185.
2 Editorial (1975) Statement on the Heimlich manoeuvre. *J. Am. Med. Assoc.* **234:** 416.
3 Heimlich H. J. (1982) First aid for the choking child—back blows and chest thrusts cause complications and death. *Paediatrics* **70:** 120.

Massive pleural effusions

DIAGNOSIS

(1) The patient is usually breathless, and may give a history of pleuritic pain.
(2) Differentiation from other causes of shortness of breath (see p. 375) is usually obvious on examination—the signs on the affected side being decreased movement, shift of the mediastinum to the opposite side, stony dullness and decreased breath and voice sounds.
(3) The diagnosis is confirmed by a chest x-ray (see below).

MANAGEMENT

(1) The effusion must be aspirated if causing distress, whatever the cause.
(2) A chest x-ray—postero-anterior and the appropriate lateral—should be taken to determine the optimal site for aspiration and to delineate structures which must be avoided, such as the diaphragm. The diaphragm is attached to the sixth rib anteriorly, the seventh rib laterally and the ninth rib posteriorly. The sixth space laterally, or eighth space posteriorly (tip of the scapula) are recommended aspiration sites.
(3) If you do need to aspirate the effusion, withdrawing fluid via a 50 ml syringe is tedious and prolongs discomfort for the patient. Therefore, insert a needle into the chest in the normal way. Attach it to the wall suction, if you have it, via a sterile underwater seal as for a pneumothorax and by a gentle negative pressure (5–10 cmH$_2$O) aspirate fluid from the chest. If wall suction is not available, an evacuated sterile bottle can be used.

Do not aspirate more than 1.5 l acutely, as otherwise you may induce reflex pulmonary oedema.
(4) Stop aspirating if:

    (i)   The patient complains of central chest pain. This means mediastinal shift is beginning to occur. This can cause rapid cardiovascular collapse and the temptation to continue must be resisted.

(ii) The patient has a haemoptysis. This means that the lung surface has been pierced. It is not usually serious but is frightening for all concerned. Unless the needle has been advanced further than necessary, the lung has re-expanded sufficiently for aspiration to be stopped.

(5) If the effusions are bilateral, aspiration of the larger effusion is usually sufficient to relieve breathlessness.

(6) Remember that aspiration of the pleural effusion can be conveniently combined with pleural biopsy, and that you need to send samples of the aspirate off for diagnostic purposes. Finally, if the pleural effusion is recurrent, the insertion of 500 mg tetracyline in 20 ml saline through your drain (after you have taken out as much fluid as possible) will provoke an inflammatory reaction and promote pleurodesis.

(7) Pleural effusions, or their treatment, may be painful. Give opiate analgesia as necessary.

REFERENCE

1   Rutowska J. (1967) An easy method of aspiration for pleural effusions. *Hospital Medicine* **2:** 370.

Adult respiratory distress syndrome (ARDS) (shock lung)[3,4,5]

DIAGNOSIS

(1) Shock lung is characterised by:

    (i)   tachypnoea;
    (ii)   deteriorating Pao_2;
    (iii) a decrease in lung compliance—usually to a level below 40 ml/cmH$_2$O;
    (iv) progressive diffuse infiltration on the chest x-ray, with associated widespread crackles, occurring in a patient who, within the preceding 48 h, has had an episode of hypotension.

(2) It is particularly likely to occur if the hypotensive episode was associated with:

    (i)   traumatised or dead tissue, as in crush injuries;
    (ii)   circulating bacterial endotoxins, as in Gram-negative septicaemia;
    (iii) fat emboli;
    (iv) amniotic fluid emboli;
    (v)   intravascular haemolysis;
    (vi) difficult or lengthy surgery;
    (vii) primary lung conditions, such as severe infections, aspiration or contusion.

(3) It arises because of an increase in:

    (i)   pulmonary capillary permeability;
    (ii)   pulmonary vascular resistance.
Both of these cause an increase in pulmonary interstitial fluid.

(4) It is associated with a normal PCWP initially. In shock lung, PCWP will be below 18 mmHg and is most reliably measured using a Swan–Ganz catheter (see p. 387) wedged in the lower half of the lung field. By contrast, in left ventricular failure, from which it must be distinguished, the PCWP is more than 25 mmHg, provided that the oncotic pressure is normal.

TREATMENT

Treatment is difficult, often prolonged, frequently unsuccessful and should be undertaken in association with your anaesthetic colleagues. It involves the following.

(1) Therapy directed toward the specific insult provoking shock lung.

(2) Early assisted ventilation. You should attempt to keep the Pao_2 around 9.3 kPa (70 mmHg) with added inspired O_2. Early introduction of continuous positive airways pressure (CPAP)[2] is helpful in maintaining oxygenation in patients with mild ARDS.

Indications for ventilation are as follows:

(i)   a patient who is getting progressively more exhausted by the effort of breathing;

(ii) respiratory rate of above 35/min;

(iii) Pao_2 of less than 9.3 kPa (70 mmHg) in spite of added O_2;

(iv) alveolar arterial oxygen differences (A-aDO_2) of greater than 6.7 kPa (50 mmHg).

The A-aDO_2 reflects the effective transfer of O_2 from the alveolus to the arterial blood. In a patient breathing room air with a Pao_2 of 20 kPa (150 mmHg)

$$\text{A-a}DO_2 = 150 - (Pao_2 + Paco_2)\, 0.8$$

and is normally less than 20. (The value 0.8 in the above equation is the respiratory quotient.)

(v)   Rising $Paco_2$. If the $Paco_2$ is above 5.3 kPa (40 mmHg), you have left things too late!

(3) Careful fluid balance. The problem is that fluid replacement is a balancing act between keeping the filling pressure of the left ventricle high enough to sustain the cardiac output, and yet low enough to minimise transmembrane fluid flux into the lung.

(i)   So which fluids should you use?

(a) blood should be replaced if the haematocrit falls below 30%.

(b) Haemaccel or plasma should be used to expand the plasma volume if necessary (see below).

    (c) Crystalloid fluids should only be used sparingly to replace losses, as these fluids will, of course, tend to leak into the lung and aggravate the underlying problem.

(ii) How do you monitor replacement? This is difficult, for the following reasons.

    (a) If your patient is on CPAP, or ventilated with PEEP, central venous pressure (CVP) readings are unreliable.

    (b) PCWP recordings only help to exclude coexistent left ventricular failure.

    (c) Therefore, clinical judgement is of paramount importance. You should strive towards a patient with warm peripheries, good urinary output, clear mental faculties and a systolic arterial pressure above 90 mmHg, but, if in doubt, err on the side of keeping your patient 'dry' rather than 'wet'.

(4) Antibiotics. As infection does not seem to play an important role in the genesis of shock lung, only use antibiotics if there is purulent sputum.

(5) Nutrition. Effective enteral nutrition, to provide 30 cal/kg/day, either via a nasogastric tube or jejunostomy, is important for both improving respiratory muscle strength and reducing the possibility of nosocomial infection.

(6) Corticosteroids. There is no evidence that these are helpful once shock lung has developed.[1] Massive doses (2 g methyl prednisolone i.v. each day for two days) may be helpful if inhalation of vomit has occurred. If there is bronchospasm, hydrocortisone and bronchodilators should be used, in the same doses as for acute asthma (see p. 81).

(7) Correction of acidosis. A low pH increases capillary leakage. Cautious correction with $NaHCO_3$ (see p. 342), with due regard to Na+ balance, should be attempted, if the pH is below 7.1.

(8) Fluid balance. Likewise, a raised urea (above 15 mmol/l) increases capillary leakage; careful attention to fluid balance and nutrition will help forestall this problem.

(9) Correction of stress ulceration. In patients who are critically ill, acute gastrointestinal bleeding can be prevented by using enteral feeding wherever possible, and sucrulfate 1–2 g t.d.s.

Rational use of these agents is based on a severity index score of illness. Each of the problems outlined below gets a score of 1.

(i)   Documented respiratory insufficiency for 24 h.
(ii)   Circulatory collapse (BP persistently <90 mmHg or requiring pressor agents).
(iii) Patients with documented sepsis.
(iv)   Patients with CCF, myocardial infarct or arrhythmias warranting therapy.
(v)   Creatinine level acutely raised to above 250 μmol/l.
(vi)   Patients with a Glasgow coma scale score <10.
(vii) Patients on high-dose steroids.
(viii) Patients with a platelet count <50,000 or prothrombin time of less than 30% of the control.
(ix)   Bilirubin >90 μmol/l with or without hepatitis.

Prophylaxis is probably only of avail in people with a score of <6, but we use it routinely.

(10) Physiotherapy. Atelectasis occurs early in the shock lung syndrome. Encouraging regular sighing or deep respirations, making sure your patient coughs and is turned frequently, are vital therapeutic manoeuvres.

(11) Extracorporeal membrane oxygenation (ECMO). A recent trial showed no increase in survival with this heroic mode of therapy.

REFERENCES

1   Bernard G. *et al.* (1987) High dose corticosteroids in patients with the adult respiratory distress syndrome. *N. Engl. J. Med.* **317**: 1565.

2   Harrison M. J. (1986) PEEP and CPAP. *Br. Med. J.* **292**: 643.

3   Leader (1986) Adult respiratory distress syndrome. *Lancet* **i**: 301.

4   Leader (1989) ARDS Times. *Lancet* **i**: 140.

5   Lloyd J. E. *et al.* (1984) Permeability pulmonary oedema. *Arch. Intern. Med.* **144**: 143.

Pulmonary aspiration syndrome[1]

Aspiration of substances into the lungs can be divided into three categories:

(1) *Toxic aspiration*. The significant fluids here are acids, alcohols, volatile hydrocarbons, oil and animal fats. These produce a chemical pneumonitis; the most important factor in the production of this pneumonitis is the acidity of the aspiration fluid: fluids with a pH below 2.5 consistently cause chemical damage. Post-partum aspiration pneumonitis, Mendelson's syndrome, is the classic example of this chemical pneumonitis.

(2) Aspiration of non-toxic materials—either liquids with a pH of >7.3 or particulate matter. Here the damage relates to the composition and/or volume of the aspirated material. Chemical pneumonitis does not occur, although secondary bacterial infection may.

(3) *Bacterial aspiration*. This is characterised by the onset of a bacterial pneumonia 24 h or so after the inhalation of an inoculum of bacteria. Poor oral hygiene is the most frequent predisposing condition, and the resultant pneumonia is usually due to a mixed bacterial infection, including anaerobes.

The remainder of this section refers solely to the chemical pneumonitis produced by toxic aspiration.

DIAGNOSIS

(1) There is usually a clear predisposing cause.

    (i) Loss of airway protective reflexes, as in comatose, anaesthetised, heavily sedated or neurologically compromised patients,

    (ii) Oesophageal disorders or decreased gastric emptying time increase the potential for aspiration.

    (iii) Iatrogenic factors, such as the presence of nasogastric tubes or n.g. tube feeding enhance the likelihood of aspiration.

(2) Chemical damage to the lungs produces bronchospasm and a massive exudation of fluid into the lungs. This causes breath-

lessness, wheezing and a cough productive of frothy pink sputum. Hypoxia, hypotension, tachycardia and the adult respiratory distress syndrome may develop (see p. 97).

(3) Chest x-ray will show patchy alveolar infiltrates. There is usually a low or normal $Paco_2$ with a low Pao_2 on blood gas analysis.

MANAGEMENT

(1) Immediately following aspiration, suction to clear the oropharynx of secretions should be undertaken. If the airway protective reflexes are thought to be compromised, your patient should be intubated.

(2) Oxygen therapy should be commenced with an MC mask, to deliver 50% inspired oxygen concentration. Continuous positive airways pressure (CPAP) is helpful as it improves the balance between ventilation and perfusion. If you cannot maintain the Pao_2 above 9 kPa (65 mmHg), consider mechanical ventilation.

(3) The wheezing should be treated with bronchodilators, as for asthma (see p. 81). The role of steroids is controversial: we give one dose of methyl prednisolone 2 g i.v., recognising that the efficacy of this is unproved.

(4) Antibiotics. Bacterial superinfection occurs within 72 h in about half of the patients with chemical pneumonitis. The infecting organisms are derived from the oropharynx, and so will be a mixed flora including anaerobes. The role of prophylactic antibiotics is unclear. In practice, we usually give metronidazole orally or rectally (see p. 351) and a penicillin (see p. 349).

(5) Fluids. Hypovolaemia, due in part to extravasation of fluids into the lungs, should be corrected. As in ARDS (see p. 97), the lung capillaries are leaky, so you have to achieve the delicate balance of a vascular volume sufficient to provide good perfusion with as low a left ventricular end diastolic pressure as possible.

(6) Remember that you should aim to prevent aspiration occurring. Always position patients with compromised airways in the semi-prone position, and be prepared to intubate as necessary. Regular antacids or H_2 antagonists to raise the pH

of gastric contents are also advisable in those who are predisposed to aspirate.

REFERENCE

1 Vender J. S. (1986) Pulmonary aspiration. In *Update in Intensive Care and Emergency Medicine*, p. 71. New York: Springer Verlag.

Community-acquired pneumonia[2]

Pneumonia is often the terminal illness in the elderly, and as such, should be managed on its merits. Pneumonia can, however, occur in otherwise healthy adults. It may strike with extraordinary rapidity, and at its most severe, someone who appears well in the morning may be dead by evening. The pathology of this particularly cataclysmic, and happily uncommon, variant is usually staphylococcal superinfection of a lung already damaged by a viral pneumonitis. In Britain, the usual pathogen in the commoner less severe presentation is *Streptococcus pneumoniae* (75% of cases).[4,5] The next most common group are those due to the so-called atypical pathogens— the main ones being *Mycoplasma*[3] and *Legionella*. As indicated above, the *Staphylococcus* is an uncommon cause, as are *H. influenza* and *Klebsiella*. In some cases, a virus alone is thought to be responsible, frequently the influenza virus.

Most cases of community-acquired pneumonia can be treated at home, but there are well-recognised markers of severity which suggest the need for admission to a high dependency unit (see (3) below).

DIAGNOSIS

(1) There may have been a preceding viral illness, which initially seeming trivial may progress to dyspnoea, fever, cough productive of yellow and often bloodstained sputum and pleuritic pain. In the severest cases, there may be progression through mental confusion and disorientation to a state of septic shock with circulatory collapse. In these circumstances, admittedly only a small proportion of the whole, you may be presented with a hypoxic, cyanosed, disorientated, peripherally cool, hypotensive patient, and in this group mortality is high.

(2) The auscultatory signs are those of widespread, often asymmetrical areas of diminished breath sounds. There may also be focal evidence of consolidation, and an accompanying pleural rub. Chest x-ray may show lobar consolidation or nonspecific diffuse lung shadowing.

(3) Assessment of severity. The following features are associated with increased mortality in community-acquired pneumonia.

    (i) Patient over 60 years old.
    (ii) High respiratory rate (>30/min).
    (iii) Low diastolic arterial pressure (<60 mmHg).
    (iv) Confusion.
    (v) Raised blood urea (>7 mmol/l).
    (vi) Low admission Pao_2 (<8 kPa).
    (vii) Very low or high white count (<4 or >30 × 10^9/l).
    (viii) Low serum albumin (<35 g/l).

MANAGEMENT

Take blood for arterial blood gases, FBP, including white cell count, electrolytes, urea and blood cultures. Also, save a specimen for serology—you must also remember to get convalescent serum. Do a chest x-ray and ECG and send sputum for Gram staining and culture. Then treat as follows.

(1) Hypoxia. Pao_2 <60 mmHg (8.0 kPa) is the rule in this type of patient. Correction should be with a high concentration of oxygen by MC mask, unless there is evidence of chronic air flow obstruction. If the Pao_2 persists below 60 mmHg (8.0 kPa) or the $Paco_2$ persists above 40 mmHg (5.3 kPa) on face mask oxygen, assisted ventilation will be required and you should consult with your anaesthetic colleagues.

(2) Infection. You will usually have to begin antibiotics before you know what the organism is.

    (i) Most patients will turn out to have *Streptococcus pneumoniae*, and will respond to penicillin. So give benzyl penicillin 1.2 g i.v. 4-hourly.
    (ii) If there is an atypical history—a disproportionate degree of systemic rather than respiratory symptoms—you should use erythromycin 500 mg 6-hourly. Likewise, if there has been no response to penicillin in 48 h, you should switch to erythromycin.
    (iii) Some authorities suggest that all community-acquired pneumonias should receive both the above drugs from the start, and this is a not unreasonable approach.
    (iv) If there has been a recent influenza outbreak, or there is

cavitation on the chest x-ray, you should treat for the *Staphylococcus* as well. Add flucloxacillin 1–2 g 6-hourly to the penicillin.

(v) If the patient is desperately ill, consider adding one of the following:

  (a) Fucidin 500 mg i.v. 6-hourly.
  (b) Chloramphenicol 1.0 g 6-hourly i.v., which is the drug of choice for *H. influenza* and is also effective against many staphylococci.
  (c) An aminoglycoside—see p. 350.
  (d) There may be a role for the quinolones, such as Ciprofloxacin, but this is as yet unclear.

(vi) If there has been any question of inhalation, add metron-idazole (see p. 351), as many of the inhaled bacteria will be anaerobes, and not all of these will be sensitive to penicillin.

(3) Physiotherapy. This is often given to help your patient cough up infected sputum. However trials have shown it to be of no benefit.[1]

(4) Circulatory collapse. In the few patients who develop circulatory collapse, the prognosis is very grave. Conventional therapy involving fluid replacement under CVP control (see p. 382) should be instituted. The only practical difference is that we suggest using predominantly colloid rather than crystalloid to support the circulation since the latter is more likely to extravasate into the already damaged lung. Insertion of a Swan–Ganz catheter, enabling you to measure pulmonary artery and pulmonary wedge pressure, will help you to manage fluid replacement in these patients. Exudation of fluid into the lungs of these patients is usually due to parenchymal lung damage. This may be clinically difficult to distinguish from left ventricular failure, but by measuring the PCWP with the Swan–Ganz catheter, you should be able to distinguish between the two (see p. 44).

(5) Steroids. Their role is equivocal; we do not use them.

As always, if your patient is critically ill, the care given by highly skilled nurses in an ITU is a critical factor in determining the outcome. You forget this at your patient's peril.

REFERENCES

1   Graham W. G., Bradley D. A. (1978) Efficacy of chest physiotherapy and intermittent positive pressure breathing in the resolution of pneumonia. *N. Engl. J. Med.* **299:** 624.
2   Harrison B. D. W. (1987) The hospital management of community acquired pneumonia. *J. R. Coll. Phys.* (Lond.) **21:** 267.
3   Leader (1991) Mycoplasma pneumonia. *Lancet* **337:** 651.
4   Lockley M. R., Wise R. (1984) Pneumococcal infections. *Br. Med. J.* **288:** 1179.
5   Macfarlane J. T. *et al.* (1982) Hospital study of adult community acquired pneumonia. *Lancet* **ii:** 255.

Gastrointestinal

Massive upper gastrointestinal haemorrhage[6]

This condition presents as:

(1) Haematemesis and/or blood per rectum (melaena). Remember, however, that melaena alone may arise from anywhere in the GI tract down to and including the caecum.
(2) Cardiovascular collapse.
(3) Postural hypotension and fainting. In the absence of any other cause such as hypotensive agents, or autonomic dysfunction, a fall in systolic arterial pressure of greater than 10 mmHg on sitting the patient up indicates an acute blood loss in excess of 1000 ml.
(4) Symptoms of anaemia—fatigue, shortness of breath and angina, which however more often result from chronic blood loss.

It is usually caused by:

(1) Bleeding peptic ulcers (possibly drug-induced—see (2) below).
(2) Acute gastric erosions. These may:

    (i)   be drug-induced (steroids, and non-steroidal anti-inflammatory drugs, such as indomethacin and salicylates being common offenders);[5]
    (ii) occur after an alcoholic binge;
    (iii) occur in any patient seriously ill for whatever reason.

(3) Reflux oesophagitis, with or without hiatus hernia.
(4) The Mallory–Weiss syndrome (traumatic oesophageal tear usually secondary to prolonged retching or vomiting).[4]
(5) Bleeding oesophageal or gastric varices (look for evidence of liver disease).

It may, however, occasionally be caused by:

(1) Gastric neoplasm.
(2) Coagulation disorder (look for bleeding elsewhere, including prolonged bleeding from puncture sites).

(3) Connective tissue disease, such as Osler–Weber–Rendu syndrome (look for telangiectasia).

MANAGEMENT

Management of this emergency always requires close collaboration between surgeons and physicians and sometimes radiologists. Ideally, every case should be treated jointly, preferably in a specially designated unit.

Restoration of blood volume

Restoration and maintenance of circulating volume and hence tissue perfusion is urgent if blood loss sufficient to cause poor peripheral perfusion has already occurred (see p. 334) or the patient has a systolic arterial pressure of below 90 mmHg and a pulse rate of above 100 beats/min. It is always necessary to take cases of gastrointestinal blood loss seriously as patients may continue to bleed in hospital. Therefore, in all cases of major bleeding (we define major bleeding as the vomiting of blood, documented melaena, poor organ perfusion or a fall in haemoglobin of more than 2 g in 24 h) take the following action.

(1) Take blood for haemoglobin, PCV, electroytes and urea, and group and cross-match 4 units of blood. Ask for a kaolin cephalin time, prothrombin time and platelet count. Remember, haemoglobin concentration may be misleading before haemodilution occurs.

(2) Set up a central venous pressure line.

(3) Replace the circulating volume. Here two basic questions must be answered.

  (i) *What with?*

    (a) Compatible blood is clearly the fluid of choice, and should be available within a few hours.

    (b) If the situation is not desperate, give 0.9% N saline while waiting. However, if there is peripheral organ failure, or persisting hypotension, and you therefore wish to give a colloid before compatible blood is available, give:

    (c) Haemaccel—we do not give more than 2000 ml in any single episode.

(d) Plasma.

(e) Dextran with an average molecular weight of 70 000 may be used; do not give doses in excess of 15 ml/kg per 24 hours as they may cause disseminated intra-vascular coagulation. Do not forget to take blood for cross-matching before giving this.

(f) In desperate circumstances 'O' negative blood may be given uncross-matched.

(ii) *How much?*

(a) Transfuse blood rapidly until the CVP rises into the upper half of the normal range (i.e. 1 cm above the manubrio-sternal joint with the patient supine, see p. 381). The patient will become warm and tranquil and the arterial pressure and pulse will return to normal. If this does not happen, it implies the patient is continuing to bleed, and you must, there-fore, continue to transfuse (while, of course, consid-ering other possible therapeutic manoeuvres). If after your initial resuscitation has been successful, the CVP drops suddenly (i.e. a fall of greater than 5 cmH₂O in less than 2 h) this should be taken as an indication of re-bleeding. Further indications such as a fresh haematemesis or fresh blood up the nasogastric tube, a fall in arterial pressure, or rest-lessness and sweating may then develop. All these will alert you to the need for further blood and action as outlined below.

(b) If you have no CVP measurements, transfuse the patient until he is warm, tranquil and has a restored arterial pressure and pulse rate. A rate of about one unit of blood per hour is reasonable to start with.

(c) In all cases look for the usual clinical signs of overload (raised JVP/CVP, crackles at the lung bases, oedema). If these occur, slow down the infusion rate and give a diuretic, e.g. frusemide 40 mg i.v. and digoxin as necessary (see p. 18).

(4) Consider passing a nasogastric tube. This has the advantage that:

(i) it rids the stomach of Guinness, pills and blood;

(ii) it may be useful in diagnosing re-bleeding;

  (iii) it may be helpful to know the pH of the stomach contents, so the appropriate dose of antacids can be given;
  (iv) the stomach can be emptied prior to endoscopy.

  However:

  (v) it is uncomfortable and sometimes distressing for the patient;
  (vi) it may cause further bleeding;
  (vii) its use is associated with an increase in respiratory complications.

  The authors do not use it routinely.

(5) In some patients, particularly the elderly who have had gradual blood loss, it is wise to give frusemide from the onset of the transfusion, as heart failure develops easily in this group.

Determining the cause

This is undertaken when initial resuscitation is under way, and may be suggested by your history and examination. In around 30% of patients, no cause will be found, despite careful evaluation. Further investigations are:

(1) Endoscopy, which should be carried out within 24 h of the patient's admission. Ensure that your patient is nil by mouth until a decision about the timing of endoscopy is taken. Although the site of bleeding will be visualised in most cases, giving comfort to physician and patient alike, early routine endoscopy has not altered the outlook in upper gastrointestinal haemorrhage.[8,13] However, now that endoscopic evidence of a blood vessel in an ulcer base is recognized to be associated with a high incidence of re-bleeding, and thus with the need for early intervention, either endoscopically or surgically, the full value of endoscopy may be greater than we presently realise.[2,3,12] It is anyway worth remembering that patients with liver disease may bleed from peptic ulcers as well as from varices, and actually seeing the bleeding site will sort out this problem for you.

(2) If the patient continues to bleed rapidly after admission, the stomach is likely to be full of blood, and endoscopy unrewarding. In these circumstances arteriography gives a high degree of diagnostic accuracy, and is probably the investigation of choice. It takes only ½ h and can be done while a theatre is

being prepared, if the surgeons consider operation is necessary. Arteriography may also be an invaluable therapeutic technique (q.v.).

Stopping the bleeding
(1) General measures:

(i)   The most important general measure is a clear hospital policy on the management of gastrointestinal bleeding. There should preferably be a designated ward where such patients are treated, so that experience of managing GI bleeds can be gained and then shared most easily.

(ii)   Tranexamic acid 1 g 6-hourly i.v. for 48 h, and then 500 mg 6-hourly, has been found to reduce mortality in upper GI bleeding, though not the frequency of recurrent haemorrhage or surgery. Until the situation is clarified, we do not advocate its routine use.[11]

(iii) Somatostatin, a potent inhibitor of acid and pepsin secretion by the stomach, has been used to stop bleeding, but a recent trial has showed it to be ineffective, except in variceal bleeding.[10]

(2) Specific sites:
● Peptic ulcer

(i)   In patients with a significant bleed (defined as the vomiting of blood, documented melaena, poor organ perfusion and a fall of Hb of over 2 g in 24 h), mortality is attributable to either continuing bleeding or, more commonly, re-bleeding. In the absence of any definitive medical therapy, early surgery or endoscopic therapy in those people likely to re-bleed is at present the only way of reducing the high mortality of this condition. Therefore in patients who are at high risk for re-bleeding (as defined below), or who have needed 4 units of blood, emergency surgery or endoscopic haemostasis should be advised unless there are compelling contraindications.[3,16]

(a) Patients over 55 years old.

(b) The presence of a spurting artery, local oozing or a protuberant non-bleeding vessel on endoscopy.[2,12]

(c) Poor organ perfusion (shock), especially if associated with confusion.

The good news is that re-bleeding is very unlikely to occur after three days.

(ii) Controlled trials of H_2 antagonists and proton blockers (such as omeprazole) have shown no clear benefit so far as prevention of re-bleeding is concerned, but they are none the less widely used!

(iii) Heat coagulation of, or the injection of a sclerosing agent into or vasoconstrictors around, a visible vessel in an ulcer base is an attractive therapeutic option for those with this facility. Recent evidence suggests that this is a better option than surgery, and we feel sure that the use of endoscopic methods will increase rapidly.[3]

● Acute gastric erosions

(i) Surgery should be avoided if possible as the condition is usually self-limiting.

(ii) Cimetidine—100 mg i.v./h in 5% dextrose, should be infused, with the aim of maintaining the pH of the stomach contents above 5.

(iii) Antacids—the best tested method of raising the pH of stomach contents is by instilling 30 ml of antacid (e.g. Maalox) hourly into the stomach. This may have advantages over H_2 antagonists.

(iv) Omeprazole 40 mg daily has been used with success, and may prove to be the treatment of the future.[14]

● Oesophageal or gastric varices[7,15]

(1) The treatment of choice is now endoscopic sclerotherapy, which should be undertaken at the same time as the diagnostic procedure. This will stop bleeding in more than 90% of patients.

(ii) Octreotide, the new synthetic analogue of somatostatin, is almost certainly as effective as urgent sclerotherapy. It will probably come to replace this as the first line therapy, and should certainly be used in those institutions in which emergency sclerotherapy is not available. The dose is 25 μg/h for at least 48 h. The infusion may need to be continued for 5 days.[10]

(iii) Vasopressin with or without nitroglycerin, and its long-acting analogue glypressin, have not been shown to have any advantage over controls, and we do not use them any more.

(iv) If octreotide and emergency sclerotherapy either fail or are not available, the Boyce modification of the Sengstaken Blakemore tube may be used.[9] Enthusiasm for this therapeutic modality is waning, but it is still a last-ditch standby.

(a) A new tube should be used on each occasion, the upper GI tract should be aspirated via a nasogastric tube, and the bed head should be elevated 6–10 in.

(b) Spray the pharynx with 2% lignocaine, test the balloons for leaks, make sure which tube connects with which balloon.

(c) With the patient in a left lateral position, pass the well-lubricated tube into the stomach, either through the nose or the mouth. You may have to use a flexible wire to stiffen the tube or alternatively put the Sengstaken Blakemore tube into the ice box of a refrigerator.

(d) Fill the stomach balloon with about 100–150 ml of radio-opaque dye to localise it (20 ml of 20% diodone in 100 ml of water) and inflate the oesophageal balloon to a pressure of 30–40 mmHg. The oesophageal balloon must not be inflated until the tube has been stabilised by the stomach balloon.

(e) With the stomach tube pulled firmly up against the oesophagogastric junction, tape it either to the patient, or preferably, a preformed traction pad.

(f) Both during insertion and when the tube is finally in place, constant low pressure (5 mmHg) suction should be applied to the accessory tube.

(g) Both balloons are left in place for 24–48 h, as necessary, then the oesophageal balloon deflated. Some authorities recommend deflating the oesophageal balloon for 10 min every 6 h in the hope of minimising the occurrence of oesophageal necrosis.

(h) The tube is left in position for another 24 h with the stomach balloon still full in case of re-bleeding. It is then removed (after emptying the stomach balloon!).

(i) No food or drink is allowed while the tube is in

place, though drugs may be given via the stomach tube.

(j) If used with care, the Sengstaken Blakemore tube will control oesophageal variceal bleeding in 90% of cases.

(k) The volumes of air and water mentioned above relate only to the Boyce modification of the Sengstaken tube; other varieties have different specifications and you should check this before using your tube.

(v) Percutaneous transhepatic portal vein catheterisation with subsequent selective injection of gel-foam into the major venous supply of the varices (left gastric and short gastric veins) is still occasionally used by some enthusiasts.

(vi) If, after a second attempt at sclerotherapy, bleeding persists, you may have to resort to emergency surgery. The presently favoured operations are:

(a) oesophageal transection;
(b) variceal plication;
(c) emergency portacaval shunt.

● Oesophageal bleeding

This may be due either to reflux oesophagitis or the Mallory–Weiss syndrome.[4]

(i) Medical measures usually suffice, but if bleeding persists surgery may become necessary.

(ii) Local arterial perfusion with vasopressin 0.2–0.4 i.u./min for up to 36 h may give temporary or sometimes permanent relief.[1]

Arteriography as a therapeutic manoeuvre[1]

(1) This has already been mentioned in connection with oesophageal or gastric varices and tears.

(2) In any other patients in whom torrential bleeding persists, and in whom surgery is neither desirable nor possible, one of two manoeuvres are helpful.

(i) If the lesion is acute and superficial, or in the territory of mesenteric perfusion, bleeding may be controlled by intra-arterial vasopressin 0.2–0.4 i.u./min given for up to 36 h.

(ii) If the lesion is chronic, arterial embolisation via the catheter is probably the treatment of choice.[17]

Stopping the bleeding by arteriography can sometimes be useful as a preliminary to surgery.

General measures

(1) The patient should be allowed to take fluids as required and offered a liberal soft nutritious diet with Aludrox 10 ml every 2 h. Both these help neutralise stomach contents.

(2) Sedation should be given to an anxious patient. Restlessness, which is often a manifestation of hypoxia, may respond to oxygen and transfusion.

(3) Measure the urinary output, as renal failure may occur in severe gastrointestinal bleeding.

REFERENCES

1   Allison D. J., Hemingway A. P., Cunningham D. A. (1982) Angiography in gastro-intestinal bleeding. *Lancet* **ii:** 30.

2   Beckley D. E., Casebow M. P. (1986) Prediction of rebleeding from peptic ulcer; experience with an endoscopic doppler. *Gut* **27:** 96.

3   Bown S. (1991) Bleeding peptic ulcers. *Br. Med. J.* **302:** 1417.

4   Foster D. N., Miloszewksi K., Losowsky M. S. (1976) Diagnosis of Mallory–Weiss lesions. *Lancet* **ii:** 483.

5   Jick H., Porter J. (1978) Drug-induced gastro-intestinal bleeding. *Lancet* **ii:** 87.

6   Langman M. J. S. (1985) Upper GI bleeding: the trial of trials. *Gut* **26:** 217.

7   Leader (1988) Management of acute variceal bleeding. *Lancet* **ii:** 999.

8   Leader (1984) Bleeding ulcers: scope for improvement? *Lancet* **i:** 715.

9   McCormick P. A. *et al.* (1990) How to insert a Sengstaken Blakemore tube. *Br. J. Hosp. Med.* **43:** 274.

10   O'Donell L. J., Farthing M. (1989) Therapeutic potential of a long acting somatostatin analogue in gastrointestinal disease. *Gut* **30:** 1165.

11   Stael C. S. *et al.* (1987) Tranexamic acid as an aid to reducing blood transfusion requirements in gastric and duodenal bleeding. *Br. Med. J.* **294:** 7.

12   Storey W. D. *et al.* (1981) Endoscopic prediction of recurrent bleeding in peptic ulcers. *N. Engl. J. Med.* **305**: 915.

13   Steer M. L., Silen W. (1983) Diagnostic procedures in GI haemorrhage *N. Engl. J. Med.* **309:** 646.

14   St J Collier D. *et al.* (1990) Acute haemorrhagic gastritis controlled by omeprazole. *Lancet* **i:** 776.

15   Westaby D. (1987) Variceal bleeding. *Gastroenterology in Practice* **8** (May).

16   Wheatley K. E. *et al.* (1990) Mortality in patients with bleeding peptic ulcers when those aged 60 or over are operated on early. *Br. Med. J.* **301:** 272.

17   Young A. E. (1981) Therapeutic embolization. *Br. Med. J.* **283:** 1144.

Lower gastrointestinal bleeding[1,3]

We define lower gastrointestinal bleeding as bleeding occurring from a site below the ligament of Trietze. The usual presentation is the passage of fresh, bright red or maroon blood per rectum. However, melaena can occur from colonic bleeding (probably due to slow transit through a sluggish colon) and fresh blood per rectum can occur from torrential upper gastrointestinal bleeding. It is therefore essential to exclude upper GI bleeding in these patients. This is most easily done by passing a nasogastric tube. If you aspirate bilious, but blood-free fluid through this, you can be confident that there is no upper GI source. If there is no bile in your blood-free aspirate, you should undertake an upper GI endoscopy to ensure that the duodenum is not the site of haemorrhage. The causes of lower GI bleeding are essentially colonic. The common causes are:

(1) Diverticular disease. About 50% of the population over 60 years have diverticular disease, so to implicate it as a source of bleeding, you really have to demonstrate a bleeding diverticulum. Bleeding usually occurs in a patient without previous symptoms from diverticular disease in the right colon. Treatment is surgical.

(2) Angiodysplasia. This vascular abnormality is an abnormal clustering of dilated submucosal veins and arteries. There is often thinning of the overlying mucosa, and the lesions are usually in the caecum and right side of the colon. They may be recognised on colonoscopy as prominent vessels, which unlike normal colonic vessels, are wiggly rather than straight.[2]

3 Colorectal cancer.

4 Ischaemic colitis.

5 Colonic polyp.

6 Inflammatory bowel disease (see p. 128).

7 Small bowel lesions, between the ligament of Trietze and ileum, are very uncommon causes of lower GI bleeding. The most frequent are tumours which may bleed, and in these patients there is usually a preceding history of abdominal pain and weight loss.[4]

MANAGEMENT

(1) Initial resuscitation is as for upper GI bleeding.
(2) Thereafter, your aim is to arrive at a diagnosis of the site of
    the bleeding. Clinical indications are unfortunately not very
    helpful. After you have excluded upper GI bleeding as
    suggested above, we recommend that the following investiga-
    tive steps should be undertaken as a matter of urgency.

    (i) Sigmoidoscopy. An estimated 10% of patients with
    lower GI bleeding have anorectal lesions visible on
    sigmoidoscopy.

    (ii) If this is negative, colonoscopy is the next best investiga-
    tive tool.[2] This should be undertaken urgently—the ear-
    lier the better. In a bleeding patient, oral preparation
    using 500 ml of 10% mannitol, 10 mg of metaclopramide,
    and plenty of water, should be commenced immediately.
    The bowel is usually clear enough to observe within 2–3 h.

    (iii) If the colonoscopy is negative, or the bleeding is too
    brisk to allow effective visualization of the colon, two
    choices are open to you:

        (a) Technetium scintiscan. This technique is useful for
        localising the site of bleeding. A decision can then
        be made to proceed to arteriography, and then to
        operate.

        (b) Mesenteric angiography. This usually identifies the
        bleeding site only if the rate of loss is greater than
        1–2 ml/min, so it is an ideal investigation in brisk
        bleeding.

(3) Having identified the site of the bleeding, the treatment is
    usually expectant or surgical. Colonoscopic electrocoagulation
    of bleeding sites, and injection of vasopressin or gel-foam
    through an appropriately located intra-arterial catheter, are
    further possibilities, although there is anxiety about inducing
    serious ischaemia of the surrounding bowel.

REFERENCES

1   Brandt L. J., Boley S. J. (1984) The role of colonoscopy in
    the diagnosis and management of lower intestinal bleeding.
    Scand. J. Gastro-enterol. **19** (Suppl 102): 61.

2   Burakoff R. (1985) A case of haematochezia. *N. Engl. J. Med.* **312:** 427.

3   Colacchio J. A. *et al.* (1982) Impact of modern diagnostic methods on management of active rectal bleeding—10-year experience. *Amer. J. Surg.* **143**: 607.

4   Katz J. (1991) A case of lower GI bleeding. *N. Engl. J. Med.* **324:** 1726.

Acute pancreatitis[1,2,3]

DIAGNOSIS

(1) Acute pancreatitis causes severe pain, usually in the epigastrium or hypochondrium, associated with vomiting.

(2) A serum amylase of >1200 i.u./l (normal value 70–300 i.u./l) in this setting is diagnostic.

(3) Lipase, catalase and phospholipase levels are not additionally helpful. Trypsin, being specific to the pancreas, may become diagnostically more important.

(4) Acute pancreatitis may be associated with the following.

    (i) Gallstones (50%). The likely cause is back pressure due to a stone blocking the common pancreaticobiliary duct.

    (ii) Alcohol (10%). Here acute pancreatitis is superimposed on chronic pancreatic damage.

    (iii) Occasionally, hypercalcaemia, hyperlipidaemia and drugs may be associated with an acute attack.

    (iv) In a quarter of cases, the cause is unknown.

(5) A raised amylase sufficient to cause diagnostic confusion can occur in small bowel obstruction, perforated duodenal ulcer, mesenteric infarction and dissection of the aorta. These can usually be distinguished clinically. Where genuine doubt exists, an abdominal ultrasound examination will usually resolve it. A laparotomy may occasionally have to be undertaken, but is associated with increased mortality and morbidity if the diagnosis turns out to be acute pancreatitis.

MANAGEMENT

(1) As the course, treatment and prognosis of mild and severe cases differ, the first step is to determine the severity of the disease. This is often difficult to assess clinically, but fortunately an objective assessment of severity is available.[4,7] The list below is of adverse prognostic factors in acute pancreatitis. If three or more of these are present at any time within 48 h of your patient's admission, a severe attack is confirmed.

(i) WBC >15 × 10⁹/l
(ii) Glucose >10 mmol/l (in a patient who is not a known diabetic).
(iii) Urea >16 mmol/l (after correction of dehydration with i.v. fluids).
(iv) Pao_2 <mmHg (8.0 kPa).
(v) Calcium <2.0 mmol/l
(vi) Albumin <32 g/l.
(vii) LDH <600 units/l.
(viii) ALT <200 units/l.

Approximately 33% of patients are classified as severe.

(2) Trypsin activation peptides (TAP), which are only present in severe disease, can now be measured. If you have this facility, the urinary TAP excretion is an accurate way of predicting activity.[5]

Having assessed the severity, any further treatment which is necessary can be based on a rational foundation.

SUPPORTIVE THERAPY

All patients with pancreatitis require basic supportive therapy, as outlined below. Further measures—(8)–(10) below—should only be considered in the severe cases.

(1) Intravenous fluids. Patients with pancreatitis have a relative fluid deficiency and require i.v. saline replacement under CVP control. If this crystalloid infusion does not restore perfusion, colloid may also be required.
(2) Bowel rest. Although in mild cases there is no specific proof that strict bowel rest helps, we advocate a policy of nil by mouth, combined with nasogastric suction in all cases.
(3) Antibiotics. We reserve antibiotics for proven infections.
(4) Analgesics. Pancreatitis is an extremely painful condition. Adequate analgesic with pethidine 50–100 mg as required should be given.
(5) Oxygen therapy. A low Pao_2 is a feature of severe pancreatitis, and respiratory failure the commonest cause of death. The cause of the hypoxia is unknown. If humidified O_2 is not effective in restoring the Pao_2 to above 60 mmHg (8.0 kPa), IPPV should be instituted.

(6) Correction of renal insufficiency. If a poor renal output (<30 ml/h) persists in spite of adequate fluid replacement, you should try to promote a diuresis by using mannitol, frusemide or dopamine (see p. 17). To ensure accurate measurement of urine output, you should catheterise the patient on admission.

(7) Correction of hypocalcaemia. This is probably secondary to the various peptides present, but is often associated with hypoalbuminaemia. It often corrects if you assiduously replace albumin (up to 40 g day may be required) in the form of plasma, plasma protein derivatives or albumin; 10 ml of i.v. calcium gluconate may also be given.

Further measures

Most of the mild cases of pancreatitis respond to the supportive measures outlined above. In the severe case, additional therapeutic manoeuvres have been tried, but, as mentioned below, found to be unhelpful.

(8) Trasylol and i.v. glucagon. Controlled trials have not supported the use of these.

(9) Peritoneal lavage with hourly 2 litre cycles of peritoneal dialysis fluid does not improve the outcome in patients with severe disease.

(10) Surgery.[6] There is now little enthusiasm for early surgery with total pancreatectomy or pancreatic debridement, which may, however, be necessary in an unresolving case as a delayed procedure. However, two studies have shown that if gallstones are involved in provoking pancreatitis, endoscopic or surgical removal of the stones within 48 h of admission is very helpful.[6] You should therefore arrange ultrasound examination for gallstones early in the course of the illness.

REFERENCES

1   Barry R. (1988) The pathogenesis of acute pancreatitis. *Br. Med. J.* **296:** 589.

2   Bateson M. C. (1986) Acute pancreatitis. *Br. Med. J.* **292:** 85.

3   Corfield A. P. *et al.* (1985) Acute pancreatitis: a lethal disease of increasing incidence. *Gut* **26:** 724.

4   Corfield A. P. *et al.* (1985) Predictions of severity in acute pancreatitis: prospective comparison of three prognostic indices. *Lancet* **ii:** 403.

5   Gudgeon A. *et al.* (1990) Trypsinogen activation peptides assay in the early prediction of severity in acute pancreatitis. *Lancet* **335:** 4.

6   Pellegrini C. (1985) The treatment of acute pancreatitis: a continuing challenge. *N. Engl. J. Med.* **312:** 436.

7   Williamson R. C. N. (1985) Early assessment of severity in acute pancreatitis. *Gut* **25:** 1331.

Ulcerative colitis[2,4]

Ulcerative colitis is characterised by widespread superficial ulceration of the colonic mucosa. It is a relapsing disease characterised
by episodes of bloody diarrhoea. The severity of any single episode
is related to the extent of colon involved, and, to a lesser degree,
the severity of mucosal ulceration. In about 70% of episodes the
colonic involvement is restricted to the sigmoid and rectum. Such
cases do not usually constitute medical emergencies. However,
more extensive involvement of the colon can give rise to a fulminant
and potentially fatal disease. Appropriate management depends on
accurate assessment of the severity of the attack.

DIAGNOSIS AND ASSESSMENT OF SEVERITY

(1) The diagnosis of ulcerative colitis is made by the association of:

   (i)   Clinical features (see below).
   (ii)   Sigmoidoscopic appearances. As the rectum is involved
          in 95% of all cases, sigmoidoscope evidence of the
          disease will almost always be present in an acute attack.
          The mucosa will be uniformly oedematous and red,
          there will be multiple small ulcers (often rather difficult
          to see macroscopically) or petechial haemorrhages, and
          free pus in the lumen of the bowel. The colonic mucosal
          wall will bleed on contact, and biopsy will provide
          histological evidence of the disease. Sigmoidoscopy must
          be carried out on all patients with a fresh attack of
          ulcerative colitis as it is the quickest and easiest way of
          substantiating the diagnosis.
   (iii) Barium enema abnormalities. In severe colitis, it is safe
          to perform a limited enema on an unprepared patient.
          Run in a small quantity of barium, remove it, and then
          insufflate a little air. This provides a good double con-
          trast enema, and will help you diagnostically, as well as
          giving an indication of the extent and severity of colonic
          involvement.
   (iv)   The absence of an infective cause for the diarrhoea.

(2) Features helpful in identifying a severe attack are:

(i) More than six liquid, bloodstained stools in 24 h. Patients with mild colitis frequently pass blood separately from faeces and it is the association of liquid faeces and blood which is important here.

(ii) Fever. A mean evening temperature of greater than 38°C.

(iii) Tachycardia. A mean pulse rate greater than 90 beats/min.

(iv) Anaemia. This is usually a combination of the anaemia of chronic disease and the anaemia of blood loss. Hb levels below 10.0 g/100 ml indicate serious disease.

(v) ESR above 30 mm/h.

(vi) Hypoalbuminaemia. Patients with ulcerative colitis may exude up to 30 g/day of protein through their raw colonic mucosa.

(vii) Electrolyte disturbances. Electrolyte and fluid loss through the inflamed mucosa may also be considerable, and hypokalaemia, hypocalcaemia and hypomagnesaemia all occur.

(viii) Abdominal pain. Pain prior to, and relieved by, defaecation is common in all grades of severity. Central abdominal pain, and colonic tenderness on palpation, usually indicate a severe attack.

(ix) Straight x-ray of the abdomen. Dilatation of the colon (>6 cm), mucosal islands, or gas under the diaphragm in a patient with severe colitis are all indications for immediate surgery. However, wherever you can see substantial faecal residue in the colon, you can assume that the bowel is normal.

(x) It should be noted that the systemic complications of ulcerative colitis (arthropathy, skin rashes, iritis and liver disease) do not necessarily relate to the severity of the bowel involvement.

DIFFERENTIAL DIAGNOSIS

Bloody diarrhoea and systemic disturbance may be a feature of:

(1) Amoebic dysentery. A history of foreign travel, characteristically foul smelling stools, the typical undermined ulcer on sigmoidoscopy and positive amoebic complement fixation test

will help you. Amoebae in the stools must be specifically
looked for as they are easily confused with white cells.

(2) Dysentery. Usually caused by Gram-negative bacteria of the
Shigella or para-typhoid groups. Send stool and a rectal biopsy
specimen for cultures and enquire after contacts. This disease
may produce rectal changes indistinguishable from ulcerative
colitis on sigmodoscopic examination, as may campylobacter
colitis. Both of the above may respond to ciprofloxacin 500 mg
b.d. orally, which you should therefore use in patients who
have associated systemic upset.

(3) Crohn's disease. Classically, Crohn's involvement of the colon
is patchy and the ulcers are deeper and serpigenous. However,
as the management of acute Crohn's colitis is essentially the
same as that of acute ulcerative colitis, the differentiation of
these two conditions is not an immediate priority.

(4) Pseudomembranous colitis. In this form of colitis, which
characteristically occurs in an ill patient who has been given
antibiotics, particularly clindamycin, yellowish adherent
plaques are seen on sigmoidoscopy. The likely causal agent is
Clostridium difficile, and the illness responds well to metronidazole 400 mg t.d.s. or vancomycin 125 mg orally 6-hourly.[1]

It is worth remembering that *Cl. difficile* may provoke a relapse
of ulcerative colitis.[1]

(5) The rectal bleeding in ulcerative colitis is not usually severe.
This, plus the characteristic sigmoidoscope findings, serve to
distinguish it from several other conditions which may present
with severe rectal bleeding, such as ischaemic colitis, diverticular disease, carcinoma of the colon and haemorrhoids.

MANAGEMENT

(1) Like most gastrointestinal emergencies, management is best
undertaken jointly by physicians and surgeons.

(2) Take blood for FBP and ESR, serum Fe and folate, albumin
and liver function tests, electrolytes including Ca^{2+} and Mg^{2+},
and urea. Do a daily, straight x-ray of the abdomen. Culture
blood and stool.

(3) Correct the metabolic disturbances.

   (i)   The fluid disturbances. Anorexia, pyrexia and enteric
         losses give rise to considerable fluid electrolyte and

protein depletion. Initial replacement should be 0.9% N
saline—preferably under CVP control. Hypoproteinae-
mia may be treated by colloid-containing fluids, for
example two units of plasma or its equivalent, each 24 h.

(ii) Electrolytes.

    (a) Na^+ deficiency is corrected as above.

    (b) Plasma K^+ is usually low. If less than 3.5 mmol/l
give 40 mmol KCl in each litre of replacement fluid.
Otherwise re-measure 6 hours later and replenish as
indicated.

    (c) If the plasma Ca^{2+} is less than 2.3 mmol/l give 10 ml
10% calcium gluconate solution (2.25 mmol) each
day.

    (d) If the plasma Mg^{2+} is below 0.8 mmol/l give 20 mmol
of 40% magnesium sulphate solution each day until
the Mg^{2+} is normal (1 g/m $MgSO_4$ = 4 mmol).

(iii) The anaemia. This is best corrected by blood transfusion.
It is reasonable to aim at a haemoglobin level of 11.0 g/
100 ml.

(iv) Nutrition. A recent controlled trial showed that there
was no difference in patient outcome when either parenteral or enteral nutrition was used. So only use parenteral nutrition if enteral nutrition is not possible.[3]

(4) Suppressing the inflammation. If there is no indication for
immediate surgery (see below), give:

(i) Prednisone 60 mg i.v./day. This is the drug of choice.

(ii) Antibiotics. The role of bacteria in either initiating or
exacerbating ulcerative colitis is unclear. Bacteraemia in
association with severe ulcerative colitis is common, and
some authorities advocate the routine use of metronidazole, penicillin and gentamicin (see pp. 348–352). Sala-
zopyrine does not confer additional benefit in an acute
attack and causes anorexia.

(5) Surgery. In most severe cases of colitis a trial of medical
management is preferable. However, if the patient is not
improving by 10 days, or, at any stage, deteriorates, total
colectomy should be undertaken. The exact timing of such an
operation has to be decided between physician and surgeon.

However, immediate surgery is always required in the presence of:

(i) Toxic dilatation of the colon. This diagnosis is suspected when prostration accompanies a distended and tympanitic abdomen and is confirmed by a straight x-ray of the abdomen. The widest diameter of the colon should be less than 6 cm. Toxic dilatation occurs only when virtually the entire epithelium of the colon has been destroyed. Mucosal islands or pieces of stripped off epithelium may hang from the colonic wall and be visible on the straight x-ray. This mucosal island sign is a further important pointer to immediate surgery.

(ii) Perforation. Colonic perforation may not cause specific symptoms or signs but is associated with a general clinical deterioration. The diagnosis is confirmed by the presence of air under the diaphragm on an upright abdominal x-ray.

(iii) Profuse haemorrhage. This is, however, extremely uncommon even in severe colitis.

(6) It is worth stressing again that treatment of this disease requires a combined medical and surgical approach. Initial treatment with prednisone neither precludes nor complicates later surgery.

REFERENCES

1 Dickinson R. J. *et al.* (1985) Double blind controlled trial of oral vancomycin as adjunctive treatment in acute exacerbations of idiopathic colitis. *Gut* **26:** 1380.

2 Lennard-Jones J. E. (1984) Medical treatment of ulcerative colitis. *Postgrad. Med. J.* **60:** 797.

3 McIntyre P. B. *et al.* (1986) Controlled trial of bowel rest in the treatment of severe acute colitis. *Gut* **27:** 481.

4 Truelove S. C., Jewell D. P. (1974) Intensive intravenous regime for severe attacks of ulcerative colitis. *Lancet* **1:** 10.

Medical conditions which may present with acute abdominal pain[6]

DIAGNOSIS

Abdominal pain may arise from stretching, violent contraction, ischaemia or infarction of the viscera, or from muscle, skin, bone, blood vessels and nerves overlying or adjacent to the abdomen. It is not, therefore, surprising that many medical conditions can give rise to abdominal pain, and cause diagnostic confusion with an acute 'surgical' abdomen. In any patient presenting with abdominal pain, a careful history and a pause for reflection while necessary investigations are being performed and, where indicated, a trial of medical therapy is undertaken, may make an occasional laparotomy unnecessary. The following group of conditions should be considered.

(1) Intrathoracic causes. As the lower six thoracic nerves supply both thorax and abdominal wall, and as the heart and pericardium rest on the diaphragm, thoracic problems often cause abdominal pain—usually in the upper abdomen. Important causes are:

    (i) myocardial infarction (see p. 11);
    (ii) pericarditis;
    (iii) pulmonary embolus (see p. 52);
    (iv) pleurisy and pneumonia;

all of which have characteristic clinical, radiographic and ECG findings. A useful clinical tip here is that if unilateral abdominal pain arises from intrathoracic causes, palpation of the other side of the abdomen does not increase pain, whereas it will if the source is intra-abdominal.[3]

(2) Intra-abdominal and retroperitoneal causes.

    (i) Acute pancreatitis (see p. 124).
    (ii) Congestion of the liver, occurring in congestive cardiac failure and acute hepatitis, both of which should be looked for.
    (iii) Acute pyelonephritis, this typically causes loin pain and

frequency, but sometimes the pain may be confined to the bladder area. Examine a fresh MSU under the microscope and send urine for culture.

(iv) Bowel ischaemia, which may be due to:

    (a) Sickle cell diseases. This should be considered in any one of African extraction with a history of jaundice. The patient may have parietal bossing and a characteristic facies.

    (b) Henoch–Schonlein purpura. Abdominal pain may occur before the other signs, such as joint pains, rash, haematuria and rectal bleeding, appear.

    (c) The vasculitic lesions of polyarteritis nodosa, systemic lupus erythematosis and other allied conditions may give rise to bowel pain. Given the clinical setting, the diagnosis is usually obvious.

    (d) The commonest cause is atheromatous narrowing of the mesenteric vessels.

(v) Constipation. This can, of itself, cause severe abdominal pain, especially in the elderly. Rectal examination and a straight x-ray of the abdomen will reveal all.

(vi) Infection.

    (a) Gastroenteritis causes colic, usually in association with diarrhoea and vomiting. A careful history will help you here. A large number of pathogens may be involved,[2,5] one of the commonest to cause confusion is *Yersinia*[1]

    (b) Worms. Tape worms can cause quite severe abdominal pain. Ova and cysts should be looked for in the stools if a history of infestation is elicited.

    (c) Primary peritonitis. This is an uncommon condition, usually occurring in patients with ascites. It is particularly liable to ocur in children with the nephrotic syndrome. Aspiration of the abdominal fluid may reveal a cloudy aspirate from which diplococci may be grown.

    (d) Typhoid.

    (e) Mesenteric adenitis.

(3) Metabolic and endocrine causes.

(i) Diabetes. You will diagnose this by finding glucose and ketones in the urine and a raised blood glucose. Of course, appendicitis can precipitate diabetic coma. However, it is reasonable to see whether treatment of the diabetes relieves the pain within 4 h or so, before proceeding to laparotomy.

(ii) Hypercalcaemia. There may be a history of constipation, polyuria, polydipsia, renal calculi and mood disturbance. Look for the typical deposits of calcium at the corneoscleral junction.

(iii) Porphyria (usually of the acute intermittent variety). The urine contains increased quantities of porphobilinogen which is oxidised to porphobilin—a brownish coloured substance—when the urine is allowed to stand for half an hour. Abdominal tenderness is usually mild and rigidity absent.

(iv) Addison's disease. This may also cause vomiting, hypotension and peripheral circulatory collapse. The patient may have the characteristic pigmentation, and the diagnosis is suggested by the typical electrolyte findings of low Na^+ and high K^+, and confirmed by measuring the plasma cortisol.

(v) Heavy metal poisoning—classically lead (look for the blue line on the gums, blood and urine lead levels and urinary corporphyrins I and III are increased). Antimony, cadmium, arsenic and mercury may also cause abdominal pain.

(4) Neurogenic causes.

(i) Compression of nerve roots by either malignancy or local degenerative lesions. The pain is usually band-like and may give rise to segmental hyperaesthesia over the abdomen and local pain over the vertebra.

(ii) Tabes dorsalis. Attacks of vomiting associated with severe epigastric pain and lasting for several days may occur in tabes dorsalis. The presence of irregular pupils reactive to accommodation but not to light (Argyll Robertson pupils) and absence of knee jerks aid the diagnosis.

(iii) Herpes zoster. Pain and paraesthesia precede the rash by a few days. It is usually unilateral and segmental and should not really cause confusion.

(5) Psychiatric cause: Munchausen's syndrome. These patients present with convincing symptoms and signs of various acute conditions often involving the abdomen, which may be covered with scars. When the patient is apprised of your suspicions, the symptoms and signs disappear and the patient rapidly takes his own discharge, usually resisting offers of psychiatric help.

MANAGEMENT

Management implies excluding those conditions mentioned above. Obviously they will not all be relevant in every case of acute abdominal pain, but it is suggested that whenever possible the following investigations should be done.

(1) A plain supine x-ray of the abdomen. A recent prospective evaluation indicates that an erect film is of no additional diagnostic help.[4]
(2) Chest x-ray.
(3) Blood film.
(4) Examine the urine for sugar, ketones, blood and pus cells.
(5) Serum amylase.
(6) ECG.

REFERENCES

1   Attwood S. *et al*. (1987) Yersinia infection and acute abdominal pain. *Lancet* **i:** 529.
2   Blacklow N. R., Cukor G. (1981) Viral gastroenteritis. *N. Engl. J. Med.* **304:** 397.
3   Cope Z. (1968) *The Early Diagnosis of the Acute Abdomen*, 13th edn. London: Oxford University Press.
4   Field S. *et al*. (1985) The erect abdominal radiograph in the acute abdomen: should its routine use be abandoned? *Br. Med. J.* **290:** 1934.
5   Gorbach S. (1987) Bacterial diarrhoea and its treatment. *Lancet* **ii:** 1378.
6   Harvard C. (1972) Medical states simulating the acute abdomen. *Br. J. Hosp. Med.* **7:** 443.

Pseudo-obstruction[1]

The problem is of a patient, usually elderly and ill from other causes, and therefore not primarily in the surgical wards, who presents with appearances which resemble acute mechanical obstruction, predominantly of the large bowel. However, no mechanical cause is found. A straight X-ray of the abdomen shows gross dilatation of the large and small bowel. Despite the lack of any mechanical obstruction, the distal large bowel may be normal in size. The pathogenesis is thought to be neuromuscular dysfunction induced by electrolyte disturbances and the metabolic problems associated with major organ failure.

The following may be contributory factors.

(1) Drugs, e.g. tricyclic antidepressants, anti-Parkinsonian drugs and anticholinergic drugs (e.g. atropine).
(2) Hypokalaemia and other electrolyte disturbances.
(3) Severe gastroenteritis.
(4) Certain spinal events, e.g. spinal fusion, prolapsed intravertebral disc and spinal fractures.
(5) Hypoxia, ureamia and dehydration.
(6) Intra-abdominal trauma—retroperitoneal bleeding may play a part.

MANAGEMENT

(1) You should correct any of the above abnormalities.
(2) Decompression will almost certainly be required. Surgical decompression is disastrous; colonoscopy is the treatment of choice, both allowing decompression and establishing conclusively the diagnosis. Sigmoidoscopy and the passing of a flatus tube may also provide some relief.
(3) Cisapride, which stimulates peristalsis by a direct action on motilin receptors of the bowel, may have a place. A starting dose of 300 mg suppositories b.d.
(4) If caecal perforation occurs, or if there is failure of conservative measures with increasing respiratory distress, caecostomy

should be performed, with the placement of a large intracaecal catheter.

REFERENCES

1   Dudley H. (1986) Pseudo-obstruction. *Br. Med. J.* **292:** 1157.

Acute gastric dilatation

DIAGNOSIS

(1) This may occur in hyperglycaemia, after childbirth, abdominal injury, application of a spinal cast and occasionally after abdominal surgery.
(2) The abdomen is distended and uncomfortable and a succusion splash can be readily elicited. Sufficient fluid may accumulate in the stomach to cause hypovolaemic shock.
(3) If reflux of the stomach contents occurs into the oesophagus the condition may be complicated by inhalation pneumonia.

MANAGEMENT

(1) Take blood for haemoglobin and PCV, electrolytes and urea.
(2) Pass a nasogastric tube and empty the stomach. Usually more than 1.5 l can be aspirated.
(3) Set up a drip, preferably with central venous pressure line and replace the fluid lost into the bowel with alternating bottles of 5% dextrose and N saline. Add 40 mmol KCl to each litre of fluid given.
(4) Check the electrolytes 6 h later and adjust the ratio of saline to dextrose and the potassium supplements in the usual way.
(5) If reflux of abdominal contents into the lungs occurs, you should be prepared for an aspiration pneumonitis (see p. 101).

Acute liver failure[7]

DIAGNOSIS

(1) Liver failure should be considered in any confused (see p. 325) or unconscious (see p. 355) patient, particularly if there are unexplained clotting abnormalities, signs of liver disease, or a history of liver disease.

(2) It may be caused by:

    (i)   Serious disease in a previously healthy patient. In this group, there are no signs of chronic liver disease, the serum albumin is often maintained, the illness is usually of less than 8 weeks duration and, in the UK, the commoner causes are:

        (a) paracetamol overdose (50%) (see p. 273).
        (b) viral hepatitis (40%: C, B, A in order of frequency).
        (c) halothane anaesthesia, idiosyncratic drug reactions, carbon tetrachloride or mushroom poisoning—particularly *Amanita phalloides*—acute fatty liver of pregnancy, Wilson's disease and the Budd–Chiari syndrome.

    (ii)   A relatively minor stress to a patient with biochemical and clinical evidence of chronic liver disease. This is the commoner cause of hepatic failure, and may be precipitated by:

        (a) gastrointestinal haemorrhage (see p. 111);
        (b) major surgery or major trauma and anaesthesia;
        (c) alcoholic hepatitis—remember that in alcohol-related liver disease, delirium tremens, thiamine deficiency producing Wernicke's encephalopathy, other B vitamin deficiencies and epileptic fits may all contribute to the disturbances in consciousness;
        (d) acute infection, including the possibility of spontaneous bacterial peritonitis;
        (e) potassium depletion and alkalosis (usually due to over-vigorous use of diuretics);

(f) drugs—sedatives, narcotics, analgesics and hypnotics.

(3) The disturbance in conscious level (encephalopathy) which often accompanies liver failure is a good indicator of prognosis, and is best graded on a 1–4 scale, as follows:

Grade 1: Mild drowsiness, impaired concentration and psychomotor function.

Grade 2: Confused and disorientated, but rousable.

Grade 3: Markedly drowsy, responding to simple commands but incoherent and often aggressive.

Grade 4: Unrousable—

  4a: Responding to painful stimuli

  4b: No response to any stimuli.

MANAGEMENT

Although the principles of management of acute and acute on chronic liver failure are similar, the objectives are somewhat different. In acute liver failure, supportive measures are used to buy time for the liver to recover. In acute on chronic failure, however, the underlying damage is not usually treatable, and reversal of the underlying cause is of paramount importance.

In all patients with liver failure take blood for a full blood picture, electrolytes and urea, blood sugar, liver function tests including prothrombin time and paracetamol levels. Take arterial blood for blood gas measurements. Save serum for markers of hepatitis A, B and C. Culture blood, urine and, when it is present, peritoneal fluid. Further management involves the following aspects.

(1) General care of the confused (see p. 327) or unconscious (see p. 356) patient. Sedation should be avoided if at all possible (see (xii) below) but if you think sedation to be necessary give phenobarbitone 100 mg i.m., diazepam 5 mg i.v. or chlormethiazole (see p. 225). Drugs included in (2) (ii) (f) above must never be given.

(2) Treatment of the cause. Specific treatments are few, exceptions being chronic aggressive hepatitis (steroids) and Wilson's disease (penicillamine). Steroids are not helpful in fulminating viral hepatitis.

(3) Stopping or treating the precipitating or contributory factors mentioned above.

(4) Minimising or correcting the multiple effects of liver cell failure:

    (i)   Minimising the protein load. The rationale behind this is that the four groups of substances which appear in increased amounts in liver failure,[1] are protein related metabolites. They are:

        (a) Ammonia. This arises largely through bacterial action on proteins in the gut, and is usually converted to urea by the liver. It causes coma in experimental animals, but not all patients dying of liver failure have a raised ammonia level.

        (b) Amines. Several amines, notably octopamine and phenylethanolamine, are present in increased amounts. It is conceivable that they act as false neurotransmitters in the brain.

        (c) Amino-acids. Amino-acid profiles are abnormal in liver disease. The amino-acid precursors of octopamine and phenylethanolamine are present in increased amounts which may account for the increased levels of these amines.

        (d) Gamma amino butyric acid, the principal inhibitory neurotransmitter in the normal brain, is greatly increased in liver failure, and is the present leading contender as the inducer of the neuropsychiatric problems in liver failure.

    (ii)   Therefore, give the following:

        (a) A low protein diet (20–30 g/day).

        (b) About 6.4 mJ (1500 kcal) as carbohydrates. This may be given either orally (e.g. 3–4 bottles of Hycal each of which contains 425 kcal) or intravenously via a central venous catheter (e.g. 1200 ml of 33% dextrose). This glucose infusion will hopefully prevent the development of hypoglycaemia, a common occurrence in hepatic failure (see (v) below).

        (c) Sterilise the gut with neomycin 1 g 4-hourly by mouth. Lactulose, in a dose just sufficient to cause diarrhoea (approx 30 ml t.i.d.), will help empty the gut, thus minimising absorbtion of protein metabolites. By altering the faecal pH to below 6, it will also beneficially alter the gut flora. Lactilol, a disaccharide analogue of lactulose which is well tolerated, is becoming more widely available.[4]

(d) Give magnesium sulphate enemas—80 ml of 50% solution twice daily—this is particularly useful if there has been gastrointestinal haemorrhage.

(e) A controlled trial of branched chain amino-acid infusion showed that while the amino-acid profile was corrected, no other benefit occurred. These may have a calorific value, but should not be used routinely.

(iii) Correcting fluid and electrolytes imbalance.

(a) Do not give more than 2 litres of fluid per day.

(b) The serum sodium is usually low (120–130 mEq/l). This is almost always dilutional, and is treated by restricting both fluids and sodium.

(c) Potassium. Dangerous hypokalaemia can occur and potassium chloride supplements are given in the usual way.

(iv) Correcting coagulation defects. These may arise for two reasons:[3]

(a) Decreased synthesis of clotting factors by the liver.

(b) Low grade disseminated intravascular coagulation, with thrombocytopenia. Fresh blood and/or fresh frozen plasma (FFP) which contains all the clotting factors are the infusion of choice. If the platelet count is low, a platelet infusion may be required. Vitamin K 10 mg i.v., although theoretically not helpful, should also be given. We no longer use heparin for the DIC.

(c) Remember that every time you damage a blood vessel, bleeding is encouraged. Therefore, be sparing of your assaults on your patients.

(v) Correcting the blood glucose:

(a) Hypoglycaemia may occur. If this is present give 25 g of dextrose intravenously, ensure that your patient is having adequate carbohydrate calories and check the blood sugar 4-hourly.

    (b) Alternatively, hyperglycaemia may be present. This rarely needs treatment—unless ketosis develops. It is treated in the usual way with insulin (see p. 163).

(vi) Correcting the effects of widespread peripheral dilatation. This may cause hypotension and/or acute renal failure. Its mechanism is obscure, and treatment difficult. You should monitor these patients with a pulmonary artery pressure line, to ensure optimal fluid balance (see p. 387). Then infuse dopamine, beginning at a dose of between 2–5 μg/kg/min. At this level of infusion it causes vasoconstriction to all arteries except those in the brain and kidney.

(vii) Combating sepsis. Amoxycillin in the usual doses 250 mg i.v. 8-hourly is safe, but if gentamicin is used, blood levels should be monitored (see p. 350). Remember septicaemia is common in acute hepatic necrosis, whatever the cause.

(viii) Minimizing the occurrence of gastrointestinal haemorrhage from acute erosions. If you have a nasogastric tube in place, give sucralfate, 1 g t.d.s. If not, give ranitidine 50 mg six-hourly i.v., which will maintain the pH of the stomach contents above 6.

(ix) Supporting respiration. Many patients with acute hepatic failure develop shock lung (see p. 97). They may therefore require early ventilation to maintain an adequate Pao_2. To minimise the chance of aspiration, you should anyway aspirate the stomach hourly through a nasogastric tube.

(x) Cerebral oedema.[5] This complication is now the commonest cause of death in acute liver failure. The oedema is difficult to control. Nursing your patient with the head up 45° may help. We find 100 ml of 20% mannitol given by bolus and repeated hourly until a water diuresis is achieved is the most successful drug therapy available. Intracranial pressure monitoring may be helpful. Steroids are not.

(xi) Lowering the concentration of circulating substances usually removed by the liver, e.g. ammonia. The following methods have been used:

    (a) exchange transfusion;
    (b) haemoperfusion over an activated charcoal column;[4]

    (c) haemodialysis;
    (d) cross circulation;
    (e) extracorporeal liver perfusion;
    (f) and increasingly, liver transplantation,[6] which offers the best hope to those who have high intracranial pressure in association with their liver failure.

(xii) The above treatments are best done in a specialist centre. You should discuss treatment with a specialist unit in each case of liver failure you manage, as the indications are changing with experience. In general these options are not helpful in acute on chronic liver failure. In your patients without previous liver disease, transfer to a specialist unit is advisable if:

    (a) There is a grade 2 or worse encephalopathy.
    (b) The prothrombin time is over 30 s and getting progressively worse. Factor V levels are also very helpful, and a level below 20%, in association with coma, is a useful guide to the need for transplantation.
    (c) Your patient is persistently hypotensive (systolic pressure <100 mmHg), hyponatraemic or thrombocytopenic.

(xiii) Sedation. Patient with acute liver failure may become disorientated and violent for many reasons and you should ensure that there is no reversible cause, such as hypoxia, before using any sedation. If sedation is essential the benzodiazepam group of drugs are safest. Diazepam, 5 mg i.v. by slow infusion usually secures peace for all. As it is metabolised by the liver, the dosage should be kept as low as possible, and repeated as infrequently as possible.

REFERENCES

1   Fraser C. L., Arieff A. I. (1985) Hepatic encephalopathy. *N. Engl. J. Med.* **313:** 865.
2   Gimson A. E. S. (1982) Earlier charcoal haemoperfusion in fulminant hepatic failure. *Lancet* **ii:** 681.
3   Kelly D. A., Tuddenham E. G. D. (1986) Haemostatic problems in liver disease. *Gut* **27:** 339.

4   Lanthier P. L., Morgan M. Y. (1985) Lactitol in the treatment of chronic hepatic encephalopathy: an open comparison with Lactulose. *Gut* **26:** 415.

5   Leader (1991) The brain in fulminant hepatic failure. *Lancet* **338:** 156.

6   O'Grady J., Williams R. (1988) Present position of liver transplantation and its impact on hepatological practice. *Gut* **29:** 566.

7   O'Grady J., Williams R. (1987) Management of acute liver failure. *Hospital Update* June, p. 481.

Acute renal failure

Acute renal failure (ARF)

Acute renal failure may be defined as a sudden rise in urea with or without accompanying oliguria (less than 400 ml/24 h in an adult). It is customary and helpful to consider ARF as:

(1) pre-renal;
(2) renal (established renal failure); or
(3) post-renal.

(1) *Pre-renal*. This is a physiological response of the kidney to poor perfusion, which may be caused by:

   (i)   Hypovolaemia—the commonest situation. This may either be absolute, owing to fluid or blood loss, or relative, as occurs for example in septicaemia, major overdoses, liver failure and pancreatitis.

  (ii)   Cardiac failure, due to any cause, including septicaemia.

In the initial stages of pre-renal failure, the kidneys' concentrating power is normal, and the urine produced is highly concentrated (see Table 2). It is essential to recognise this since restoring perfusion will avert established renal failure (ATN, see below).

Table 2   Urine differences in pre-renal and established renal failure

	Pre-renal failure	Established renal failure
Urine/plasma osmolal ratio	>1.5:1	1.1:1
Urine/plasma urea ratio	>10:1	<4:1
Sodium mmol/1	<10	>20

(2) *Renal*. Renal damage per se is characterised by considerable deterioration in renal function and concentrating power. The urine produced, therefore, is dilute, and serves to distinguish renal from pre-renal failure (see Table 2). Established renal failure may be due to the following causes.

   (i)   Acute tubular necrosis (ATN). The pathogenetic mechanism is unclear.[6] However, causes include:

(a) Persistent impairment of renal perfusion.

(b) Drugs and chemicals, including non-steroidal anti-inflammatory agents, antibiotics, such as the aminoglycosides, radiocontrast mediums,[2] low molecular weight dextrans and many others.

(c) Circulating pigments, including haemoglobin (haemolysis), bilirubin or myoglobin.

(d) Myoglobin release occurs in the syndrome of rhabdomyolosis.[1] While still seen in association with crush injuries, we now see it more frequently in drug abusers, including those that take cocaine.[7] Patients with rhabdomyolosis and ARF have higher than usual levels of uric acid and phosphate, and very high levels of muscle-derived creatinine phosphokinase (often greater than 12 000 U/l).

(e) Frequently, several causes co-exist.

(ii) Acute interstitial nephritis. Causes include:

(a) drugs—non-steroidal anti-inflammatory drugs, diuretics, rifampicin, ampicillin and sulphonamides are among those implicated;

(b) infections, such as leptospirosis, Legionnaires' disease and the haemorrhagic renal syndrome.

(iii) Acute glomerulonephritis.

(a) This may be secondary to bacterial infection (usually streptococcal or staphylococcal), or part of a systemic disease such as PAN (now the commonest cause), SLE, Goodpasture's syndrome and, increasingly, HIV.

(b) Because of the response to immunosuppression, it is important to diagnose PAN, SLE and Goodpasture's syndrome promptly, using the appropriate serological tests (antinuclear cytoplasmic antibody (ANCA), ANF and anti-GBM antibodies) and renal biopsy.

(iv) Haemolytic uraemic syndrome (HUS),[4] including thrombotic thrombocytopenic purpura. This is characterised by micro-angiopathic haemolytic anaemia.

(v) Tubular obstruction, due to myeloma, insoluble drugs (sulphonamides), uric acid nephropathy, often in association with the treatment of lymphoreticular disorders, and oxalate crystals.

(vi) Hypercalcaemia.

(vii) Acute on chronic failure. A trivial insult, such as minor salt depletion, infection or the consumption of non-steroidal anti-inflammatory agents, to a chronically diseased kidney may produce acute renal failure.

(viii) Vascular problems. Occlusion of the renal arteries, on the basis of atheromatous renal artery stenosis, is an increasingly recognised cause of ARF in elderly smokers, often with a previous history of TIA, myocardial infarct or peripheral vascular disease. The diagnostic giveaway is the unequal renal size (one kidney has had renal artery stenosis longer than the other). Urgent angioplasty may be curative.

(3) Post-renal

Obstruction to urine flow, with consequent reduction in renal function, may occur in the ureter and urethra.

(i) *Ureter*: calculi, retroperitoneal fibrosis and tumours, most commonly of cervix or bladder. Bear in mind the possibility of obstruction to a single functioning kidney.

(ii) *Urethra*: prostatic hypertrophy or urethral stricture. If the obstruction is relieved, prompt and rewarding return of renal function can be achieved.

DIAGNOSIS

The diagnosis of ARF, as defined, is biochemical. The signs and symptoms of fluid overload and uraemia, drowsiness, nausea and twitching are often overshadowed by the underlying cause.

(1) The history may give clues of longstanding renal disease, such as polyuria and nocturia and there may be stigmata of chronic renal failure such as hypertension, anaemia, pigmentation, pruritus, or renal bone disease with characteristic radiological changes of periosteal resorption of the distal phalanges. In such cases, the kidneys, when visualised, may either be large (polycystic or hydronephrotic) or small and shrunken. If there has been no previous renal disease, the kidneys are of normal size.

(2) The biochemical changes usually present are as follows.

(i) Raised urea. ARF is usually accompanied by a catabolic state, and the urea deriving from excessive protein breakdown can only accumulate—serum creatinine is also raised to a relatively lesser degree.

(ii) Raised potassium. Potassium, released from cells by acidosis, catabolism and the sick cell syndrome accumulates and may cause fatal cardiac dysrhythmias.

(iii) Low sodium. This is usually caused by fluid overload (dilution) as opposed to true sodium depletion.

(iv) Low HCO_3. Metabolic acidosis is due to inadequate secretion of non-volatile anions (e.g. SO_4 and PO_4), inadequate renal tubular generation of HCO_3, and inadequate formation of NH_3, by the distal tubules. H+ ion formation may also be increased in this situation by poor tissue perfusion, lactate accumulation and tissue damage.

(3) Haematological changes.

(i) A normochromic normocytic anaemia may suggest that there is underlying chronic renal failure.

(ii) In the HUS there is an anaemia and thrombocytopenia, and fragmented cells are seen in the blood film. Clotting factors are usually normal.

(4) Therefore, take blood for electrolytes, urea, FBP (including platelets), clotting factors, blood cultures, serum calcium and blood glucose. Send urine, if necessary obtained by catheterisation, for Na+ urea and osmolality (see Table 2). This only requires a few millilitres of urine, takes a short time to do, and must be insisted upon. Take a straight x-ray of the abdomen to evaluate renal size and visualise calculi, and a chest x-ray.

MANAGEMENT

This is aimed initially at diagnosing and correcting reversible or predisposing factors, i.e. poor renal perfusion or post-renal obstruction. If these measures do not restore renal function (i.e. established ARF is present), further treatment is as indicated below.

(1) The metabolic sequelae of kidney failure are dealt with until renal function is restored. This is usually necessary before the diagnostic process is complete.

(2) The workload of the kidney is reduced by minimising tissue breakdown and hypoperfusion.

(3) A specific diagnosis of the cause of ARF is made and appropriate therapy is given. You must obviously stop any drugs which accumulate in renal failure (aminoglycosides, digoxin, opiates,) or which are potentially damaging; if appropriate, treat glomerulonephritis as soon as possible with immunosuppressives, and dilate identified renal artery stenosis. Other specific therapy is not usually relevant to immediate management.

Management is continued as follows.

(1) Weigh the patient if possible.

(2) Rule out a pre-renal cause.

    (i)   Assess the patient for renal underperfusion. Heart failure is usually obvious and requires conventional treatment. Hypovolaemia causing general tissue underperfusion may also be evident clinically, i.e. cool peripheries, tachycardia, hypotension (particularly postural hypotension), plus disturbances of consciousness. If there has been substantial fluid loss, there may be reduced skin turgor, and eye ball tension will be low. A dry mouth and tongue are significant only in the absence of mouth breathing. The urine shows the characteristics of pre-renal failure. However, assessment of hypovolaemia can be extremely difficult, particularly if it is relative hypovolaemia, so if there is any doubt, the CVP, and left ventricular end diastolic pressure, must be measured (see pp. 381 and 387) If this confirms hypovolaemia, appropriate fluid (saline, blood or plasma) must be given rapidly until the CVP is in the upper range of normal (p. 383). Occasionally this manoeuvre restores urine flow even when the urine has shown the characteristics of established renal failure, but in this situation restoration of tissue perfusion must be carried out with the greatest attention to signs of impending fluid overload.

    (ii)   If correction of hypovolaemia or obstruction does not lead to brisk diuresis, renal damage has occurred, and established renal failure is present.

(iii) Remember that hypovolaemia may be due to a hypoproteinaemic state, such as the nephrotic syndrome, in which case circulating volume may be restored with 1 litre of salt-free albumin.

(3) Rule out a post-renal cause.

(i) Catheterise the bladder to ensure that urethral obstruction is not present. If the bladder is empty, insert 200 ml of 0.02% aqueous solution of chlorhexidine, and withdraw the catheter.

(ii) A straight x-ray and renal ultrasound examination is an effective and simple way of excluding obstruction higher up the renal tract, as well as showing the size and number of kidneys.[8]

(iii) When obstruction is confirmed, the surgeons or radiologists must be contacted without delay, as it is now usually possible to relieve the obstruction in the x-ray department with percutaneous nephrostomies.

Management of established ARF

(1) The precipitating condition will need treatment on its own merits.

(2) (i) Dopamine 2.5 μg/kg/min may initiate a diuresis, and by promoting the polyuric phase of renal failure, curtail the duration of the illness. Although no clinical trials of its efficacy have been undertaken, we think it a valuable asset.

(ii) Alternatively, mannitol 25%, 50 ml i.v. over 2 h, or frusemide 500 mg i.v. over 1.5 h may initiate a diuresis.

(iii) Mannitol can precipitate acute cardiac failure in patients who are already overloaded, frusemide must never be given to patients who are still hypovolaemic, as it may reduce tissue perfusion still further.

(3) Fluid balance. Fluid intake should be 500 ml plus fluid lost the previous day (bearing in mind diarrhoea, vomiting and leaking fistulae, and adding 500 ml/day for each degree of fever). A weight loss of up to 0.5 kg/day indicates appropriate fluid replacement and is due to tissue loss. Gross fluid overload is an indication for dialysis.

(4) Nutrition. Starvation is a major cause for continuing catabolism in ARF and every attempt should be made to provide 12.6 MJ (3000 kcal) as carbohydrate or fat per day. This will reduce the urea load and promote healing. High-calorie fluids, such as Caloreen 16.7 kJ (4 kcal)/g or Hycal 1.0 MJ (244 kcal)/100 ml, given with due attention to the necessity for fluid restriction, are suitable sources.

In low-potassium, high-carbohydrate diets, 20 g of protein/day is allowable. Parentrovite forte 10 ml i.v. or equivalent should be given daily. If the patient is being dialysed, a 60 g protein, high-calorie diet can be given, and constitutes one of the advantages of dialysis. Intravenous fluids should only be given if oral or nasogastric feeding is impossible. A CVP line inserted with due regard to sterility helps, as the solutions you will infuse are highly irritant to small veins; 50% dextrose 4.2 MJ (1000 kcal)/500 ml and 10% Intralipid 2.1 MJ (550 kcal)/500 ml are the most concentrated calorie sources and contain no electrolytes. Intravenous feeding may induce acute carbohydrate intolerance (common anyway in ARF) and blood glucose levels should be checked regularly.

(5) Potassium. This is often high and may reach a dangerous level (more than 7 mmol) which requires treatment.[5]

(i) The best emergency therapy is 10 ml of 10% calcium chloride i.v. This decreases the excitability of membranes rather than actually reducing the serum K^+.

(ii) Intravenous infusion of 500 ml 20% dextrose containing 25 units insulin over 2 h will reduce serum K^+ temporarily.

(iii) If there is acidosis and the patient is not overloaded, 75–100 mmol $NaHCO_3$ i.v. over 2 h will reduce serum K^+.

(iv) Ion-exchange resins, either orally or rectally, can be used for the less urgent situation. Calcium zeocarb 225 (15 g t.i.d.) is perhaps the best.

(6) Sodium. As discussed above, low serum Na usually indicates Na dilution and redistribution and is not an indication for saline infusion. Unless there is gross loss of electrolytes, none should be given in the oliguric phase of ARF. In practice, small quantities (less than 30 mmol of Na^+ or K^+/day) are unavoidable if nourishing food is provided.

(7) Acidosis. It is rarely possible to correct the acidosis, aside

from correcting tissue perfusion and oxygenation. Life-threatening acidosis (pH <7.1) is an indication for dialysis as $NaHCO_3$, the appropriate corrective fluid, will exacerbate fluid overload. The $NaHCO_3$ may, of course, be given as part of any replacement fluid necessary (see p. 154).

(8) Infections. Whatever the cause of ARF, septicaemia is highly likely—common organisms being *Pseudomonas pyocyanea, Bacterium proteus, Escherichia coli* and *Bacteroides*. Before the results of the blood cultures are available it is wise to start a broad spectrum, preferably bactericidal antibiotic regime, e.g. ampicillin 500 mg 6-hourly, and flucloxacillin 250 mg 6-hourly. If a change of antibiotics is indicated, they may be used as follows.

(i) The aminoglycosides. Gentamicin is the traditional choice, but because it probably has less nephrotoxicity netilmycin is our present choice. Both require you to monitor blood levels. The initial dose of gentamicin is 1–1.5 mg/kg in a single dose; that of netilmycin is 2–3.5 mg kg. Further doses are given according to blood levels (see p. 350). Remember that frusemide enhances the toxicity of gentamicin.

(ii) Cefotaxime 2–4 g 8-hourly i.v., or chloramphenicol 500 mg 6–hourly may be used safely, and without blood level monitoring. Cefoxitin may also be used.

(iii) Azlocillin, 4 g/day in two divided doses may be used.

(iv) Fungal infections may supervene and should be looked for in blood cultures. The likely organism is *Candida* acquired endogenously, and oral amphotericin lozenges 1 q.d.s., should be given prophylactically. (For the treatment of candidal septicaemia, see p. 352).

(v) If *Bacteroides* is found, metronidazole or chloramphenicol should be used (see p. 349).

(vi) Do not give tetracyclines as they raise the blood urea.

(9) Drugs. Many are excreted unchanged by the kidney. Before giving any drug to a patient in renal failure, make sure you know the appropriate dose. Drug levels are often available now—avail yourself of them. Metaclopramide 10 mg (1 ml) is a safe antiemetic and diazepam a suitable sedative. Paracetamol is probably the safest mild analgesic to use. Pethidine can be used with care. Give a normal loading dose, and then titrate according to response. Morphine is best not used, as

the main metabolite, the 6-glucuronide, accumulates in ARF, and is very active. Scrutinise the drug sheet daily, as a deterioration in either renal function or the patient's general state may be drug-related.

(10) Bleeding. Because platelet function is impaired, and your patient is often very ill, bleeding, especially from the gastrointestinal tract, is common. Prophylactic sucrulfate may help here (see p. 144) or use an H_2 antagonist.

(11) Pulmonary oedema. This is due to a combination of fluid overload leading to a raised left ventricular end diastolic pressure (see p. 43) and leaky capillaries, as in the ARDS (see p. 97). As indicated below, dialysis will be required, but you should first institute treatment as outlined in the relevant sections (see p. 45). Vasodilators, such as glyceryl trinitrate, are particularly useful, and intermittent positive pressure ventilation may buy you time.

(12) General. The patient with ARF has a physically and psychologically debilitating illness. You must try to keep up his or her morale (yours as well). Keep the patient as mobile and active as possible. Always have a therapeutic reason for any invasive techniques, both for the patient's peace of mind and for reasons of infection. Remember that the quality of nursing care is a major determinant of the ultimate outcome, and will be improved if the nurses understand what is happening (as much as you do).

(13) Dialysis. Haemodialysis, continuous arteriovenous (CAVHD) or venovenous haemofiltration (CVVHD)[3] or peritoneal dialysis facilitates control of uraemia, allows a more liberal diet and tides the patient over while the kidneys recover. Indications for dialysis are seldom absolute, but the following are general guidelines.

(i) cardiac failure, or fluid overload, in an oliguric patient;
(ii) serum K+ greater than 6.5 mmol/l;
(iii) blood urea >35 mmol/l;
(iv) blood pH <7.1;
(v) to create room for i.v. feeding if this is deemed necessary.

A deteriorating trend in your patient may require you to commence dialysis before the above figures are reached. Peritoneal dialysis, CAVHD or CVVHD can be carried out in the ITU of a hospital which does not have an associated renal unit, which may be an advantage if your unit is skilled in handling patients with renal disease. Otherwise it can be lethal, and it is always prudent to consult with your nearest renal unit.

REFERENCES

1   Better O. *et al.* (1990) Early management of shock and prophylaxis of acute renal failure in traumatic rhabdomyolysis. *N. Engl. J. Med.* **322:** 825.

2   Brezis M. *et al.* (1989) A closer look at radiocontrast induced nephropathy. *N. Engl. J. Med.* **320:** 179.

3   Brown E. *et al.* (1988) Continuous arteriovenous haemodialysis. *Br. Med. J.* **297:** 242.

4   Kavi J. *et al.* (1989) Causes of haemolytic uraemic syndrome. *Br. Med. J.* **298:** 65.

5   Leader (1989) Hyperkalaemia—silent and deadly. *Lancet* **ii:** 1240.

6   Levinsky N. (1977) Pathophysiology of acute renal failure. *N. Engl. J. Med.* **296:** 1453.

7   Roth D. (1988) Acute rhabdomyolysis associated with cocaine intoxication. *N. Engl. J. Med.* **319:** 673.

8   Webb J. (1990) Ultrasonography in the diagnosis of renal obstruction. *Br. Med. J.* **301:** 944.

Section V

Endocrine

Diabetic ketoacidosis and coma[1,7]

Diagnosis

(1) Diabetic ketoacidosis usually presents with polyuria and drowsiness (pre-coma) which may in a surprisingly short time, but usually over a day or more, progress to coma.

   (i) The patient usually shows signs of:

      (a) sodium and water depletion—dry slack skin, tachycardia and hypotension, particularly posturally induced;

      (b) acidosis—deep sighing respirations;

      (c) ketosis—foetor and vomiting.

   (ii) The clinical picture is sometimes confused with salicylate poisoning, which also shows reducing agents on Benedict's test. However, ketones, unlike salicylates, are volatile and are removed by boiling the urine. In any case the demonstration of a substantially raised blood glucose (>20 mmol/l) clinches the diagnosis.

   (iii) A notable symptom of diabetic pre-coma is abdominal pain, particularly in children. This and the finding of shifting areas of tenderness may obscure the signs of acidosis, ketosis and dehydration which are also usually present.

   (iv) The picture is utterly unlike that of hypoglycaemic coma. The only thing they have in common is that they may both occur in diabetes. If there is any doubt never give insulin. Instead give 50 g of glucose i.v. as a diagnostic test. This will do little harm to the patient in hyperglycaemic coma (although it may cause a sharp rise in serum K^+) whereas insulin can kill a hypoglycaemic patient or cause severe irreversible brain damage.

(2) It should be thought of in any patient drowsy or unconscious following:

   (i) surgery or other trauma;

   (ii) myocardial infarction;

   (iii) cerebral infarction.

(3) It may be precipitated by an infection, which should always be looked for and treated as necessary.

(4) It may rarely be caused by acute pancreatitis.

MANAGEMENT

If possible, the patient should be managed in an intensive care or high dependency unit.

(1) The aim of management is to correct:

(i)   fluid loss—the average loss is 90–120 ml/kg;

(ii) electrolyte losses—especially potassium (average loss 3 mmol/kg) and sodium (average loss 7–10 mmol/kg);

(iii) hyperglycaemia;

(iv) acidosis.

(2) The fluid loss, causing hypovolaemia and the symptoms mentioned above, should be corrected gradually (with half the total loss being replaced in the first 12–24 h). Too rapid correction of hyperglycaemia causes gross osmotic swings, and too rapid correction of the acidosis causes pH differences between the CSF and blood, both of which are potentially hazardous, and may contribute to the cerebral oedema which occasionally complicates treatment of this condition. So:

(i)   Put up a drip. As in all hypovolaemic states a central venous pressure line is preferable, as it allows replacement of adequate (and often large) volumes of fluid with safety.

(ii) Take blood for electrolytes and urea, Hb and PCV and arterial pH. Check for ketonaemia by dipping a ketostix in plasma. This separates off the non-ketotic forms of diabetic acidosis (see below).

(iii) Give i.v. fluids as quickly as possible until the CVP is normal and the patient is well perfused (usually 3–4 litres are necessary within the first 4 h). Thereafter slow down the infusion rate to supply normal maintenance requirements and then keep the patient well perfused. Give all the fluid as 0.9% N saline until the blood sugar is below 13 mmol/l, and thereafter change to 5% dextrose. Some advocate colloid infusion, rather than crystalloid infusion, in the initial resuscitation of diabetics.[2]

The case for their use remains unproven; we keep to the conventional crystalloid regime, using colloids only if hypotension persists after initial fluid replacement. Potassium will also be required (see below).

(iv) There are two commonly used regimens for giving insulin.[5] The easiest is to give a continuous low dose infusion of soluble insulin. Make up a concentration of 1 unit insulin/ml by adding 50 units of soluble insulin to 50 ml of N saline (NOT dextrose which is acidic and may inactivate the insulin) and infuse at an initial dose of 6 units/h. A constant infusion pump is ideal, but a paediatric giving set is a useful alternative. This dose of insulin causes an average fall in blood sugar of 4–5 mmol/l/h, which is the rate of fall you should aim for. A less preferable regime is to give 0.1 units/kg soluble insulin i.m. each hour, following a loading dose of 20 units i.m.

It is unusual for patients to require more than six units of insulin per hour. If they do, think of:

(a) infection;
(b) other endocrine problems, such as thyrotoxicosis or Cushing's syndrome;
(c) drug interaction; this is a particular problem in diabetic labour when very high doses—30 units i.v./h—may be required to maintain normoglycaemia if high doses of steroids or β-adrenergic agonists are being given.[6]

(3) While this is going on, if your patient is not conscious, consider inserting a urinary catheter. You will need this to ensure that an adequate urine flow is established (acute renal failure is very rare in diabetes possibly because the osmotic diuretic effect of glycosuria protects the kidney). Do not rely on urine glucose to monitor progress—frequent blood glucose measurements are essential for this purpose. Remember to remove the catheter as soon as the patient is better (hopefully within 24 h)—taking a catheter specimen of urine for culture as you do so.

(4) Next, consider the following.

(i) Electrolyte losses. The polyuria preceding coma will have resulted in sodium and potassium depletion. Although the initial sodium is usually normal, the previous urinary losses have been hypotonic with respect to plasma. Hence, 5% dextrose may be given early in treatment (see (2) (iii) above). The initial plasma potassium may be high because of the intracellular acidosis, but will fall rapidly as the blood glucose falls and as the acidosis is corrected. Thus, even if the initial potassium is high you are highly unlikely to run into problems with hyperkalaemia. The reverse is usually the case. K^+ 20 mmol may be given with the first litre of fluid and the first dose of insulin provided the T waves on the ECG are not peaked, and provided urinary output is adequate; 40 mmol K^+ given with each ensuing litre of fluid is usually sufficient. Occasionally even more may be required as shown by serial plasma K^+ estimations. The K^+ should be kept at 4.5 mEq/l.

(ii) Acidosis. Although acidosis is itself dangerous, the routine administration of HCO_3 to patients with a pH of more than 7.1 is not recommended because of the risk of:

(a) paradoxical increase in CSF acidosis alluded to above;
(b) further increasing K^+ flux into cells.

When the pH is less than 7.1 give 50 mmol of HCO_3 over 2 h. If the pH is still below 7.1, give a further 50 mmol in the next 4 h. Remember to give extra K^+; we suggest 40 meq K for each 50 mmol of HCO_3

(iii) The precipitating cause. Do an ECG, and if possible have a continuous ECG display to detect any arrhythmias or evidence of hyper- or hypokalaemia. Look for infection, especially in the chest (chest x-ray) and urinary tract (urine microscopy and culture). Take blood cultures, routinely and start the patient on a broad spectrum antibiotic, such as ampicillin 500 mg q.d.s., unless there is a definite reason not to suspect infection.

(iv) If your patient is comatose, aspirate the stomach contents through a nasogastric tube, as many patients in diabetic coma have dilated, atonic stomachs, the contents of which may cause inhalation pneumonia. If there is no gag reflex, you should protect the lungs with a cuffed endotracheal tube prior to aspirating the stomach.

(v) Continuing hypotension is almost certainly due to hypo-volaemia. If it persists despite adequate fluid replace-ment, consider other causes of hypotension and treat accordingly.

(vi) General nursing care of the comatose patient.

(5) If you use the insulin regime suggested above, the blood glucose is likely to be halved within 4 h—hourly estimates of blood glucose, 2-hourly estimates of K^+ and 2-hourly esti-mates of arterial pH are necessary until you are certain you are going in the right direction. Thereafter, hourly glucose and 4-hourly K^+ are sufficient.

(6) As a result of these and your other clinical measurements, you may have to adjust:

(i) Sodium—by altering the ratio of 5% dextrose to N saline.

(ii) Potassium—if the serum K^+ is normal, continue with the same dosage; if low, increase the dosage, and if high, stop the K^+ immediately but repeat the measurement as a high K^+ at this stage is extremely uncommon.

(iii) Bicarbonate—if the pH is rising gradually, further administration of HCO_3 is unnecessary. If it is still dangerously low, i.e. less than 7.1, and not rising you may have to give more HCO_3. Give this slowly (i.e. 75 mmol in the next 4 h).

(iv) Fluid—you have probably not given the total replace-ment within 4 h, but remember to watch the patient's neck veins and lung bases as well as the CVP to ensure you do not give too much.

(v) PO_4—hypophosphataemia of a significant degree (PO_4 <0.32 mmol/l) occasionally occurs in diabetic ketoaci-dosis. It causes general debility and anergy, and may be corrected by infusing 9 mmol of monobasic potassium phosphate in 0.5% saline over 12 h, and repeating as necessary. However, there is little evidence that this speeds the process of recovery.[3,4]

(7) Four hours later repeat the measurements. By now the patient should be considerably improved, and probably out of coma. If she is not it may be for the following reasons.

(i) The patient's initial metabolic disturbances were very severe and are not yet corrected.

(ii) There may be an undetected precipitating cause of coma. Estimate the serum amylase and calcium at this stage, or before if there is a suggestive history of pancreatitis.

(iii) The patient may have one of the following complications of the condition or its treatment:

    (a) Hypoglycaemia—check that the blood glucose is not below 4.5 mmol (80 mg%).

    (b) Cerebral oedema.[8] Subclinical brain swelling, as seen on a CT scan, often occurs during the treatment of diabetic coma; overt cerebral oedema can occur. Its aetiology is uncertain, but it may be related to too rapid lowering of blood glucose or replacement of fluid loss with hypotonic solutions. This allows a high osmotic gradient to develop between extra and intracellular compartments.

    (c) Hypokalaemia and/or gastric dilatation.

    (d) Major artery thrombosis.

    (e) Addison's disease—diabetic ketosis may precipitate an Addisonian crisis in a patient with pre-existing adrenal insufficiency. Check the arterial pressure.

(8) Improvement in blood sugar levels often precedes improvement in other metabolic variables. Thus, the patient may be normoglycaemic but still nauseated or vomiting and ketotic. For this reason it is suggested that the insulin infusion rate should be reduced to 3 units/h, and that 5% dextrose (1 litre over 8 h) is given, as soon as the blood glucose is less than 11 mmol/l. This regime is continued until the patient can eat and drink normally. She should then start maintenance subcutaneous insulin. Assessing control by urine testing no longer has a place in the management of acute diabetic emergencies, and regimes of the sort outlined above are probably the easiest way of controlling any diabetic who cannot eat and drink, e.g. those undergoing surgery or labour (see p. 172).

(9) Remember that the gross hypovolaemia associated with hyperglycaemia can mask signs of infection. These may become apparent when your patient's fluid deficiencies have been corrected, so always re-examine the patient carefully at this stage. Diabetic ketoacidosis per se can cause a brisk leucocytosis, so is not in itself a reliable sign of infection.

REFERENCES

1   Foster, D. W., McGarry D. J. (1983) The metabolic derangements and treatments of diabetic ketoacidosis. *N. Engl. J. Med*. **309**:159.

2   Hillman K. M., (1982) Crystalloid infusion in diabetes. *Lancet* **ii:** 548.

3   Knochel J. (1985). The clinical state of hypophosphataemia. *N. Engl. J. Med*. **313:** 447.

4   Leader (1981) Treatment of severe hypophosphataemia. *Lancet* **ii:** 734.

5   Leader (1977) Insulin regimens for diabetic ketoacidosis. *Br. med. J*. **1:** 405.

6   Thomas D. J. B. *et al*. (1977) Salbutamol induced diabetic ketoacidosis. *Br. Med. J*. **2:** 438.

7   Wheatley T. *et al*. (1987) Diabetic emergencies. *Hospital Update* January, p. 31.

8   Winegrad A. I. *et al*. (1985) Cerebral edema in diabetic ketoacidosis. *N. Engl. J. Med*. **312:** 1184.

Hyperosmolar non-ketotic diabetic coma[1,2]

DIAGNOSIS

(1) Diabetic coma may occur without ketonuria in the following circumstances.

    (i)   When diabetic coma is complicated by acute renal failure. Here the patient has ketonaemia and is acidotic.

    (ii)   Diabetic coma with lactic acidosis (see p. 171).

    (iii) Hyperosmolar non-ketotic diabetic coma. This is really rather a bad term, because diabetic ketoacidosis is also hyperosmolar—not, however to the same degree. These patients have no ketones in the urine or blood, are not acidotic and do not, therefore, overbreathe.

(2) In (1) (iii) above the patients frequently are elderly and have an insidious onset of illness over weeks. The illness may be provoked by thiazide diuretics or anti-convulsants. It may present with either focal or diffuse neurological signs with or without an accompanying cerebrovascular accident. The blood glucose is often very high (around 60 mmol/l) causing an osmotic diuresis in which large amounts of potassium, sodium and water are lost. The ensuing hypovolaemia is usually obvious clinically and is associated with pre-renal uraemia. There is proportionately greater loss of water than salt, and the serum sodium is often raised—above 155 mmol. The combination of a raised sodium, urea and glucose causes very high serum osmolality, which may exceed 400 mosmol/kg (serum osmolality in mmol/kg = 2(Na + K) + urea + glucose, all in mmol/l). This in turn causes severe intracellular dehydration—one of the factors responsible for coma. There is a good correlation between osmolality and the conscious state, as indicated below.

Plasma osmolality (mmol/l)	conscious state
310–330	Alert
330–350	Obtunded
350–370	Stuporose
370–420	Comatose

(3) The pathogenesis of this illness is not fully established, but recent evidence suggests that these patients may have just sufficient circulating insulin to control lipolysis thereby preventing the development of ketones but not enough to prevent hyperglycaemia.

The prior use of thiazide diuretics, which have an additional hyperglycaemic effect, is common.

(4) Fifty per cent of these patients will have an obvious, and often serious precipitating illness, such as infection, stroke, myocardial infarction or recent surgery.

MANAGEMENT

Take blood for haemoglobin and PCV, electrolytes and urea, blood glucose, serum amylase and calcium and plasma osmolality. Then treat as follows.

(1) Correct the dehydration, hyperosmolality and sodium and potassium depletion. As mentioned in (2) above, the fluid and electrolyte loss in hyperosmolar coma is usually greater than that in ketotic coma. Loss of 25% of the total body water is common. You should aim to replace half this loss in the first 12 h, and the rest in the ensuing 24 h. The problem is, with what? As so often, there is controversy. Some experts advocate using the same fluid and electrolyte regime as in ketotic diabetic coma (see p. 162). However, the conventional advice is to replace the water and sodium deficit with 0.5 N saline from the onset. A sensible compromise is to use 0.5 N saline if the initial serum sodium is above 150 mmol/l, or if the sodium rises above 150 mmol/l at any stage during treatment, but otherwise to give isotonic saline as for ketotic coma. Remember when calculating fluid deficits that in old people the total body water is only 50%, not the more usual 60% of body weight.

(2) Correct hyperglycaemia. It might be thought that the lack of acidosis allows full sensitivity to insulin. This is often, but by no means always, the case. Insulin should be given as described for ketotic diabetic coma (see p. 163), the response being checked with repeated measurements of the blood glucose, and the rate of administration adjusted accordingly.

(3) Venous and arterial thromboses are very likely to occur in this

situation, so some advocate heparinising the patient for 2–3 days (see p. 18). There is, however, no certain evidence that this is helpful.

(4) Treat any underlying or precipitating causes, such as infection or acute pancreatitis.

(5) After the acute episode has passed these patients often have mild diabetes which can be controlled with diet alone or small doses of oral hypoglycaemic agents.

REFERENCES

1   Arieff A. I., Carroll H. J. (1972) Nonketotic hyperglycaemic coma. *Medicine* **51:** 73.

2   Gill G. V., Alberti K. G. M. (1985) Hyperosmolar non-ketotic coma. *Practical Diabetes* **2:** 30.

Non-ketotic diabetic acidosis

The acidosis of diabetic pre-coma and coma is not always caused exclusively by ketones. It may occasionally be due to other anions; formic acid in methyl alcohol poisoning; alpha keto-glutaric acid in liver failure; phosphate and other anions in renal failure; and lactic acid, which is much the most common. For this reason it is important to check that ketones are actually present in the plasma of a diabetic with acidosis. If ketones are absent, then these other serious underlying conditions should be looked for.

Urgent surgery in diabetics[1]

There is an increased mortality in surgery undertaken in poorly controlled diabetics. Every diabetic has a 50% chance of undergoing surgery in their lifetime. As 5% of these are emergency operations, this is a problem which you may well be asked to attend to. In any diabetic requiring emergency surgery, you should:

(1) Discontinue the prevailing mode of therapy.
(2) Give 1 litre of 10% dextrose 12-hourly with 20 mmol K^+ added (see (6) below).
(3) Infuse insulin through an infusion pump, at a dose dependent on the initial blood sugar, and adjusted to keep the sugar between 5 and 10 mmol/l (see Table 3).
(4) You should do a preop. sugar, intraoperative sugars at hourly intervals, and 3–4-hourly postop. sugars, and alter your infusion rate accordingly.

Table 3

Sugar level	Insulin infusion
5 mmol/l	1 unit/h
5–10 mmol/l	2 units/h
>10–20 mmol/l	3 units/h
> 20 mmol/l	4 units/h

(5) Continue the regime until the patient is eating again, and then switch back to the previous regime (provided, of course, this was controlling their diabetes adequately!).
(6) You should also monitor the K^+ level. If the K^+ level is >5 mmol/l stop the K^+ infusion. If the K^+ is 3.5–5 mmol/l add 20 mmol K^+ to each litre 10% dextrose. If the K^+ is <3.5 add 40 mmol K^+ to each litre of 10% dextrose.
(7) There are some circumstances where you will need higher levels of insulin infusion:

   (i)   If your patient has a severe infection.
   (ii) In cardiac surgery (the bypass pump may be primed with dextrose).

(iii) If an adrenergic agent is being used at the same time.

(iv) If your patient is having parenteral nutrition.

(v) If your patient is on suppressive doses of corticosteroids.

(8) Remember that if your patient is in diabetic ketoacidotic pre-coma, initial control of the metabolic state may:

(i) relieve the abdominal pain and vomiting which you thought was 'surgical' in origin;

(ii) make any necessary surgery much safer.

So always allow a few hours for correction of this (see p. 162) before undertaking surgery.

For elective surgery a somewhat different approach is permissible.

(1) Insulin-dependent diabetics.

(i) Admit the day prior to surgery.

(ii) If they are not already on a twice daily regime of a mixture of medium- and short-acting insulin, change them to this.

(iii) On the preoperative day, give the evening dose of medium- and short-acting insulin as normal.

(iv) On the operative day, proceed as for emergency surgery with i.v. insulin and glucose.

(2) Non-insulin-dependent diabetics (NIDDS)

● Diet controlled

(i) If fasting sugar is <7.0 mmol/l you will not require to take any special action.

(ii) If major and therefore prolonged surgery is anticipated, however, or if the fasting sugar is >11.0 mmol/l, proceed as for emergency surgery with i.v. insulin and glucose.

● Tablet controlled

(i) Stop the tablets the day before surgery, 3 days before in the case of long-acting sulphonylurea such as chlorpropamide.

(ii) Assess control on day of admission, and then proceed as for diet controlled patients above.

REFERENCE

1   Gill G. *et al.* (1989) Surgery and diabetes. *Hospital Update* May, p. 327.

Hypopituitary coma[1]

DIAGNOSIS

(1) Hypopituitary coma may be precipitated in a patient with long-standing pituitary failure by infection, trauma (including surgery) myocardial infarction or cold, sedatives and hypnotics. It may also occur following an acute insult to the pituitary gland, e.g. surgery, head injury, haemorrhage or post-partum haemorrhage.

(2) The clinical picture is one of gonadotrophin, thyroid and adrenal deficiency. These deficiencies have usually developed gradually, as have the patient's symptoms. Thus, there is a history of somnolence, sensitivity to cold and increasing confusion, progressing over a few weeks to coma. On examination, the skin is strikingly pale and dry, but of fine texture. Pubic and axillary hair is usually absent and the prematurely wrinkled features of hypogonadism may be obvious. The breasts and genitalia are atrophic. There is a general lack of pigmentation, and blood pressure, temperature and pulse rate are often below normal. If, in addition, the posterior pituitary is involved, polyuria due to a lack of ADH may cause dehydration. These multiple endocrine deficiencies all contribute to the coma, as indicated below.

MANAGEMENT

Estimate the blood glucose with BM stix and take blood for full blood count, electrolytes and urea, blood glucose, serum thyroxine, TSH, blood cortisol, growth hormone and arterial blood gases.

(1) Consider treatment of the possible causes of coma, of which the most common are:

    (i) Adrenocortical deficiency. Many of the problems outlined below are primarily caused by adrenocortical insufficiency and at least 100 mg of hydrocortisone must be injected i.v. without delay (see p. 186). This may initiate a diuresis if water intoxication has occurred, or protect the patient from water intoxication if saline and water depletion require large volumes of intravenous fluid.

(ii) Hypothyroidism. Attempts to raise the metabolic rate with tri-iodothyronine (T_3) while other causes of coma are still operative exacerbates coma, and this should not be given until treatment of other causes of coma is under way. A suitable regime for the administration of T3 is: 0.01 mg 8-hourly for three doses; and then 0.02 mg 12-hourly for two doses; 0.1 mg twice daily thereafter. The drug is most usually given via a nasogastric tube, but can be given intravenously if the appropriate preparation is available.

(iii) Hypothermia (see p. 289).

(iv) Electrolyte disturbances. Two patterns of electrolyte disturbance may occur.

(a) Water intoxication. This is by far the most common, and arises because, in the absence of cortisol, the patient's capacity to mount a water diuresis is depressed. If the posterior pituitary is intact, the inappropriate secretion of ADH associated with myxoedema may also be a factor.[2] Water-intoxicated patients may complain of weakness, headache, nausea and blurring of vision. Tendon reflexes are exaggerated and muscle cramps occur. Drowsiness progresses to confusion, convulsions and coma. The serum sodium is usually less than 120 mmol/l, there may be hypokalaemia, and the urea is usually low (below 6.0 mmol/l). Intake of all fluids should be stopped, unless there is oliguria. This is frequently all that is necessary. However, if oliguria is present, if the patient is in pre-coma, or convulsions have occurred, give 2 N saline at about 40 ml/h until the urine flow has been more than 45 ml/h for at least 3 h. Because of the risk of water intoxication, you should not give hypotonic fluids to patients in hypopituitary coma until adequate replacement of cortisol and thyroxine has been achieved.

(b) Salt and water depletion. This is uncommon. The serum Na+ may be low, but the urea will be high and the patient hypovolaemic. When it is due to polyuria secondary to ADH deficiency, give 5 units of aqueous pitressin subcutaneously and sufficient N saline to make good previous salt losses. However, it is more commonly due to vomiting and diarrhoea occurring in a patient with cortisol deficiency. N saline infusions will again be required.

(v) Hypoglycaemia. Give 25 g of dextrose i.v. (see p. 184).

(vi) A central venous pressure line will help considerably in the management of these electrolyte disturbances and you should insert one whenever possible.

In addition the following may be contributary.

(vii) Hypoxia. Give 50–60% oxygen by face mask. If this is inadequate as judged by the Pa_{O_2}, some form of assisted respiration is indicated.

(viii) Hypotension. This is usually due to steroid insufficiency and/or hypovolaemia and responds to hydrocortisone and adequate fluid replacement.

(2) Investigation and treatment of the cause.

(3) When coma has been relieved and the crisis is passed, daily replacement therapy will be necessary.

(4) Diabetics who have been hypophysectomized for treatment of diabetic retinopathy are extremely sensitive to insulin—changes of a few units either way may lead to severe hypoglycaemia or ketoacidosis.

REFERENCES

1   Garrod O. (1967) Hypopituitary coma. *Hospital Medicine* **2**: 300.

2   Robertson G. (1989) Syndrome of inappropriate anti-diuresis. *N. Engl. J. Med.* **321:** 538.

Pituitary apoplexy[1,2]

Pituitary apoplexy occurs when sudden haemorrhage and/or necrosis cause sudden expansion of a pituitary tumour.

DIAGNOSIS

(1) The condition presents with a characteristic array of symptoms and signs. There is a sudden onset of headache, visual impairment or loss and ophthalmoplegia. The patient becomes stuporous and may lapse into a coma. Neck stiffness may be present.
(2) A lumbar puncture should not be performed as this presentation is also consistent with temporal lobe herniation.
(3) Skull x-ray nearly always shows enlargement of the sella.
(4) CT, or preferably MRI, scan of the head may show parasellar haemorrhage and suprasellar mass effect.

MANAGEMENT

Since the patient may die within hours, neurosurgical help should be sought urgently. The relief of pressure by a transnasal decompression of the sella is the procedure of choice. In the interval give dexamethasone 6 mg i.v. every 6 h together with the usual measures as necessary to support circulation and ventilation.

REFERENCES

1 Lewin I. *et al.* (1988) Pituitary apoplexy. *Br. Med. J.* **297:** 1526.
2 Riskind P. N. (1986) A case of pituitary apoplexy. *N. Engl. J. Med.* **314:** 229.

Acute lactic acidosis[1,2]

Lactic acid, which is formed from pyruvate as the end-product of anaerobic glycolysis, is in equilibrium with pyruvate. The position of equilibrium is determined mainly by tissue oxygenation. The lactate level, normally less than 1 mmol/l, will rise in the following circumstances.

(1) With a rise in the pyruvate concentration. Here the pyruvate lactate ratio is normal (1:10) and the patient is not acidotic. For reasons that are not understood this occurs in the setting of hyperventilation such as may occur after a stroke or pulmonary embolus. The prognosis for these patients is that of their underlying disease, which should be treated in the normal fashion.

(2) With poor tissue oxygenation. Here lactate has risen ten times or more relative to pyruvate (the absolute level of lactate is >5 mmol/l) and the patient is acidotic. There are two separate categories:

    (i) The decreased tissue oxygenation may be evident. The patient is seriously ill. The oxygen supply to the tissue is severely compromised, as in septic, cardiac or hypovolaemic shock, or hypoxia for any reason. In this group the excess blood lactate falls with therapy directed at reversing the underlying 'shock' state. (This group is the type A lactic acidosis of Cohen and Wood.)

    (ii) Lactate production may be increased, or lactate removal decreased without any obvious oxygen supply problems. Thus, the patient initially appears to be well perfused, with a normal Pao_2. The reason for this form of lactate disturbance, despite an apparently adequate oxygen supply, is not clear. In this group of patients (type B lactic acidosis of Cohen and Wood), there may be no obvious antecedent illness, but more commonly, there is an identifiable provocative factor. The most important of these is that the patient may have been taking phenformin, suffer from ethanol intoxication, have had a rapid sorbitol or fructose infusion, or have severe liver disease. Occasionally the acidosis develops in patients who seem to be recovering satisfactorily from an event such as a myocardial infarct, and an increase in lactate may occur during the first few hours of treatment of diabetic ketoacidosis. In this group, the serum lactate levels are uninfluenced by oxygen therapy, and the serum bicarbonate often fluctuates wildly, and with apparently only little relation to HCO_3 infusion. The decreasing use of phenformin has resulted in a decline in incidence of type B lactic acidosis as metformin is only very rarely associated with lactic acidosis.

DIAGNOSIS

(1) Lactic acidosis should be suspected in acidotic (and therefore hyperventilating) patients if a large number of anions remain unaccounted for (the anion gap).[3,4] The sum of the anions that we conventionally measure (Cl^- and HCO_3^-) normally approximates to the sum of the serum cations ($Na^+ + K^+$). Thus, if the anion gap $(Na^+ + K^+) - (Cl^- + HCO_3^-)$ is greater than 18 mmol/l, and is not accounted for by ketones, salicylates, uraemia, methanol, ethylene glycol or paraldehyde, all of which can give rise to a metabolic acidosis with a large anion gap, [2] lactic acidosis may well be present.

(2) The presence of lactic acidosis should, of course, be suspected in a diabetic patient who is acidotic but who has no, or only few, circulating ketones.

(3) It has been found that the PO_4 level is usually high in lactic acidosis. An average level of 2.9 mmol/l has been recorded, whereas in the metabolic acidosis of diabetic coma, the average is 1.6 mmol/l.

(4) A lactate level of >5 mmol is arbitrarily considered as diagnostic. The average level in 285 cases of type B acidosis was 16.9 mmol/l, with an average anion gap of 37 mEq/l.

MANAGEMENT

• Type A lactic acidosis

The excess lactate here is only one of degree, as most 'shock states' are accompanied by increased lactate levels. The treatment is that of the 'shock state' underlying the problem (see p. 334).

• Type B lactic acidosis

This involves:

(1) Investigation for any underlying conditions. Include a full blood count, electrolytes and urea, blood culture, blood glucose, serum amylase and calcium, ECG, microscopy and culture of urine arterial blood gases, and blood lactate level. Blood should be taken for grouping, and serum saved for cross-matching. Unsuspected hypovolaemia may be revealed by a low central venous pressure. A drug history may reveal that phenformin has been consumed.

(2) Treatment of the underlying condition is obviously of prime importance.

(3) Correction of the acidosis. Acidosis (pH <7.1) has a negative inotropic effect, and persistent acidosis will lead to shock and eventual death. It thus seems rational to treat the acidosis vigorously and early, in an attempt to halt this progression. Several measures have been advocated, although none has been subjected to a controlled trial, and it is increasingly clear that optimizing perfusion and the correction of any underlying problems is the best way of doing this.

(i) $NaHCO_3$. Fortunately, the enthusiasm for giving large doses of $NaHCO_3$ is waning.[5] This practice has the same hazards in lactic acidosis as it does in diabetic ketoacidosis (see p. 164). So, if the pH is below 7, give 2 mmol/kg body weight over the first hour, and then aliquots of 50 mmol over ½ h, if deemed essential and your patient is not improving, to raise the plasma $NaHCO_3$ to 14 mmol/l, over the next 24 h. You should also ensure that your patient's ventilation is sufficient to blow off any excess CO_2 generated by the hydrogen ions buffered by your $NaHCO_3$.

(ii) Methylene blue 5 mg/kg given as an infusion to buffer excess lactate.

(iii) Haemodialysis and peritoneal dialysis have both been used, without any great enthusiasm or success.

(iv) Dichloroacetate. This is a powerful activator of pyruvate dehydrogenase, and induces a striking decrease in lactate concentration. It should be given at a dose of 50 g/kg body weight, infused in 0.9 N saline over 30 min.[6]

(v) Thiamine 100 mg twice daily should be given, as this

dramatically relieves lactic acidosis in the few patients who have associated thiamine deficiency.

(4) Hypoxaemia should be corrected using 50–60% O_2 by face mask.

REFERENCES

1   Alberti K. G. M. M., Nattrass M. (1977) Lactic acidosis. *Lancet* **2:** 25.
2   Bihari D. J. (1986) Metabolic acidosis. *Br. J. Hosp. Med.* **35:** 89.
3   Dinubile M. (1988) The increment of the anion gap—over-extension of a concept. *Lancet* **ii:** 951.
4   Gabow P. *et al.* (1980) Diagnostic importance of an increased serum anion gap. *N. Engl. J. Med.* **303:** 854.
5   Ryder R. (1987) The danger of high dose $NaHCO_3$ in biguanide induced lactic acidosis. *Br. J. Clin. Pract.* **41:** 730.
6   Stackpoole P. W. *et al.* (1983) Treatment of lactic acidosis with dichloroacetate. *N. Engl. J. Med.* **309:** 390.

Hypoglycaemic pre-coma and coma[2,3]

DIAGNOSIS

(1) Hypoglycaemia must be considered in any confused, disorientated, aggressive or excitable person, especially if they are known to be diabetic on insulin, or taking sulphonylureas.

(2) Hypoglycaemia may be precipitated by alcohol, typically coming on about 12 h after a binge. The combination of alcohol and hypoglycaemia may be a difficult diagnostic problem to grapple with (sometimes literally) and is of medico-legal significance.

(3) Coma is an emergency par excellence. You have to act quickly if irreversible brain damage is to be prevented. It is characterised by pallor, a moist skin, dilated pupils and possibly tachycardia.[3]

(4) The significance of these signs may not strike the observer and hypoglycaemia must be considered and excluded in any unconscious patient. BM stix are adequate for this purpose and if they show a glucose content of less than 2.3 mmol/l (40 mg/100 ml) treatment should be given without waiting for the blood glucose result, for which blood must first be taken.

(5) The only thing that hypoglycaemic coma and hyperglycaemic coma have in common is that in both the patient may be diabetic and unconscious. BM stix reliably distinguish the two. If you are still doubtful give dextrose i.v. (see below). It will do little harm to a patient in hyperglycaemic coma and will usually restore consciousness in patients with hypoglycaemic coma.

(6) Occasionally hypoglycaemia may present with focal neurological signs such as hemiplegia or focal fits.

(7) **NEVER** give insulin as a 'diagnostic test' for a patient in coma. In hypoglycaemia it is usually fatal and invariably disastrous.

MANAGEMENT

(1) Take blood for blood glucose, before initiating any treatment.

(2) If the patient can drink, give 25 g dextrose in orange juice.

(3) If the patient is comatose, give 25 g dextrose i.v. (50 ml of 50% dextrose) and when the patient rouses, a further 25 g to drink.

(4) Glucagon may be given in the following circumstances.

    (i)   If the patient cannot be restrained for long enough to give an i.v. injection safely, give glucagon 1 mg i.m., which raises blood sugar to within the normal range in 5–10 min, although its action is short-lived.

    (iv) Sulphonylureas reduce hepatic release of glucose, probably as a consequence of their effect on raising insulin levels. Glucagon promotes hepatic glyconeogenesis, and so it would seem logical to use it in sulphonylurea-induced hypoglycaemia.[1] As so often, there is disagreement, as glucagon also stimulates insulin release. We therefore only use glucagon (1 mg by i.m. injection, repeated 6-hourly as necessary) in patient whose hypoglycaemia is proving difficult to control with glucose infusions.

(5) Recovery is usually complete in 10–15 min but may occasionally take up to 1 h, despite adequate blood glucose levels.

(6) When the crisis is over, consider the cause.

(7) In patients rendered hypoglycaemic by long-acting insulins, or whom you suspect of taking really large doses of any insulin, after you have undertaken the initial therapy as outlined above, you should put up a 10% or 20% dextrose drip, and keep this running for at least 48 h. This is to prevent the real danger of hypoglycaemia recurring over the ensuing 24–48 hours. The same strictures apply to hypoglycaemia induced by the sulphonylureas. The blood sugar, as monitored by BM stix, should be maintained between 5 and 10 mmol/1.

(8) In any case, recovery of consciousness should be buttressed by a good meal.

REFERENCES

1   Ferner R. *et al*. (1988) Sulphonylureas and hypoglycaemia. *Br. Med. J*. **296:** 949.

2   Jarrett R. J. (1971) Blood glucose homeostasis. *Br. J. Hosp. Med*. **6:** 499.

3   Leader (1985) Hypoglycaemia and the nervous system. *Lancet* **ii:** 759.

Addisonian crisis

Addisonian crisis may be primary, due to destruction or atrophy of the adrenal gland, or secondary, due to failure of the hypothalamic–pituitary–adrenal axis. The usual cause of secondary hypoadrenalism is the previous administration of exogenous steroids. Since, theoretically, only the glucocorticoid secretion is under pituitary control, mineralocorticoid deficiency should occur in primary but not in secondary hypoadrenalism. In fact, there is a tendency for the whole adrenal cortex to atrophy after long-term steroid ingestion and mineralocorticoid deficiency may be assumed to be present in secondary hypoadrenalism.

DIAGNOSIS

(1) The diagnosis should be considered in any hypotensive patient, who may also be vomiting, especially if they have received steroids within the past year. The signs of chronic adrenal insufficiency may or may not be present, so do not necessarily expect a pigmented, asthenic patient.

(2) It may be precipitated by infection, myocardial or cerebral infarction, trauma (including surgery), parturition or any metabolic stress. It may complicate septicaemia caused by pyogenic organisms—usually the Meningococcus—and is said to be due to haemorrhage into the adrenals. However, the majority of these patients are probably suffering from septic shock, for the plasma cortisols when measured are usually appropriately high.

(3) It is a useful, if cynical, maxim that in the above situation no one should be allowed to die with unexplained hypotension or coma without first receiving 200 mg of hydrocortisone i.v.

MANAGEMENT

The patient is depleted of sodium, potassium and water and may be hypoglycaemic. Take blood for baseline haemoglobin and PCV electrolytes and urea, blood glucose and plasma cortisol and ACTH.

If you suspect Addison's disease, you should perform a short synacthen test before giving any steroid replacement, so that you can retrospectively confirm your diagnosis. Take a resting sample for cortisol analysis, then give 250 µg of tetracosatrin i.m. or i.v., and take cortisol samples ½ and 1 h later.

Arrange an abdominal x-ray, which may show adrenal calcification. Then manage as follows.

(1) Steroid replacement. Give 100 mg hydrocortisone sodium succinate i.v. and 100 mg i.m. and then 50 mg i.m. 8-hourly. Although hydrocortisone is essentially a glucocorticoid, it has sufficient mineralocorticoid activity when used in the above dosage to make it the drug of choice in both primary and secondary adrenal failure. However, some authorities suggest that a mineralocorticoid, such as deoxycorticosterone 10 mg i.m., should be given in any case where there is profound hypotension or clinical shock.

(2) Estimate blood glucose by BM stix. If less than 2.3 mmol/l (40 mg%), give 25 g of glucose orally or i.v. without waiting for the blood sugar results.

(3) Put up a drip, preferably with a CVP line. Give at least 1 litre of N saline in the first hour, and then as necessary to keep the CVP within the normal range.

(4) Consider the cause.

   (i)   Do an ECG which may demonstrate myocardial infarction or suggest hypokalaemia.

   (ii) Look for signs of infection. Do not start a broad-spectrum antibiotic as routine. However, if the patient is pyrexial without obvious cause, investigations should include a chest x-ray, urine microscopy and blood cultures and then start on a broad-spectrum antibiotic parenterally. Bear in mind that hyperpyrexia does occur occasionally as a feature of Addisonian crisis.

(5) By now the electrolyte results should be available.

   (i)   Hyponatraemia needs further treatment with normal saline.

   (ii) Potassium supplements may be necessary.

   (iii) Further fluid replacement will depend on how much salt and water depletion has occurred. The commonest cause of continuing hypotension is hypovolaemia. Therefore, if in doubt, set up a CVP line and replace accordingly (see p. 381).

(6) Repeat the blood electrolytes 8-hourly if rapid fluid replacement is necessary. Water intoxication can easily occur in these patients if hypotonic saline is given, and the serum sodium should not be allowed to fall below 125 mmol/l.

REFERENCE

1   Clayton R. (1989) Diagnosis of adrenal insufficiency. *Br. Med. J.* **298:** 271.

Myxoedema coma[1,2,3]

DIAGNOSIS

(1) Patients usually present during the winter months, being particularly susceptible to hypothermia. It may, therefore, complicate conditions where hypothermia is common, such as strokes or chlorpromazine overdose.

(2) Before coma supervenes the patient may have been mentally dulled or psychotic.

(3) Usually the patient has the classic appearance and signs of myxoedema, except the delayed relaxation time of deep tendon reflexes which cannot be elicited. Hypotension and bradycardia are invariable.

(4) If coma has occurred, two-thirds of patients die. This may be due to insufficient appreciation of the multiple factors which contribute to myxoedemic coma (2(i)–(vii) below).[4]

(5) Onset of coma may be accompanied by convulsions, which are treated in the usual way (see p. 224).

(6) It is, on occasions, difficult to know whether a patient in coma has myxoedema or not, especially as both thyroxine and tri-iodothyronine may be low in any very ill person. If you are in genuine doubt, it is worth treating as for myxoedema coma, as you are not likely to do any harm in the short term.

MANAGEMENT

(1) Measure blood glucose with BM stix and take blood for full blood count, electrolytes and urea, blood glucose, cortisol, thyroxine or tri-iodothyronine and blood gases.

(2) Treat the following as indicated.

    (i) Hypoadrenalism. This will be present in all cases of myxoedema coma associated with hypopituitarism. As the pituitary status in any given patient with myxoedema coma may not be known, all should be given 100 mg hydrocortisone i.v. stat. and then 50 mg i.m. 8-hourly.

    (ii) Hypothyroidism. Whether to give l–tri-iodothyronine

(T_3) or thyroxine (T_4) or both, and how much of each you should give is a subject steeped in controversy. The effect of T_3 begins in 4 h so, whereas T_4 takes longer to act. However, T_4 replacement is easier and more reliable, and its action is smoother. We think a reasonable policy is to give both, as outlined below.

(a) l–tri-iodothyronine (T_3). Give 5 μg 8-hourly, either by nasogastric tube or i.v. if a suitable preparation is available.

(b) In addition, give T_4 200 μg i.v. stat. and then 100 μg i.v. daily thereafter for two doses. The dosage of both the above should be halved if you are confident that your patient is suffering from ischaemic heart disease.

(iii) Hypoventilation. This may give rise to hypoxia alone or hypoxia and hypercarbia. Measure the blood gases. if the Pa_{CO_2} is raised (40 mgHg, 5.3 kPa) ventilation will be required, ventilation may also be required if the Pa_{O_2} cannot be kept above 60 mmHg (8.0 kPa) give O_2 via a face mask.

(iv) Hypothermia. Do not warm the patient rapidly. This may cause cardiovascular collapse. Simply use lots of blankets (see p. 290).

(v) Hypoglycaemia. If this is present, give 25 g of dextrose i.v. as frequently as necessary.

(vi) Hypotension. If the above measures do not restore the blood pressure, give plasma expanders—blood, Haemaccel, or plasma, whichever is available. If hypotension persists after hypovolaemia is corrected, as verified by a CVP line, it may be necessary to use an inotrope (see p. 17).

(vii) Hyponatraemia. This is nearly always caused by dilution and redistribution, possibly due to inappropriate ADH secretion. The appropriate treatment is fluid restriction. Attempts to correct hyponatraemia by hypertonic saline infusions merely exacerbate fluid retention. However, if the serum sodium is less than 120 mmol/l and the patient is now oedematous, it is possible that hyponatraemia may be contributory to the coma. In this situation give 50 ml increments of 5 N saline hourly (65 ml) and watch the CVP, lung bases and the effect on the serum sodium carefully.

REFERENCES

1   Evered D., Hall R. (1972) Hypothyroidism *Br. Med. J.* **1:** 290.
2   McClellan A. (1987) Thyroid emergencies. *Hospital Update* May: p. 375.
3   Perlmutter M. (1964) Myxoedema crisis of pituitary or thyroid origin. *Am. J. Med.* **36:** 883.
4   Royce P. C. (1971) Severely impaired consciousness in myxoedema. *Am. J. Med. Sci.*; **261:** 46.

Thyrotoxic crisis[3,4]

DIAGNOSIS

(1) The signs of breathlessness, anxiety, tremor, severe eyelid retraction and uncontrolled atrial fibrillation are virtually diagnostic. The thyroid gland is usually enlarged and obviously hyperactive, and the patient hyperpyrexial.

(2) However, patients can occasionally present with:

    (i)   a rapidly progressive weakness leading to drowsiness and coma;

    (ii) an acute psychosis;

    (iii) abdominal pain and vomiting, simulating an acute abdominal crisis.

(3) It is usually precipitated by an infection, surgery, diabetic ketosis, or by prematurely stopping antithyroid treatment. It may occasionally occur following [131]iodine therapy for thyrotoxicosis, if the gland has not been suppressed beforehand with iodine, or amiodarone therapy.

MANAGEMENT

(1) Take blood for a full blood picture, electrolytes, blood glucose, and serum thyroxine, and save serum for tri-iodothyronine estimation should this be required later.

(2) Hyperthyroidism. Give:

    (i)   potassium iodide 200 mg i.v. over 1 h and then 100 mg q.d.s. orally per day; this is reduced when the hyperthyroidism comes under control and its beneficial effect lasts not longer than 2 weeks;

    (ii) carbimazole 20 mg 6-hourly, or failing this, propylthiouracil 250 mg 6-hourly by mouth (or stomach tube if necessary). It is best to give the carbimazole or propylthiouracil 1 h before giving the potassium iodide, as this will ensure that the blockade of organification of iodine is established before the potassium iodide is given.

(3) anxiety. If possible, the patient should be nursed by himself in a quiet, semi-dark room.

   (i)   If anxiety is severe, an acute psychosis may supervene which usually responds to propranolol. The oral dose is 80 mg t.d.s., but it may be given i.v. 2 mg over 5 min, and then 80 mg 8-hourly if the patient is initially too sick to swallow. Propranolol should also be given to control the tachycardia of thyrotoxicosis, which contributes to the failure. It should not, however, be used if there is pulmonary or peripheral oedema unless there is associated atrial fibrillation (see (4) below).[2] If propranolol aggravates heart failure, as may occasionally be the case, atropine 0.4–1.0 mg i.v. should be given.

   (ii) In addition, you may need to give chlorpromazine 100 mg i.v. This also helps treat hyperpyrexia.

(4) Left ventricular failure.[5] This is caused by uncontrolled atrial fibrillation or tachycardia, and is treated along the usual lines with diuretics and oxygen (see p. 45). In addition, propranolol, in the dosage described above, rapidly reduces the ventricular rate and restores sinus rhythm, thereby controlling the failure. Digoxin has no influence on the ventricular rate in this situation but is given as it increases the force of myocardial contraction.

(5) Hyperpyrexia. Some degree of fever is always present and does not necessarily indicate infection. Use fans, and tepid sponges, together with chlorpromazine as above. Aspirin increases the metabolic rate, displaces thyroxine from prealbumin, and should not be used. If the above measures are ineffective, propranolol given as above may cause dramatic improvement.

(6) Dehydration. This may occur from hyperventilation and sweating as well as insufficient fluid intake. CVP recordings are especially valuable in this situation as hypovolaemia may be complicated by heart failure. Give 20% or 33% dextrose i.v. as extra calories are needed to supply increased metabolic demands. In addition, cautious replacement of sodium losses will also be necessary. Do not attempt to raise the serum sodium by giving hypertonic saline as this may precipitate pulmonary oedema. Repeat the electrolytes after 12 h.

(7) Adrenal insufficiency. Hypotension and vomiting may be due to adrenocortical insufficiency which is unmasked by the

metabolic stress. Take blood for plasma cortisol and give 100 mg of hydrocortisone i.v. without waiting for the result, followed by 50 mg 6-hourly.

(8) Hypoxia. Occasional patients have a severe associated myopathy. This may give rise to ventilatory failure (see p. 71), so monitor the blood gases, and be prepared to institute IPPR as necessary.

(9) Thromboembolic complications. These appear to be common, and serious. Give heparin (see p. 18).

(10) Thyrotoxic crisis may be fatal and in severe cases it may be necessary to anaesthetise, paralyse and ventilate the patient in an attempt to reduce metabolic requirements.

(11) The use of haemoperfusion over a polyacrylamide gel column has been advocated in intractable thyrotoxic crisis. This technique looks promising and is worth considering.[1]

Effective therapy of the precipitating cause is a major determinant of the ultimate outcome.

REFERENCES

1 Herrman J., Ruddorff K. H., Gockenjan G. (1977) Charcoal haemoperfusion in thyroid storm. *Lancet* **i:** 248.

2 Ikram H. (1977) Haemodynamic effects of beta-adrenergic blockade in hyperthyroid patients with and without heart failure. *Br. Med. J.* **1:** 1505.

3 Mackin J. F., Canary J. J., Pittmann C. S. (1974) Thyroid storm and its management. *N. Engl. J. Med.* **291:** 1396.

4 McClellan A. (1982) Thyroid emergencies. *Hospital Update* May, p. 375.

5 Skelton C. L. (1982) The heart in hyperthyroidism. *N. Engl. J. Med.* **307:** 1206.

Acute hypercalcaemia[1,2,3]

Most patients who require urgent treatment for hypercalcaemia either have an underlying malignancy or primary hyperparathyroidism. In both these circumstances, the prominent cause of the hypercalcaemia is calcium resorption from bone, which has important therapeutic implications (see (4) below). Other rarer causes are the milk-alkali syndrome, sarcoidosis and vitamin D intoxication (for differentiation see reference 2.).

DIAGNOSIS

Polydypsia, polyuria, abdominal pain, disorders of behaviour, profound muscle weakness, vomiting and pyrexia may progress to cardiovascular collapse and coma. The inevitable fluid loss is accompanied by the loss of both magnesium and potassium. Acute renal failure, due in part to this hypovolaemia, may occur. A fatal cardiac arrhythmia may terminate the condition. The serum calcium in these cases is usually more than 4 mmol/l (16 mg/100 ml). Conjunctivitis due to local calcific deposits on the corneo-scleral junction is a most striking physical sign. It is best seen with a hand lens and strong lateral lighting. The ECG shows a shortened QT interval.

MANAGEMENT

(1) Take blood for haemoglobin, PCV, electrolytes (including Mg^{2+} and Cl^-, if you can get it) and urea, serum calcium, phosphate and alkaline phosphatase albumin, plasma osmolality and plasma proteins. Perform an ECG.

(2) The objectives of treatment are then to correct dehydration, which will lead to an appreciable improvement in both symptoms and calcium levels, and then to give a drug which will bring the calcium down to normal levels within 24–48 h. Faster reduction seems to be dangerous.

(3) Rehydration. This is the single most important measure in the treatment of hypercalcaemia. Rehydrate your patient with

isotonic saline and 5% dextrose, giving potassium and magnesium supplements as necessary—a CVP line is valuable. You may need 4–5 l of N saline in the first 24 h. It is wise to add 20 mEq of K^+ and 10 mEq of Mg^{2+} to each litre, and monitor both K^+ and Mg^{2+}. This rehydration will invariably lower the serum Ca^{2+}. Once your patient is rehydrated, the addition of frusemide 40 mg/i.v, 6-hourly, has an additional calciuric, and therefore serum calcium-lowering, effect.

(4) Biphosphonates. These agents, which inhibit calcium resorption from bone, have transformed the treatment of hypercalcaemia. Give pamidronate 30 mg in 1 litre of 0.9 N saline i.v over 4 h, or if you cannot get this, disodium etidronate 7.5 mg/kg in 250 ml 0.9 N saline i.v. over 2 h daily for 3 days. Either of these will almost always lower the calcium to normal.

(5) These above measures will almost always suffice. If they do not, try:

    (i) Plicamycin (formerly called mithramycin) 25 μg/kg i.v. over 3 h in a solution of 5% dextrose or by a bolus. This is usually effective within 12–36 h.

   (ii) Salmon calcitonin can be used in a dose of 200 MRC units i.m. or i.v 6-hourly.

(6) If you think that the hypercalcaemia is due to either a haematological malignancy (such as myeloma) or sarcoid or vitamin D intoxication, steroids should be used, either hydrocortisone 100 mg i.v. 6-hourly, or prednisolone 60 mg/day.

(7) As soon as the cause of the hypercalcaemia has been identified, specific treatment should be started.

REFERENCES

1   Drug and Therapeutics Bulletin (1990) Treating cancer associated hypercalcaemia **22** (October): 85.

2   Fraser P., Watson L., Healy M. (1976) Further experience with discriminant function in the differential diagnosis of hypercalcaemia. *Postgrad. med. J.* **52:** 254.

3   Heath D. (1989) Hypercalcaemia in malignancy. *Br. Med. J.* **298:** 1468.

Tetany

DIAGNOSIS

(1) Tetany is usually diagnosed by observing the characteristic carpopedal spasm of the hands (and sometimes feet). This is usually heralded by circumoral paraesthesiae and may be accompanied by excessive neuromuscular irritability (the basis of Chvostek's sign).

(2) Is less easily recognised when it presents itself as laryngospasm, psychosis or generalised convulsions. Carpopedal spasm usually accompanies these manifestations, but if not, can usually be elicited by inflating a sphygmomanometer cuff above the systolic arterial pressure for 3 min.

The condition may be caused by:

(1) Hypocalcaemia. This occurs after thyroid/parathyroid surgery, following a prolonged 'forced' diuresis, in malabsorption and in rickets and osteomalacia, sometimes immediately after vitamin D therapy is started. If it is unrelieved, laryngeal spasm and generalised convulsions ensue. Psychotic behaviour may be prominent. Treatment may be divided into those patients with:

    (i) Mild hypocalcaemia (moderately symptomatic patients with a corrected calcium of >2.0 mmols/l). Give oral effervescent calcium (Sandocal) two tablets 6-hourly.

    (ii) Severe hypocalcaemia (severely symptomatic, or corrected calcium <2.0 mmols/l). Give 10% calcium gluconate i.v.: 20 ml of this contains 176 mg of Ca^{++}, and you usually require 15 mg Ca^{++}/kg body weight. Give 20 ml in the first 10 min, and the rest by slow infusion over the next 12 h. Then proceed to 1 alpha OH cholecalciferol 2–4 μg/day. Monitor the serum Ca^{++} and PO_4^{--} and Mg^{++}.

(2) Hypomagnasaemia.[1] This almost always co-exists with hypocalcaemia, and can also cause a positive Chvostek's sign and convulsions. Unless you have definitive evidence that the magnesium level is normal, you should give 0.25 mmol mag-

nesium chloride /kg i.v. over 4 h in 1 litre of 0.9 N saline, in conjunction with the calcium gluconate (1 mmol of magnesium chloride hexahydrate = 200 mg).

(3) Hyperventilation: see p. 376.

(4) States of alkalotic hypokalaemia. Usually seen when dehydration caused by vomiting is 'corrected' with infusions containing bicarbonate. Treatment is with potassium supplements, plus i.v. calcium gluconate as above.

(5) Rapid correction of chronic acidosis causes a decrease in ionised calcium and hence tetany. This is treated by giving calcium, as in (1) above.

REFERENCE

1   Levine B. (1984) Magnesium, the mimic/antagonist of calcium. *N. Engl. J. Med.* **310:** 1253.

Neurological

The completed stroke[9,19]

The World Health Organisation definition of stroke is 'rapidly developing clinical signs of focal disturbance of cerebral function, with symptoms lasting for 24 h or longer, or leading to death, with no apparent cause other than of vascular origin'.

Stroke causes the death of 16% of men and 8% of women, and is the third most common cause of death in the UK. Predisposing factors to stroke are:

(1) inherent biological traits—old age, male sex;
(2) physiological characteristics—hypertension, hypercholesterolaemia, diabetes, obesity;
(3) behaviours—lack of exercise, smoking, excess alcohol, and in women taking the contraceptive pill;
(4) social characteristics—it is commoner in Afro-Caribbeans and in those living in more socially deprived circumstances.

In a population of 300 000 (served by the average Acute General Hospital in the UK), there will be about 400 new strokes each year, with an additional 100 recurrent strokes. Many of these patients will be admitted to hospital.

DIAGNOSIS

Strokes may be due to:

(1) Cerebral infarction (80% of strokes in most series). The vessels may be occluded by thrombosis in situ, or by embolic material arising from:

    (i)   The heart. Embolism is said to be rarely due to fibrillation alone unless the mitral valve is abnormal or the left atrium enlarged. Emboli arise from infected or calcified heart valves or from a prolapsing mitral valve.[5] Mural thrombi associated with myocardial infarction may become detached. Emboli from these sites may occlude vessels elsewhere and peripheral pulses must be checked.

    (ii)   Neck vessels—commonly from atheromatous plaques at the origin of the internal carotid artery. A bruit may be heard but if stenosis is tight a bruit may be absent or contralateral.

(iii) Thrombosis in situ. This usually occurs on atheromatous sections of the intracranial vessels. Thrombosis accounts for most internal capsular infarcts and also for most brainstem strokes, where occlusion of small end-vessels causes ischaemic scars (lacunes; so called because they look like small black dots at post-mortem). Lacunes, 70% of which are associated with hypertension, may cause a wide variety of syndromes but may recognisably present as:[1]

   (a) pure motor stroke affecting the face and arm on one side, or arm and leg on one side (not the face alone or one limb alone);
   (b) pure sensory stroke with the same distribution as above;
   (c) dysarthria with a clumsy hand;
   (d) ataxic hemiparesis without dysphasia or parietal signs.

Cerebral infarction secondary to thrombosis is not always caused by atheromatous disease; other causes such as arteritis (collagen disease), syphilis, the contraceptive pill, migraine, polycythaemia and other hypercoagulable states should be excluded.

In all forms of infarction aside from lacunes, premonitory episodes of neurological deficit are not uncommon, meningism is rare, the CSF is not usually xanthochromic and unless there is massive infarction, there is no shift of midline structures within the first 24 h. These features help to distinguish infarction from haemorrhage, a distinction which can only reliably be confirmed by a CT scan. However, a recent study has further refined our ability to distinguish clinically between the types of stroke using a score derived from eight clinical features.[10]

(2) Cerebral haemorrhage (15% of strokes—the residual 5% are patients who present as strokes, but turn out to have other lesions.)[17] The haemorrhage may be:

   (i) Primarily intracerebral (10%). Bleeding in people with hypertension usually occurs from minute, thin-walled aneurysmal dilatation of intracranial arteries—Charcot–Bouchard aneurysms. Occasionally, bleeding occurs from vascular malformations in normotensive patients.

In about three-quarters of cases the bleeding spreads from the brain substance into the subarachnoid space and the resulting meningeal irritation gives rise to vomiting, headache and neck stiffness. Within the first 24 h the haematoma, in about three-quarters of cases, causes a shift of midline structures. CT scan reliably detects haemorrhage and, if this is readily available, lumbar puncture should not be performed because of the slight risk of coning.

(ii) Primarily subarachnoid (5%). The bleeding occurs from an aneurysm (65%) or A–V malformation (5%) directly into the subarachnoid space. In 20% no cause is found, and in these the prognosis is good.[18] The symptoms, which characteristically start abruptly, are those of meningeal irritation, with or without loss of consciousness. There may often have been warning leaks, causing severe headaches lasting a day or two, in the weeks preceding the more serious bleed.[15] Focal neurological deficits may be present due to arterial spasm or extension of haemorrhage into the brain. The combination of a focal neurological deficit in a patient with signs of subacute bacterial endocarditis strongly suggest mycotic aneurysm. Blood in the subarachnoid space may be identified by CT scan, and if so lumbar puncture is unnecessary.

If the CT scan is unavailable or unrevealing, a lumbar puncture should be carried out—remember that occasionally an early LP will show normal CSF since it may take 12 h for xanthochromia to appear in the lumbar CSF. All bloody CSF should be centrifuged so that subarachnoid bleeding identified by the xanthochromic supernatant may be distinguished from a traumatic tap where the supernatant is clear. Remember that mild degrees of xanthochromia may not be visible to the naked eye, and spectrophotometric analysis should be asked for if you are uncertain as to whether there is xanthochromia or not.[7] Remember also that xanthochromia persists for 3 weeks after a subarachnoid haemorrhage, so its presence does not necessarily imply a recent event. When a subarachnoid haemorrhage has been identified the patient should be discussed urgently with your neurosurgical colleagues. The aim should be to transfer patients for 4-vessel angiography with a view to clipping of any aneurysm. Other therapeutic interventions which have been advocated are discussed later (see p. 208).

In any unconscious patient other causes of unconsciousness must be excluded (see p. 355). In addition the following conditions may cause diagnostic confusion.

(1) Subdural haematoma. A history of head injury, while typical, may be lacking, especially in patients with pre-existing cortical atrophy. Percussion of the skull may reveal lateralised tenderness sufficient to arouse deeply stuporose patients, and also an area of dullness over the haematoma.[3]

Inequality of the pupils and a fluctuating but overall deteriorating level of consciousness, with progressive focal neurological signs, are all highly suggestive. There may be a shift of midline structures and the diagnosis may be confirmed with CT scan. However, if subdural haematomas are bilateral, there may be no mass effect, and if isodense, may be undetectable on CT scan. The very normality of the CT scan in a clearly deteriorating patient is in itself suspicious, and an MRI scan should be done or the CT scan should be repeated.

(2) Extradural haematoma.

(3) Brain tumour: 3–5% of clinically diagnosed acute strokes turn out to be due to a tumour. This should be revealed by a CT scan.

(4) Brain abscess. This usually occurs in the setting of purulent lung disease, infected ears or nasal sinuses, or in patients with a right-to-left intracardiac shunt. Ring enhancement is typically seen on CT scan but may be difficult to distinguish from a brain tumour. Surgical aspiration (to make the diagnosis and identify the organism) together with appropriate antibiotic therapy is usually all that is necessary.[12]

(5) As we have suggested earlier, the differentiation from strokes of the mass lesions described in (1)–(4) above can only be made confidently with a CT scan. CT scans are not everywhere readily available, but in any 'stroke' patient with:

(i) a history on admission which is either unclear, or suggestive of a gradually evolving focal deficit, particularly if the progression has been in a continuous rather than stepwise fashion;

(ii) a history of taking anti-haemostatic drugs (you will want to know whether to stop these or not);

(iii) a deficit which progresses in a way uncharacteristic of stroke;

(iv) a progressing neurological deficit during the initial period of hospitalisation, or brainstem instability;

(v) and when you are considering the use of aspirin;

you should consider the desirability of obtaining a scan.[17] In effect, many units now scan most people admitted with a diagnosis of stroke.

(6) Hemiplegic migraine. A history of preceding or accompanying visual disturbance, a throbbing headache which is associated with nausea, and photophobia usually in a young person in association with a normal CSF clinches the diagnosis.

(7) Epileptic attacks, particularly those associated with residual paralysis (Todd's paralysis) may also temporarily be mistaken for strokes.

MANAGEMENT

The main purpose of the investigation is to determine whether any treatable causes (see below)—unfortunately the minority—are present. The history and clinical findings may help.

(1) The investigation of choice is a CT scan. This will with a high degree of reliability distinguish between a stroke and other lesions, as well as between haemorrhagic and other types of stroke. It is clearly impractical, and some would say not good medicine, to get a CT scan on all patients. Fortunately, there are now reasonable guidelines on which to act, which have been outlined in (5) above. The other circumstances in which we recommend getting a CT scan are:

(i) If you are contemplating anticoagulant, or antiplatelet therapy, you need to ensure that the lesion is not haemorrhagic[3] (see section (2) p. 202).

(ii) If you have diagnosed a cerebellar lesion, as surgery may be helpful here, and brainstem compression is of particular anxiety (see section (2) p. 208).[6]

(2) If subarachnoid haemorrhage is suspected, CT examination is the investigation of choice. If this facility is not available, CSF examination should be undertaken, but is, of course, contrain-

dicated where there are signs or symptoms of raised intracranial pressure.

(3) Arteriography may be required to localise the space-occupying lesion if a CT scan is not available, and is anyway indicated in the further investigation of subarachnoid haemorrhage, as well as in any patients in whom a significant carotid stenosis is deemed to be treatable. Full blood picture and ESR, VDRL and FTA-ABS may detect the rare cases of collagen disease, syphilis or polycythaemia, which are treated on their merits. A KCCT and PT will exclude a bleeding tendency, and a glucose level will tell you if there is co-existent diabetes.

(4) Duplex scanning, which is a highly effective non-invasive way of detecting carotid stenosis, should be undertaken in those patients with TIA or with minor hemispheric stroke in whom carotid endarterectomy is contemplated (see p. 218).

(5) A skull x-ray is only worth while if there is a question of head injury.

General measures

(1) General care of the helpless and or comatose patient (see p. 356).

(2) Treatment of complications which may follow a stroke.

  (i) Dehydration. This is avoided by feeding fluids through a nasogastric tube if the patient has a cough reflex, and if not, by giving fluids intravenously.

  (ii) Deep vein thrombosis: 5000 units of calcium heparin subcutaneously 8-hourly for 14 days, starting within 48 h of the stroke substantially reduces the morbidity from DVT.[13]

  (iii) Hypothermia (see p. 289).

  (iv) Hyperthermia (temperature >40°C (104°F)). This usually occurs in conjunction with a pontine lesion. If severe it may itself cause depression of consciousness; consequently, cooling the patient with tepid sponging is occasionally associated with marked improvement.

  (v) Diabetes. This may be precipitated by an intracranial catastrophe, and is anyway a predisposing factor to stroke. There is evidence that raised sugars further compromise brain function, and you should keep the blood sugar between 4 and 8 mmol/l, using a sliding scale of insulin (see p. 172).

(vi) Fits. These need treatment in the usual way (see p. 224).

(vii) Hypertension. This may be a transient phenomenon, settling within a few hours of the stroke. If it persists (i.e. a diastolic pressure above 120 mmHg) it would seem logical to reduce this to a level appropriate to the patient's age. However, following a stroke, the auto-regulatory capacity of blood vessels in the brain may be impaired for a period of about 3 weeks. This means that, in contradistinction to normal, the flow in the diseased area becomes pressure-dependent. Lowering arterial pressure will thus reduce flow to this area. Against this is the danger of continuing hypertension damaging resid-ual healthy brain. We advocate, as a compromise, gentle reduction of arterial pressure until the diastolic is less than 110 mmHg and the systolic less than 170 mmHg. This should be accomplished by conventional oral hypo-tensive thereapy.

(viii) Hypertensive encephalopathy. The considerations in (vii) above do not apply if there is evidence of hyperten-sive encephalopathy (see p. 48).

(ix) Cerebral oedema. Seen as low attenuation with mass effect on CT scan, it reflects the volume of ischaemic tissue. It may occasionally cause papilloedema. There is no evidence that dexamethasone affects the oedema surrounding infarction or that it alters the mortality or morbidity following stroke. Dexamethasone is, however, extremely effective in reducing oedema surrounding tumour or abscess and may be given as 6 mg 6–hourly. An acute rise in intracranial pressure may be treated by a bolus of 20% mannitol 1–2 g/kg i.v. over 5–10 min. Unfortunately, the effect is only temporary, and this regime may need to be repeated. It is rarely appropriate to resort to other measures, such as hyperventilation.

(x) There has been a flurry of activity aimed at reducing the amount of, and improving the viability of the ischaemic tissue around either an infarct or haemorrhage. The role of aspirin, anticoagulation and surgery is discussed else-where. Calcium channel antagonists,[21] prostacyclin, thrombolytic therapy[11] and routine haemodilution have either been proved to be unhelpful, or need to be established through rigorously controlled trials.[2] However, if your patient has a haematocrit above 49, it seems reasonable to reduce this by venesection, while keeping up an adequate circulating volume.[22]

Specific measures

In general determining the cause of a completed stroke has little immediate therapeutic spin-off. However, in the following situations specific therapy may be helpful.

(1) *Primary subarachnoid haemorrhage* (see above). There is real danger of re-bleeding in this group, maximal between 7–10 days, and neurosurgical advice should be sought as soon as the diagnosis is made.

    (i) Early treatment with an antifibrinolytic agent such as epsilon amino caproic acid (EACA) 24 g orally per day, or tranexamic acid, has not been found to be helpful.[23]

    (ii) However, the calcium antagonists nimodipine in a dose of 60 mg 4-hourly, started as soon after diagnosis as possible, does seem to improve outcome.[16]

    (iii) Beta-blockers are also said to be helpful. We remain to be convinced.[24]

    (iv) Surgery to prevent re-bleeding should always be considered in this group, particularly in the patient with little neurological impairment. There is now some enthusiasm for surgery in deeply unconscious patients, and so it is wise to discuss all patients with a diagnosed subarachnoid haemorrhage with the neurosurgeons.[8]

(2) *Cerebellar haematoma.*[6] This merits separate mention as it is amenable to surgery. Unfortunately progression to coma and death is rapid due to brainstem compression. In the short interval before coma the patient may complain of occipital headache and vertigo. There is a gaze palsy to the side of the haemorrhage. Mild ipsilateral lower motor neurone VIIth nerve palsy and dysarthria are common, but only a minority show nystagmus or ipsilateral ataxia. Contralateral hemiplegia does not occur, so the finding of a gaze palsy without limb paralysis is a useful pointer. Diagnosis is by CT scan.

(3) *Embolism.* Where the emboli have come from either a clot in the ventricle, following, for instance, a myocardial infarct (see

p. 60) or in a patient with valvular disease, whether or not they have associated atrial fibrillation, anticoagulation with heparin and warfarin should be started. There is controversy as to when, with most authorities now recommending starting within 48 h, provided that a CT scan at that time shows that the infarct is not haemorrhagic. If the infarct is haemorrhagic, delay anticoagulation for at least two weeks.

(4) Low dose aspirin certainly reduces the incidence of stroke following TIAs;[2] the evidence that it helps to prevent further stroke in patients with atrial fibrillation (in the abscence of valvular disease—see (3) above) is reasonable;[20] the evidence that this effect extends to all those who have had an infarct is not so strong,[20] but we use it in a dose of 75 mg/day in all the above circumstances. We do not routinely perform a CT scan prior to starting aspirin at this dose, as we consider the risk of provoking haemorrhage very small indeed. We acknowledge that this is controversial, and we await the results of studies to confirm us in our belief.

(5) When any of the causes considered under differential diagnosis are found, appropriate therapy should be instituted.

REFERENCES

1   Bamford J. (1991) Classification and natural history of clinically identifiable subtypes of cerebral infarction. *Lancet* **337:** 1521.

2   Grotta J. (1987) Current medical and surgical therapy for cerebrovascular disease. *N. Engl. J. Med.* **317:** 1505.

3   Guarino J. R. (1981) Auscultatory percussion of the head. *Br. Med. J.* **1:** 1075.

5   Leader (1985) Cerebral embolism. *Lancet* **i:** 29.

6   Leader (1988) Cerebellar stroke. *Lancet* **i:** 1031.

7   Leader (1989) Xanthochromia. *Lancet* **ii:** 658.

8   Leader (1987) Intracerebral haematoma from aneurysmal rupture: operation in moribund patients? *Lancet* **ii:** 1186.

9   Leader (1991) Treatment for stroke. *Lancet* **337:** 1129.

10 Leader (1984) Stroke: was it haemorrhage or infarction? *Lancet* **i:** 204.

11 Leader (1990) Non-coronary thrombolysis. *Lancet* **335:** 691.

12 Leader (1988) Treatment of brain abscess. *Lancet* **i:** 219.

13 McCarthy S. *et al.* (1986) Low dose subcutaneous heparin in

the prevention of deep vein thrombosis and pulmonary emboli following acute stroke. *Age Ageing* **15:** 84.

14 Norris J. W., Hachinski V. C. (1982) Misdiagnosis of a stroke. *Lancet* **i:** 328.

15 Ostergaard J. (1990) Warning leaks in subarachnoid haemorrhage. *Br. Med. J.* **301:** 190.

16 Pickard J. *et al.* (1989) Effect of oral nimodipine on cerebral infarction and outcome after subarachnoid haemorrhage. *Br. Med. J.* **298**. 636.

17 Sandercock P. *et al.* (1985) Value of computed tomography in patients with stroke. *Br. Med. J.* **290:** 193.

18 Shepard R. H. (1984) Prognosis of spontaneous subarachnoid haemorrhage of unknown cause. *Lancet* **i:** 777.

19 Stroke Octet (1992) *Lancet* **339:** 342 (8 February and subsequent issues).

20 Stroke Prevention in Atrial Fibrillation Study Group (1990) *N. Engl. J. Med.* **322:** 863.

21 Trust Study Group (1990) Randomised, double blind, placebo controlled trial of nimodipine in acute stroke. *Lancet* **336:** 1205.

22 Thomas D. J., Marshall J., Ross Russell R. W. (1977) Effect of haematocrit on cerebral blood flow in man. *Lancet* **2:** 941.

23 Vermeulen M. *et al.* (1984) Antifibrinolytic treatment in subarachnoid haemorrhage. *N. Engl. J. Med.* **311:** 432.

24 Walter P. *et al.* (1982) Beneficial effects of adrenergic blockade in patients with subarachnoid haemorrhage. *Br. Med. J.* **284:** 1661.

Transient ischaemic attacks (TIAs)[4,6]

DIAGNOSIS

These are episodes of transient neurological deficit due to vascular disease. They may be recurrent, sometimes only last a few minutes, and are due to temporary reduction in blood supply to part of the brain. The importance of recognising TIAs is that they are followed by major stroke with a frequency of about 5% per annum, particularly if the TIA is in the carotid territory.

They may be caused by:

(1) Emboli arising from atheroma of the vertebral and carotid arteries, or their branches, or from the heart. This is the single most important cause of TIA.

(2) In the setting of borderline local cerebral perfusion, transient reduction in overall cerebral blood flow may cause significant, albeit temporary, local ischaemia. This can occur on the basis of:

    (i) A fall in perfusion pressure due to:

        (a) hypotension (e.g. hypotensive drugs);
        (b) decreased cardiac output (e.g. arrhythmias).

    (ii) Increased viscosity:

        (a) a PCV of above 49%;
        (b) paraproteinaemia.

(3) Transient reduction in local blood flow:

    (i) Hypertension. Focal neurological deficit may occur as part of hypertensive encephalopathy (see p. 48).
    (ii) Migraine. Complicated migraine may occasionally cause hemiplegia characterised more by dysaesthesiae than weakness, or a third or sixth nerve palsy (ophthalmoplegic migraine). It is usually possible to elicit a history of previous attacks of 'classical' migraine.
    (iii) Mechanical effects on flow.

        (a) Neck movements may cause occlusion of the vertebral arteries with ensuing posterior cerebral and brainstem ischaemia. Failure of autoregulation of the posterior cerebral circulation may cause the structures so supplied to be vulnerable to changes of the systemic circulation. This may play a role in 'vertebral basilar insufficiency'.

(b) Subclavian steal. In this uncommon condition movement of one arm diverts blood from the vertebral arteries causing symptoms of transient brainstem ischaemia.

(4) Lack of nutrients, which presumably cause focal symptoms on the same basis as (2) above:

(i) Anaemia. Haemoglobin of less than 7 g/100 ml may be the sole cause of TIA.

(ii) Hypoglycaemia. This may rarely present itself with a focal neurological deficit.

In a proportion of cases no cause can be found, presumably because of lysis of the vascular obstruction, or because the vessel involved is too small to be identified.

(5) TIAs should be differentiated from:

(i) Focal epilepsy. In focal epilepsy, the patient often complains of positive symptoms (e.g. paraesthesiae, spontaneous movements). These are uncommon in TIAs.

(ii) Todd's paralaysis. This is the transient focal weakness that occurs after an epileptic seizure.

(6) Attacks resembling TIAs may be the initial symptoms of cerebral tumours. These are presumably caused by alteration of circulation in the adjacent brain.

Examination, therefore, must include careful auscultation of the head, heart and neck, measurement of lying and standing arterial pressure and the pressure in each arm and assessment of peripheral vasculature. A 24-hour continuous ECG, plasma glucose, lipid profile and cholesterol and full blood picture and ESR may establish an underlying cause which should be dealt with accordingly. A prolapsing leaflet of the mitral valve may give rise to a loud mid-systolic click or be silent. It can, however, be detected by echocardiography,[7] which will also detect stenotic or infected heart valves.

MANAGEMENT

There are several uncontroversial aspects of management. These include:

(1) Control of hypertension. The diastolic pressure should be slowly reduced to less than 100 mmHg, using conventional oral hypotensive agents. Reduction of arterial pressure may be all that is required to control TIA.

(2) Control of blood glucose.

(3) Reduction of PCV to below 45% by repeated small (200 ml) venesections, and replacement of the blood removed with crystalloid, although the initial enthusiasm for this therapeutic manoeuvre is diminishing.

(4) Reduction of hypercholesterolaemia or hyperlipidaemia, and the control of other risk factors, such as smoking.

(5) Prophylactic anticoagulants following emboli arising from the heart (see p. 19).

(6) The control of any cardiac arrhythmia.

(7) Aspirin, in a dose of 300 mg/day, has been shown to reduce the frequency of stroke after TIAs. Trials are in progress to see whether a smaller dose will suffice, and either 150 mg or 75 mg/day can be used in the case of GI intolerance.[4]

(8) Carotid endarterectomy.[1,2,5] There is now clear evidence that surgery on patients with symptomatic high grade carotid stenosis (>70%) is highly effective in preventing subsequent stroke. So you should investigate patients with a carotid bruit and symptoms with either Doppler ultrasonography or digital subtraction imaging. Those with significant stenosis should be referred to a vascular surgeon. In those with lesser degrees of stenosis, the situation is less clear. We give this group of patients aspirin 75 mg/day. It is important to remember that patients with TIAs often have evidence of vascular disease elsewhere—indeed the commonest cause of death in patients with TIAs is myocardial infarction—and the aspirin may also prevent other vascular problems.

(9) Formal anticoagulation. There is no evidence that this is superior to aspirin, but see p. 209.

REFERENCES

1   Kistler J. *et al.* (1991) Carotid endarterectomy—specific therapy based on pathophysiology. *N. Engl. J. Med.* **325:** 505.

2   Leader (1991) Operating to prevent stroke. *Lancet* **337:** 1255.

3   Sandercock P. (1988) Aspirin for strokes and transient ischaemic attacks. *Br. Med. J.* **297:** 995.

4   Sandercock P. (1990) Management of transient ischaemic attacks. *Hospital Update* September, p. 725.

5   Thomas D. *et al.* (1991) Carotid endarterectomy. *Br. Med. J.* **303:** 985.

6   Warlow C. (1985) Transient ischaemic attacks—current treatment concepts. *Drugs* **29:** 474.

7   Wynne J. (1986) Mitral valve prolapse. *N. Engl. J. Med.* **314:** 577.

Closed head injury[1,7]

DIAGNOSIS

(1) Of the 1.1 million patients who present annually to accident and emergency departments following head injury only a few have impairment of consciousness. Although the diagnosis of head injury is seldom in doubt, it needs to be considered in every unconscious patient. Witnesses should be sought to help dispel any residual doubt.

(2) Evidence of head injury may be revealed in an unconscious patient by careful examination of the head and neck. Blood and/or CSF in the external auditory canal or behind the tympanic membrane indicates a basal skull fracture. An anterior fossa fracture may be indicated by CSF rhinorrhoea or periorbital haematomata. Vitreous haemorrhage may occur following a whiplash injury, especially in children.

(3) Head injury may occur in the setting of other conditions, some of which may also cause coma, for example acute alcoholic intoxication. In this situation, as in all cases of head injury with loss of consciousness, the skull should be x-rayed. A skull fracture cannot be diagnosed clinically, is a powerful indicator of the severity of injury, and may be associated with occult intracranial pathology.

(4) Consideration should be given to injury elsewhere, particularly in the neck (see p. 216).

MANAGEMENT

Head injuries may give rise to unconsciousness and death because of the contusion and haemorrhage sustained at the time. However, events subsequent to the injury also account for considerable morbidity and mortality. Whatever the cause, the key problem is the development of cerebral oedema, which in turn compromises cerebral blood flow. As suggested above, this cerebral oedema is all too frequently aggravated by extracranial and potentially reversible factors, such as hypoxia, hypovolaemia and hypotension, fits and infection. Due attention must be given to these secondary events, which, while not requiring specialist neurosurgical input, are at least as important as the consequences of the primary injury.

Therefore management should include the following steps, in order of priority.

(1) Check the airway. If adequate ventilation is in any doubt, either because of brainstem involvement or because of inhaled vomit, blood or a chest injury, intubate and ventilate.

(2) Check the arterial pressure and perfusion. Hypotension usually occurs from blood loss from injuries elsewhere, but occurs occasionally for central reasons. Treatment is with volume expansion and pressor agents as necessary (see p. 17).

(3) Control seizure activity (see p. 224).

(4) Examine the neck. If there is local pain, evidence of trauma or loss of power or sensation in the limbs, do not move your patient until a lateral neck x-ray has excluded cervical instability.

(5) Pain. Paracetamol 250–500 mg each 6 h, DF 118 or Co-codamol 1–2 tablets 4-hourly, or dihydrocodeine 30 mg parenterally 6-h are probably the safest options. Do not give stronger opiates or sedatives. Metaclopramide 10 mg 8-hourly is useful for nausea.

(6) When the above are satisfactorily controlled, assess the level of consciousness using the Glasgow coma scale. Three elements of behaviour are scored.

  (i) Eye opening

	Score
No response to any stimulus	1
To pain (infraorbital pressure)	2
To verbal command (loud shout!)	3
Spontaneous, with blinking	4

  (ii) Motor response (to infraorbital pressure)

	Score
No response	1
Abnormal extension (extension of both arms and legs)	2
Abnormal flexion	3
Weak flexion (flexor withdrawal response to nail-bed pressure)	4
Localising (able to use a limb to locate and resist supraorbital pressure)	5
Obeys command	6

The arms are usually more responsive than the legs; in the case of different patterns in arms and legs, always record the best response.

(iii) Verbal response

	Score
Nil	1
Incomprehensible (mumbling, no recognisable words)	2
Inappropriate (intelligible words, often profanities; no phrases)	3
Confused (phrases, but disorientated and confused in content)	4
Fully orientated	5

Information derived from these observations should be recorded on a chart. Severe head injury is defined as a Glasgow coma scale score of less than 8. Whatever the initial score, any deterioration in the level of consciousness implies progression of the neuronal damage. This calls for an urgent reappraisal of the situation, usually by a more experienced colleague.

(7) Now that most doctors are aware of the general supportive measures outlined above, improvement in the outcome of head-injured patients will depend on the early recognition and treatment of intracranial haemorrhage. The traditional diagnostic pointers appear late, so the central issue you have to grapple with is 'Which head-injured patients require a CT scan?' Fortunately there are now clear guidelines.

You should consult your neurosurgical colleagues, with a view to getting both their advice as well as a CT scan, if your patient has any of the following.[1]

(i)   Fractured skull with confusion or worse impairment of consciousness, focal neurological signs, fits, or any other neurological symptom or sign.

(ii) Coma continuing after resuscitation, even if there is no skull fracture. (Coma is defined as not obeying commands, not speaking, not opening eyes—that is, a Glasgow coma score of 8 or below.)

(iii) Deterioration in the level of consciousness or development of other neurological signs.

(iv) Confusion or other neurological disturbance lasting more than 6 h, even without skull fracture.

    (v)   Compound depressed fracture of the vault of the skull.

    (vi)   Suspected fracture of the base of the skull.

           This in essence means that most patients admitted because of their head injury will require a CT scan and, if that is suggestive of intracranial haematoma, transfer to a neurosurgical unit.

(8) It is therefore important to have clear criteria for admission of patients following head injury. The following are widely accepted:[1]

    (i)   Confusion or any other depression of consciousness at the time of examination.

    (ii)   Skull fracture.

    (iii) Neurological symptoms or signs or both.

    (iv) Difficulty in assessing patient, for example because of ingestion of alcohol, epilepsy or other medical conditions which cloud consciousness.

    (v)   Lack of a responsible adult to supervise the patient and other social problems.

A short period of amnesia after trauma (<5 min), in the absence of a skull fracture, and with full recovery, is not in itself an indication for admission.

(9) Skull fractures are usually only picked up on x-ray, and so a further question is 'Who needs a skull x-ray?'[5,6]

    (i)   Any patient falling into categories (ii)–(vi), in (7) above.

    (ii)   Any patient falling into categories (i), (iii), (iv) in (8) above.

    (iii) Any patient with scalp bruising or swelling or suspected penetrating injury.

    (iv) Any patient with CSF fluid or blood from the nose or the ear.

(10) These guidelines apply equally to children and adults.[8] Those patients who do not require skull x-ray, or in whom there are no other indications for admission and the x-ray shows no fracture, can be safely discharged to the care of a responsible adult.

Further management

Those patients requiring admission should be managed as follows.

(1) No sedation should be given, unless absolutely unavoidable.
(2) Antibiotics. Avoid using prophylactic antibiotics. Benzylpenicillin 1 000 000 units i.v. 6-hourly, or co-trimoxazole 960 mg b.d. in patients with penicillin allergy, should be given in the following circumstances.

    (i)   Basal or compound vault fractures.
    (ii) Suspected or proven meningitis.

(3) Steroids should not be used
(4) Restlessness is a warning sign. Your patient should not be sedated without:

    (i)   excluding, and treating as necessary, hypoxia, hypotension, metabolic derangement, a full bladder, or pain due to other injuries;
    (ii) excluding, and treating as necessary, any of the causes of secondary deterioration in conscious level described below.

When you have accomplished all the above, you will have ensured that you are providing optimal conditions for the recovery of the brain. You must also ensure that you can detect any complications before they cause any secondary brain damage. The mainstay of the admission is therefore careful neurological observations, using the Glasgow coma scale, which should be recorded hourly for the first 24 h.

If a deterioration in the conscious level occurs, the following possibilities should be considered.

(1) Hypoxia—check the arterial blood gas tension, respiratory rate, chest x-ray. Start oxygen as necessary.
(2) Poor perfusion. Check the pulse, blood pressure, and that your patient is not anaemic. Exclude bleeding from other injuries, particularly intra-abdominal injuries.[2]
(3) Metabolic derangements—exclude dehydration. Check electrolytes, urea and sugar levels. Consider the possibility of drug overdose.
(4) Missed intracranial haematoma—review the CT scan, and consider a further scan.
(5) Fits. Seizures may not have been witnessed. If, 1 h after controlling them, the conscious level has not improved, consult a neurosurgeon.
(6) Meningitis. If this is suspected, do not do a lumbar puncture

before CT scan has excluded the presence of raised intracranial pressure. Appropriate treatment is with penicillin and chloramphenicol, or a third generation cephalosporin (see p. 368).

(7) If none of these is found, the likely problem is increasing cerebral oedema, with the concomitant rise in intracranial pressure (ICP). Normal ICP is between -3 and $+15$ mm/Hg, and the pressure rises to over 20 mmHg in half the patients with severe head injury during the first 72 h after injury, and there is a strong correlation between the level of ICP and mortality. There is at present no very effective treatment for raised ICP, but short-term benefit may be obtained either by:

   (i)   Hyperventilation—dropping the Paco$_2$ to 3.3–4 kPa (25–30 mmHg).

   (ii)   Intravenous mannitol 0.5–1.0 g/kg as a bolus over 10–30 min.

(8) Remember that there are circumstances when continuing treatment is not justified. Severe head injuries in the elderly,[3] and patients with very low Glasgow coma scales have very poor outcomes,[4] and you should be aware of this when instituting therapy.[4]

REFERENCES

1   Bullock R. (1990) Head injuries. *Br. Med. J.* **300:** 1576.
2   Butterworth J. *et al.* (1980) Detection of occult abdominal trauma in patients with severe head injuries. *Lancet* **ii:** 759.
3   Galbraith S. (1987) Head injuries in the elderly. *Br. Med. J.* **294:** 325.
4   Gibson M. (1989) Aggressive management of closed head trauma—a time for reappraisal. *Lancet* **i:** 369.
5   Guidelines for Initial Management after Head Injury in Adults. (1984) *Br. Med. J.* **288:** 983.
6   Leader (1990) Head to head over Harrogate. *Lancet* **335:** 695.
7   Richards P. (1986) Severe head injury: the first hour. *Br. Med. J.* **293:** 643.
8   Teasdale G. *et al.* (1990) Risks of acute traumatic intracranial haematoma in children and adults; implications for managing head injuries. *Br. Med. J.* **300:** 363.

Syncopal attacks (faints)

DIAGNOSIS

Syncope, or faint, is defined as loss of consciousness due to transient impairment of cerebral blood flow leading to cerebral ischaemia. A faint is heralded by a feeling of light-headedness. Objects and sounds then appear distant, and there is a progression to loss of consciousness. The progression of symptoms may be aborted if the sufferer lies down.

The patient will be strikingly pale, with a weak slow pulse and hypotension. (in healthy young adults a systolic blood pressure of <50 mm/Hg will provoke syncope). The pathophysiology of syncope is either through reflex stimulation of the vagus nerve, through drugs or disease impairing the autonomic nervous system, through conditions which directly impair cardiac output, or a combination of the above.

The common causes of syncope are:

(1) Vaso-vagal. Vagal activity produces a bradycardia and fall in blood pressure which is associated with peripheral vasodilatation. Vaso-vagal attacks (simple faints) occur in adolescents and young adults who are otherwise entirely healthy, and are often provoked by emotional or painful stimuli. They are always postural, with the symptoms starting while standing or sitting, and are more frequent after sleep deprivation and fasting.

(2) Cardiogenic syncope. Cardiac output reduction sufficient to cause syncope occurs in three main ways:

    (i)   acute tachy- or brady-dysrhythmias;
    (ii) obstruction to flow as in aortic stenosis;
    (iii) low output states—as in pericardial effusions or pulmonary embolism.

(3) Orthostatic hypotension—many circumstances in which there is a fall in arterial pressure on standing of >25 mmHg may cause syncope. Such a fall may be due to:

    (i)   drugs, particularly hypotensives and tranquillisers;
    (ii) autonomic neuropathy, as in diabetes mellitus;

      (iii)   fluid depletion, as after haemorrhage or in steroid deficiency;

      (iv)   malignant vaso-vagal syncope. This increasingly frequently recognized group of patients faint without any warning or stimulus. The tilt test, in which the patient is tilted head up, with foot support, to an angle of 60° for 45 minutes, and develops symptoms associated with bradycardia and hypotension, is diagnostic.[3]

(4) Cough and micturition syncope.

      (i)   Micturition syncope—in which men may faint while micturating—usually happens at night, and is due to a combination of postural hypotension, reflex vagal activity induced by a full bladder, and impaired venous return due to straining.

      (ii)   Cough syncope. Coughing raises intrathoracic pressure, impairs venous return and may thus cause syncope.

(5) Carotid sinus syncope, defined as asystole of 3 s or more, or a fall in systolic arterial pressure of more than 50 mmHg, when the carotid sinus is stimulated. This is due to atherosclerotic disease at the carotid bifurcation, causing excessive carotid sinus sensitivity.

Cerebral ischaemia is one of the many triggers for a convulsion. Faints if prolonged can therefore provoke a secondary hypoxic convulsion. Such patients should not be considered to have epilepsy.

Some other conditions which cause transient alteration of consciousness include:

      (i)   epilepsy (see p. 224);
      (ii)   severe hypertension (see p. 48)—remember that transient losses of consciousness may be due to sudden elevation, as well as sudden drops, in arterial pressure;
      (iii)   hyperventilation (see p. 376);
      (iv)   cataplexy;
      (v)   paroxysmal vertigo;

although in these last two, consciousness is not truly lost.

MANAGEMENT

All that needs to be done in the simple faint is to lie the patient flat, or with the head slightly down, relieve any compression of the neck and maintain an airway. As indicated above, a careful history and full examination is mandatory if serious conditions are not to be missed. Investigations should include haemoglobin, blood glucose, chest x-ray, ECG and consideration, if the attacks are repeated, of 24 hour ambulatory monitoring of ECG and or EEG. Unfortunately, even after these worthy endeavours, a definitive diagnosis is usually possible in only about 50% of patients.[1,2,3] The encouraging thing is that in patients with no clear diagnosis, the prognosis appears excellent.

REFERENCES

1   Hubbard W. (1989) Syncope *Cardiology in Practice* June, p. 43.
2   Kapoor W. N. (1990) Evaluation and outcome of patients with syncope. *Medicine* **69:** 160.
3   Leader (1991) Explaining syncope. *Lancet* **338:** 353.

Fits[3]

The common generalised tonic clonic convulsion is usually self-limiting. All that is required is to see that the patient has an airway (turn the patient on his side and remove false teeth), does not bang against furniture or roll into the fire. The patient should not be actively restrained; well-meaning attempts to separate the teeth are unnecessary, frequently traumatic and not advised. Repeated tonic clonic seizures without recovery between attacks or one seizure lasting more than 5 min—status epilepticus—is an emergency because irreversible brain damage may occur. This occurs on the basis of hypoxia, hyperpyrexia and hypotension as well as continuing electrical activity, which itself may cause neuronal damage. In this context, it is salutary to remember that after about 20 min of continuous seizures, the metabolic demands of the brain exceed the delivery of substrate.

MANAGEMENT

General

As your patient is unconscious, you should institute the general measures necessary for the care of the unconscious patient (see p. 356).

Specific

  (1) Suppressing the fits is the first priority.

      (i)   The drug of choice is one of the benzodiazepines.[1] Give either clonazepam 1–2 mg i.v. or diazemuls 10 mg i.v. Repeat the dose if seizure activity has not ceased within 5 min. Diazemuls, diluted in 5 or 10% dextrose may be given by slow i.v. infusion at a dose of 1.5–3.0 mg/kg/day. The same strictures probably apply to clonazepam. Benzodiazepines can produce respiratory depression, particularly if your patient has had a recent dose of another anticonvulsant drug.

      (ii) If the benzodiazepines fail to control the fits, phenytoin sodium should be used. Infuse 15–20 mg/kg of ready-made infusion fluid—250 mg/5 ml over 45 min. This infusion will produce a phenytoin level of >10 μg/ml for 24 h. This drug has the advantage of not impairing the conscious level and thus allowing an early neurological assessment. Phenytoin sodium must not be added to any other i.v. infusion as an acid precipitate may form.

In the unlikely event that seizures are not controlled by the above measures, alternatives include :

(iii) Chlormethiazole. Use 500 ml of an 0.8% solution over 6–8 h. This drug may also cause hypotension and respiratory depression, and if you have to use it for more than 12 h your patient should be looked after in a high-dependency area.

(iv) Intramuscular paraldehyde 5 ml into each buttock is still an occasional useful standby, particularly if intravenous drugs cannot be used. Since it is painful, its use should be avoided unless the patient is unconscious. It is generally given using glass syringes since it is said to dissolve plastic. In practice it is safe to use modern plastic syringes provided it is given immediately. It may also be given i.v. A 6% solution is made up in a glass bottle (30 ml in 500 ml dextrose saline). A rapid bolus of 25 ml of this solution is given, and repeated to a maximum of 100 ml. Decreasing doses, again as rapid boluses, are given over the next 5 h (25, 20, 15, 10, 5 ml). Paraldehyde rarely causes respiratory depression.

(v) Thiopentone. This drug may rarely cause laryngospasm, depresses the conscious level and respiration, and should only be used when facilities for assisted ventilation are readily available. The initial loading dose is 5 mg/kg i.v. Then give 1–3 mg/kg/h, maintaining a maximum blood thiopentone concentration of 60–100 ml/l.

If after all the above endeavours, the fits are not controlled, you may have to paralyse as well as ventilate your patient. This will allow you to gain control of the situation. You should realise that the abnormal brain activity, which may still be continuing in your paralysed patient, is itself a cause of continuing neuronal damage. Attempts to control this, probably with a combination of phenytoin and chlormethiazole, should continue under continual EEG surveillance.

(2) Determining the cause.

    (i)   In patients with epilepsy, status may be caused by either a deficiency or, rarely, an excess of their anticonvulsants. Always do urgent anticonvulsant estimations to determine the patient's blood levels.

    (ii)   If status is the first manifestation of seizures, a tumour is often present, and a CT scan should be performed.

    (iii) Hypoglycaemia (p. 183) hypocalcaemia (p. 196), hypomagnesaemia, hypoxia and hyponatraemia may provoke seizures. Hyponatraemic seizures are best treated by an initial infusion of 50 ml of 29.2% saline, repeated thereafter at a rate designed to raise the serum sodium by 3 mmol/h.[4] To monitor these problems, you will need to do BM stix, blood glucose, plasma calcium, electrolytes and urea, and arterial blood gases.

(3) After the fits have been controlled.

    (i)   Examine the patient including the mouth carefully, as injuries during the fits are common.

    (ii)   Then allow the sleep which occurs after fits to continue.

    (iii) Initiate maintenance therapy with one of the major anticonvulsants such as carbamazepine or phenytoin: i.v. phenytoin may be given as a loading dose as above (never give it by i.m. injection as it is absorbed erratically).

(4) Pseudostatus. Just occasionally, patients who present with apparent status in fact have pseudostatus epilepticus, a condition mimicking status, but in which the seizures are psychogenic. These patients usually have a long history of bizarre behaviour, normal EEGs and abnormal response to anticonvulsants. It is usually clear that consciousness is preserved during the attacks, and there is often vocalisation and odd behaviour. A sympathetic approach, in conjunction with your psychiatric colleagues, is the best treatment. You must clearly avoid the hazards of additive anticonvulsant therapy.[2]

REFERENCES

1   Greenblatt D. J., Shader R. I., *et al.* (1983) Current status of the benzodiazepines. *N. Engl. J. Med.* **309:** 354.

2   Leader (1989) Pseudostatus epilepticus. *Lancet* **ii:** 485.
3   Ward C. (1987) Status epilepticus. *Hospital Update* March, p. 190.
4   Worthley L., Thomas P. (1986) Treatment of hyponatraemic seizures with intravenous 29.2% saline. *Br. Med. J.* **292:** 168.

Spinal cord compression

DIAGNOSIS

(1) The diagnosis may be suggested by a history of back pain, paraparesis, sensory loss and incontinence, associated with paraesthesiae or root pain brought on or exacerbated by movement. Physical examination may establish a sensory motor, or reflex level which is a guide to the level of compression.

(2) Sudden cord lesion in the absence of trauma may be caused by either intramedullary or extramedullary pathology. While the attempt to distinguish the two is an interesting clinical exercise, the conclusions are frequently wrong particularly when the onset of symptoms is acute. The distinction is made by MRI or myelography, one of which should be performed immediately (see below).

Clinical points we have found useful include:

(i) well-localised spinal tenderness, as revealed by percussion, suggests epidural abscess;

(ii) previous and remote neurological episodes, e.g. retrobulbar neuritis, suggests demyelinating disease;

(iii) a previous and ill-advised lumbar puncture performed in a patient with deranged coagulation suggests extradural haematoma;

(iv) extradural tumours are most commonly metastatic. The primary site should always be looked for.

MANAGEMENT

Cord compression sufficient to cause symptoms and signs for more than a few hours causes irreversible cord damage, and is therefore a medical emergency. Your neurosurgical colleagues should be consulted as soon as the diagnosis is suspected and investigations carried out in conjunction with them. X-ray of the spine may reveal erosion of pedicles or vertebral bodies suggesting extradural lesions, but myelography, or increasingly MRI, will be required for definitive diagnosis.

Acute ascending polyneuritis[5]

DIAGNOSIS

(1) The diagnosis is made from a characteristic history of onset of weakness which involves first the legs, then the arms and may spread to involve the bulbar muscles, face and respiratory muscles, although this sequence may be reversed. Symptoms often start 5–12 days after a mild virus or bacterial infection, an operation or vaccination, and progresses rapidly to peak within 3 weeks. Commonly, weakness may be preceded by paraesthesiae and mild sensory loss. Sometimes muscle tenderness is also present. Deep tendon reflexes become absent.

(2) Differentiation is from other causes of acute weakness.[2]

    (i)   Acute poliomyelitis. The paralysis, which is nearly always asymmetrical and confined within muscle groups, is generally preceded by mild meningitic symptoms by 3–4 days. In addition, sensory signs are never found in 'polio'.

    (ii)   Other causes of acute polyneuritis are distinguished by examination or simple tests. These may be either

        (a) axonal (e.g. drugs and porphyria);
        (b) demyelinating (e.g. diphtheria);
        (c) inflammatory (e.g. the vasculitides);
        (d) toxic-botulism causes generalised weakness but the onset is typically ocular bulbar, and characteristically associated with severe constipation.

    (iii)   Focal cord lesions, such as cauda equina compression or a myelopathy. These will give you a clear motor, reflex or sensory level. Sensory loss may first occur in the sacral region, which you must therefore examine carefully.

    (iv)   Myasthenia (see p. 233).

    (vii)   Acute myopathies.

    (viii) Tick paralysis is an important consideration in some countries, including the USA and Australia. The less accessible parts of the anatomy should be carefully searched since removal of the offending tick is followed by dramatic return of power.

(ix) A similar syndrome occurs in association with Lyme disease (see p. 300). However, there is often a mild pleo-cytosis in the CSF, which should alert you to the real diagnosis. Serological tests will confirm your suspicion.

(3) Cerebrospinal fluid usually contains a raised protein and normal cell count at some stage of the illness but may be normal initially. A urine VMA should always be performed in children because of the association with neuroblastoma. Nerve conduction velocities are significantly slowed at least in some portions of the nerves (since this is a disease of segmental demyelination), and may be undertaken to confirm the diagnosis.

MANAGEMENT

(1) Steroids and plasma exchange. Steroids seem to confer no benefit.[3] In two recent well-controlled trials, plasma exchange was shown to speed recovery, and should be used as early as possible in the course of the illness.[1,4] A satisfactory method of performing this exchange consists of removing roughly one plasma volume/exchange (that is, 40–50 ml/kg) for five exchanges over 7–14 days. Additional management is entirely supportive, artificial ventilation being indicated urgently if paralysis of intercostal muscles or the diaphragm occurs. This happens in about a quarter of all patients during the first 3 weeks of the illness.

(2) Intravenous immune globulin. There is recent evidence that immune globulin is as effective as plasma exchange in speeding recovery. The suggested dose is 0.4 g/kg daily for 5 days, starting as soon as possible after diagnosis.[6] We await further confirmation of the efficacy of this approach.

(3) The power of the respiratory muscles may be assessed clini-cally in the first instance by asking the patient to count in exhalation. The patient takes a maximal inspiration, and begins to count off seconds from a clock until he is forced to take another breath. Power is impaired if the patient cannot go beyond 15 s. While respiration is jeopardised this test should be performed hourly. Serial measurements of vital

capacity should be made at 2-hourly intervals. Most authorities would now recommend elective ventilation if the vital capacity falls to a litre (in an adult).

(4) You should measure the arterial blood gases, but even if they are normal, do not be complacent, as respiratory failure can occur very rapidly with little previous distress or deterioration in the counting ability or the blood gases. Equipment for endotracheal intubation should be at hand—together with a ventilator (preferably out of sight).

(5) Respiratory embarrassment may also occur if bulbar paralysis is unrecognised. Nasal secretions and saliva accumulate in the pharynx, and intubation followed by tracheostomy with a cuffed tube may be required in order to protect the airway.

(6) Autonomic disturbances, such as gastrointestinal stasis, arrhythmias, spontaneous fluctuation of the blood pressure and pulse rate may occur—hence the need for meticulous ECG monitoring required in these patients. Acute bradyarrhythmias contribute a major share of the mortality. If these, or dropped beats, occur, a transvenous cardiac pacemaker should be passed as a matter of urgency.

(7) Full recovery of muscular function often occurs after total paralysis. The main factor influencing survival is meticulous and full nursing care with special attention to tracheostomy toilet, prevention of bed sores, muscle contractures, wrist and foot drop and evacuation of bowels and bladder. Regular suppositories and an in-dwelling bladder catheter may be necessary.

(8) There is a grave danger of pulmonary emboli developing in these patients. Start s.c. heparin as soon as possible (see p. 18) plus TD stockings and passive physiotherapy.

REFERENCES

1 Behan P. (1987) Plasma exchange in neurological diseases. *Br. Med. J.* **295:** 283.

2 Cros D. (1990) Guillain–Barré syndrome—a severe variant. *N. Engl. J. Med.* **323:** 895.

3 Hughes R. A. C., Newsom-Davis J. M., Perkin G. D. *et al.* (1978) Controlled trial of prednisolone in acute polyneuropathy. *Lancet* **2:** 750.

4   Hughes R. A. C. (1985) Plasma exchange for Guillain–Barré syndrome. *Br. Med. J.* **291:** 615.
5   Leader (1988) Guillain–Barré syndrome. *Lancet* **ii:** 65.
6   Ropper A. (1992) The Guillain–Barré syndrome. *New Engl. J. Med.* **326:** 1130.

Myasthenia gravis[3]

DIAGNOSIS

(1) The diagnosis is made from a history of characteristic weakness after continued exertion, without the associated muscle pain of physiological fatigue. In mild cases, power is normal after a period of rest, but then declines abnormally quickly on exercise. In more severe cases weakness is constant. The weakness may be generalised or confined to particular groups of muscles, e.g. the extraocular muscles or bulbar muscles. The onset of easy fatiguability is usually insidious—occurring only at the end of the day—but occasionally it is acute. Fatiguability is demonstrated by continued use of specific muscles for a short period of time. There is no sensory loss and the reflexes are nearly always preserved.

(2) The anti-acetylcholine receptor antibody, present in 90% of cases, is specific to myasthenia. If this is not available, or is negative in patients strongly suspected of having myasthenia, the diagnosis may be confirmed by the Tensilon test, which should always be performed with an assistant and resuscitative facilities at hand. Decide which muscle groups are weakest. Choose the three most evident and also measure the forced vital capacity (FVC). Give edrophonium (Tensilon) 2 mg i.v. stat., preceded by 0.6 mg of atropine, and if there is no sweating, salivation, lachrimation, colic or muscle fasciculation during the next minute give a further 8 mg i.v. Re-assess the three muscle groups and re-measure the FVC within the next minute. The effect is rapid and short-lived, so you have to observe the patient closely. Frequently the response is equivocal—some muscle groups responding dramatically and others not at all. If the overall response is indecisive repeat the test later in the day and try to gauge the general trend. If there is still genuine doubt, the effect of Tensilon on the motor response to repetitive nerve stimulation can be studied. If any unpleasant cholinergic side-effects occur during the test, they may be aborted by atropine 1.0 mg i.v.

MANAGEMENT

(1) Start pyridostigmine (Mestinon) 30 mg every 6 h, and gradually increase to 30 mg 3-hourly, then 60 mg 3-hourly up to 120 mg 3-hourly, the dose being adjusted to provide maximum response without side effects. Oral, subcutaneous and intramuscular preparations are available as necessary.

(2) If swallowing is affected, place a nasogastric tube for feeding and drug and food administration.

(3) Steroids, azathioprine, plasma exchange, cyclosporin and thymectomy have been advocated by some in the early stages of the disease—consult your local neurologist about these.[2]

Myasthenic crisis (too little treatment)

DIAGNOSIS

The myasthenic crisis is an exacerbation of weakness which most often occurs in an already diagnosed myasthenic patient. It is less frequent than formerly, now that treatment regimes are based on immunosuppression rather than anticholinesterases. However, it may occur in a previously undiagnosed patient, being precipitated by stress, emotion, infection or trauma, or by drugs which block neuromuscular transmission,[1] e.g. streptomycin, gentamicin, kanamycin and clindamycin. Anaesthetists are fully conversant with the prolonged action of suxamethonium or curare in these patients.

Management

Give edrophonium (Tensilon) as outlined above (see p. 233). An immediate improvement in muscle power indicates that the patient requires further anticholinesterase therapy, in addition to any other therapy he or she may already be receiving. Therefore, proceed as outlined for management of myasthenia. While pyridostigmine is taking effect it may be necessary to support respiration with a ventilator. Occasionally severe weakness requiring ventilatory support persists despite maximal therapy. In this situation plasmapheresis may be life-saving, and should be used urgently if response to anticholinesterases is inadequate.

Cholinergic crisis (too much treatment)

DIAGNOSIS

(1) Cholinergic crisis is precipitated by excessive anticholinesterases. It occurs typically ½–2 h after the previous dose.

(2) The initial warning symptoms and signs are colic, sweating,
salivation and fasciculation. These symptoms are sufficiently
clear and drug-related for it to be extremely rare for further
progression to develop. However, deliberate over-adminis-
tration may proceed via nervousness, drowsiness and confusion to ataxia, dysarthria, hypertension and bradycardia
culminating in coma, which may be interrupted by convulsions, and finally death. The warning signs may be masked if
atropine or atropine-like drugs are given with the anticholinesterases. Helpful physical signs may be small pupils (less than
3 mm in diameter) and fasciculation which persists to a late
stage.

(3) It is obviously crucial to distinguish a cholinergic crisis from a
myasthenic crisis, which is the commonest cause of acute
weakness in a myasthenic patient. If there is still doubt after
the history and examination give edrophonium (Tensilon)
2 mg i.v. with a ventilator at hand. If there is objective
improvement, the weakness is due to a myasthenic crisis. If
there is no response or a deterioration the diagnosis is a
cholinergic crisis.

Management

(1) Stop pyridostigmine and any other anticholinesterases.

(2) Give atropine sulphate 0.6 mg i.v ½-hourly to a maximum of
8 mg.

(3) Maintain respiration. If acute respiratory failure occurs the
patient is ventilated in the usual way. If acute respiratory
failure has not occurred the power of the respiratory muscles
may be assessed clinically by having the patient count in
exhalation and measuring the vital capacity (see p. 230). This
should be done hourly. In addition the blood gases should be

measured regularly (the $Paco_2$ should be checked at least 6-hourly) and should also be done immediately if any deterioration of the counting test occurs.

(4) Reformation of cholinesterase should be assessed by response to the edrophonium test, which should be performed 2-hourly until a positive response of increase in muscle power occurs. At this point a small dose of oral pyridostigmine (e.g. 30 mg) should be tried.

REFERENCES

1   Argov Z. (1979) Disorders of neuromuscular transmission caused by drugs. *N. Engl. J. Med.* **301:** 409.
2   Drachman D. B. (1987) Present and future treatment of myasthenia gravis. *N. Engl. J. Med.* **316:** 743.
3   Scadding G. K., Harvard G. W. H. (1981) Pathogenesis and treatment of myasthenia gravis. *Br. Med. J.* **2:** 1008.

Generalised tetanus[4]

DIAGNOSIS

(1) The typical case is entirely characteristic and quite unforget-
table. The history is of dysphagia and stiffness and pain in the
muscles of the neck, back and abdominal wall. The stiffness
often occurs first in the facial muscles, leading to trismus
(lockjaw) and risus sardonicus. Examination reveals hyper-
tonia, usually greater in the extended legs than in the arms,
together with painless trismus. In all but the milder cases the
rigid posture is interrupted by paroxysms in which extension
of the back, neck and legs and flexion of the shoulders and
elbows is accompanied by the characteristic grimaces. These
last up to 20 s and are painful. The increase in tone persists
between paroxysms, thus distinguishing tetanus from strych-
nine poisoning and rabies. If the time between the onset of
the first symptom and the first spasm is no more than a few
hours, a severe course is likely. In such circumstances, the
disease usually peaks within 4–5 days, plateaus for a similar
period, and wanes over the ensuing month or so.

(2) The attack may be modified by previous immunisation—the
spasm remaining localised to the site of infection.

(3) The site of entry should be sought. Apart from obvious
puncture wounds and infected umbilical stumps, this includes
ruptured tympanic membranes usually associated with an ear
discharge. Before treatment is instituted, the patient should
be watched for a period of 10–15 min while he or she is lying
relaxed in a quiet and darkened room. This, combined with
your other observations, will enable you to categorise your
patient—this in its turn gives you a general guideline as to
how intensive your treatment will need to be. The categories
are outlined below.

Grade 1: Mild increase in tone, but no dyspnoea or respiratory
difficulty. Sedation will probably suffice in this group.

Grade 2: More pronounced increase in tone, with some impairment
of breathing or swallowing, but with no generalised spasms. Here,
tracheostomy as well as sedation may be needed.

Grade 3: Any patient with generalised spasms will require curarisation and artificial ventilation. In Britain, most cases fall into this category. Your initial observations will also provide a baseline upon which the effects of treatment may be assessed.

MANAGEMENT

Management of these cases involves the following aspects:

(1) Suppressing the organism and its toxin.

   (i) Give human tetanus immunoglobulin (Humotet 100 i.u./ kg intramuscularly (**never** intravenously)—a previous test dose being unnecessary. In the event of unavailability of human immunoglobulins, you should still give the heterologous anti-tetanus serum (ATS). Give 0.2 ml as a test dose, and if there is no reaction within ½ h, give 5000 units of ATS i.m. Intrathecal human tetanus immunoglobulin has been shown to be of benefit if given in early tetanus. The dose is 250 i.u. instilled intrathecally.[3]

   (ii) Antibiotics. Metronidazole 500 mg orally, or 1.0 g rectally 8-hourly, has recently been shown to be more effective than the traditional benzyl penicillin 1 megaunit 6-hourly.[1]

   (iii) Excise all dead tissues surrounding the wound (if any) not less than 1 h after the patient has been protected by ATS and metronidazole. The wound is kept open and irrigated with hydrogen peroxide (or 1 × 4000 potassium permanganate solution) three times a day.

(2) Treating increase in tone. If the patient is developing rigidity, alternate chlorpromazine 0.5 mg/kg and phenobarbitone 1.0 mg/kg 3-hourly. It is usually necessary to give these intravenously. The aim is to achieve a state of light sleep for most of the time. If this regime is ineffective add diazepam 0.2 mg/kg i.v. or diazemuls repeated 4-hourly as necessary or as a continuous infusion (see p. 224) of 3–10 mg/kg/day, or meprobamate 400 mg orally every 4 h. Remember that patients with rigidity have increased fluid and calorie requirements. If these drugs in combination do not produce relaxation, curarisation and artificial ventilation (IPPR) are indicated (see below).

(3) Treating spasms. Spasms are painful and dangerous as they may cause hypoxia and crush fractures of the spine and must

be controlled by curarisation and IPPR.[2] Spasms occur in response to a stimulus. This may be a distended bladder, faecal impaction or bronchial mucus and effective control of spasms may be secured by eliminating these stimuli rather than by increasing the dose of drugs. Swallowing also may precipitate spasms. For this reason, if the disease is likely to be severe (the shorter the incubation period, which may vary from 1 day to several months, the more severe the disease is likely to be) a nasogastric tube should be passed early rather than late. While close attention to care is important, intervention must be kept to an absolute minimum. The single spasm which needs to be treated urgently—for example, laryngospasm—may respond to chlorpromazine 100 mg i.v.

Thus, to summarise, curarisation and IPPR are indicated:

(1) If increase in tone is uncontrolled and makes breathing difficult.
(2) If laryngospasm occurs. *This is an absolute indication*. Laryngospasm may be precipitated by attempts to pass a nasogastric or endotracheal tube and these procedures should not be attempted in the interval between the first episode of laryngospasm and the ensuing tracheostomy.
(3) In every patient who has generalised spasm. Complete muscle relaxation and IPPR may necessitate transfer to a specialised unit, for the chances of a successful outcome depend largely on meticulous and intensive nursing care which may be necessary for 6 weeks or more. To the usual hazards of this sort of treatment are added other more specific complications to which patients with tetanus are especially liable, e.g. hyperpyrexia and bacterial shock, autonomic imbalance and arrhythmias. If these autonomic disturbances occur, they are probably best treated with small doses of labetolol, a short-acting agent which has some alpha as well as beta activity. In addition, heavy sedation as well as paralysis is probably beneficial.

REFERENCES

1   Ahmadsyah I., Salim A. (1985) Treatment of tetanus: an open study to compare the efficacy of procaine penicillin and metronidazole. *Br. Med. J.* **291**: 648.

2 Edmondson R. S., Flowers M. W. (1979) Intensive care in tetanus: management, complications and mortality in 100 cases. *Br. Med. J.* **1**: 1401.
3 Leader (1980) Tetanus immune globulus: the intrathecal route. *Lancet* **2**: 464.
4 Weinstein L. (1973) Tetanus. *N. Engl. J. Med.* **289**: 1293.

Brain death

The advent of prolonged ventilation has given rise to a group of patients with brain death. The non-functioning brainstem is followed, usually within a few days, by asystole, despite continued ventilation. Thus, given certain vital pre-requisites, a patient with a non-functioning brainstem can be certified as dead. This is an important diagnosis for two reasons.

(1) It allows ventilation to be discontinued, and thus minimises distress to relatives and carers.
(2) It allows organ donation to proceed.

The diagnosis of brain death cannot be considered until certain conditions have been excluded.

(1) Intoxication with narcotics, hypnotics or tranquillisers. This entails a specific enquiry and, if necessary, a full drug screen. Since there is insufficient knowledge about the effects of therapeutic concentrations of phenobarbitone (when used as an anticonvulsant) when associated with brain injury, the assessment of brainstem function for the diagnosis of brain death should be deferred until blood levels of phenobarbitone are below 10 mg/l, the lower limit of the therapeutic range.
(2) Hypothermia. The core (rectal) temperature should be more than 35° C.
(3) Action of relaxants—neuromuscular blocking agents. If in doubt—for example, following operation—this can be excluded by finding deep tendon reflexes, spinal withdrawal reflexes or by using a peripheral nerve stimulator.

In addition the cause of the patient's state must be known. This means both:

(1) excluding metabolic disturbances. Measurement of electrolytes (including Ca^{2+}) and urea, blood glucose and blood gases, including pH; and
(2) that there should be a positive diagnosis of a disorder which can cause irreversible damage. When severe trauma or major intracerebral haemorrhage has occurred, tests for brain death need not be delayed. However, when brain death is suspected

after severe hypoxia, cardiac arrest or cerebral or fat embolism it is prudent to wait for 24 h before making the first assessment.

DIAGNOSIS

The diagnosis should be made by two consultants or a consultant and senior registrar (at least 5 years post registration) with expertise in the field working either together or separately. Needless to say, neither should belong to a transplant team if organ donation is anticipated. The tests should be carried out twice with the interval between being adequate for the reassurance of all directly concerned.
The tests are as follows.

(1) Absent verbal response, spontaneous movements and pupillary light reflex. The pupils may be either mid-point or dilated. The essential factor is that they are unreactive to light.
(2) Absent corneal reflex.
(3) Absent oculo-cephalic reflex (see p. 358).
(4) Absent vestibulo-ocular reflex (see p. 358). Any wax obscuring the eardrum must first be removed. Then slowly instill 20 ml of ice-cold water into the external auditory canal. No eye movement (or other response) should occur. If the drum is obscured by local trauma this test can be omitted but the diagnosis of brain death can still be made if all the other conditions are fulfilled.
(5) No gag or cough reflex on stimulation by catheter of the pharynx or trachea, respectively.
(6) No reaction to a noxious stimulus in the area of distribution of the cranial nerves. This may be conveniently applied by firm supraorbital pressure.
(7) No ventilatory response to hypercarbia. This is most conveniently assessed by ventilating the patient with pure oxygen for 10 min followed by 5% CO_2 in O_2 for 5 min. The patient is disconnected from the ventilator and observed for 10 min while delivering oxygen at 6 l/min by catheter into the endotracheal tube. This procedure will ensure that the Pa_{CO_2} will be at least 6.65 kPa while the patient is not exposed to additional hypoxia. If the patient has previous chronic respiratory failure and may normally exist on hypoxic drive, expert

advice should be sought and the test carried out with careful blood gas analysis.

A checklist of these reflexes with recorded response is a useful aide memoire and entry for the notes. Provided all these conditions are fulfilled:

(1) other tests such as an EEG or arteriography are unnecessary and may only confuse distressed relatives.
(2) the decision to withdraw ventilation can be taken. The timing of this becomes increasingly irrelevant provided that all those concerned with the patient appreciate that he or she is already dead. In one institution it is the practice to issue a death certificate at this stage—while the patient is still being ventilated—in order to drive the point home. The timing must be balanced between unseemly haste and subsequent recrimination on the one hand and the needless prolongation of relatives' uncertainty and suffering on the other.

REFERENCES

1   Pallis P. (1982–) ABC of brainstem death. (Series of articles: the first in *Br. Med. J.* **285:** 1409.)

Sickle cell anaemia

Sickle cell anaemia[1]

Sickle cell crisis does not occur in AS genotypes; it may be found in mixed haemoglobinopathies, such as SC disease or S thalassaemia but more commonly it occurs in the homozygous sickle cell genotype. Distribution of the disease is throughout West and Central Africa, the West Indies and North America, and the Mediterranean littoral; your patient will probably come from one of these areas. The disease is well recognised in its indigenous areas, and indeed may account for some of the ancient African myths.[3]

The basic problem is that deoxygenated haemoglobin tends to form gel precipitates in the red cell, causing them to sickle. Sickling is not necessarily irreversible, but the sickle cell is more sensitive to haemolysis, has a short life and, by increasing the viscosity of the blood, decreases flow in capillaries and small arterioles. People suffering from sickle cell disease spend large portions of their life in a stable state, with mean haemoglobins of 9.0 g/100 ml. A crisis can be defined as a sharp turn or definite change in the course of the disease, with development of new signs and symptoms.

Whatever the nature of the crisis, it is usually provoked by some stress, often an infection. This may be a urinary tract infection, diarrhoea and vomiting, pneumonia, or, in the tropics, malaria. Other provoking factors are exposure to cold, anaesthesia, operations and pregnancy.

Five patterns of sickle cell crisis are described.

(1) Vaso-occlusive (the commonest type).[2] Here hyperviscosity causes sludging, stasis and infarction of the involved tissue. The symptoms are of a sudden onset of excruciating pain, often widespread, but most intense in one specific area. The commonest sites are the lumbosacral spine, chest, large joints and abdomen, where an intra-abdominal surgical crisis may be simulated. Because of the pain, your patient may be in agony. There may be widespread muscle and bone tenderness, an anaemia, a mild fever and the white cell count is often raised to 20 000–60 000, even in the absence of infection. There may be a mild unconjugated hyperbilirubinaemia.

(2) Haemolytic crisis. Intravascular hypoxia causes a massive

haemolysis. There will be profound anaemia (Hb 3–4 g/100 ml) and other features of haemolysis such as reticulocytosis, low haptoglobin levels and a raised indirect bilirubin.

(3) Sequestration syndrome. In this situation there is a sudden massive painful enlargement of the liver and spleen, probably on the basis of vaso-occlusive ischaemic damage to these organs. There is an acute fall in PCV, and haemoglobin often falls to 2–3 g/100 ml. This type of crisis is restricted to children and pregnant women, and presents as cardiovascular collapse.

(4) Reticulocytopenic ('aplastic') crisis. Transient cessation of red cell production, usually caused by parvovirus infection,[5] may precipitate profound anaemia. Unlike the haemolytic crisis, the reticulocyte count will be reduced. This type of crisis again usually occurs in children.

(5) Megaloblastic crisis. Severe anaemia or pancytopenia may be precipitated by an inadequate intake of folic acid; daily requirement is greatly increased in haemolytic disorders.

Patients often have features of more than one of the above groups.

There is, at present, no effective specific treatment which reverses sickling, although many remedies are being tried. The outcome of the sickle crisis largely depends on effective treatment of the underlying cause, which must be diligently sought.

TREATMENT

Take blood for FBP, a sickling screening test, blood gases, liver function tests, electrolytes and urea. Do blood and urine cultures and where appropriate viral studies. Do an MSU and stool culture if there is diarrhoea. Do a chest x-ray and an ECG.

(1) The results of your history, examination and of the above tests should allow you to determine the underlying cause of the particular episode of crisis. This must be treated on its merits. If your patient is febrile, or there is other reason to suspect infection, give a broad spectrum antibiotic such as amoxycillin 250 mg 8-hourly because of the frequent association of crisis and infection. You should also keep your patient warm.

(2) Rehydration. These patients are often fluid-depleted, a factor which increases blood viscosity and thus hypoperfusion.

Appropriate fluid, usually a mixture of 0.9% N saline and 5% dextrose should be infused, under CVP control if necessary, until the patient is adequately perfused. The specific fluids you infuse will depend on the problem provoking the illness, and also on the results of your initial serum electrolytes.

(3) Acidosis. Acidosis may be associated with a crisis, probably due to poor tissue perfusion. Acidosis also exacerbates sickling—thus it seems logical to reverse any acidosis present by giving $NaHCO_3$ as part of the infusion fluid, in amounts which you can calculate from the formula on p. 342.

(4) Oxygen. Hypoxia also aggravates sickling and if the Pao_2 is less than 80 mmHg (kPa), it is reasonable to give 100% oxygen by face mask to correct this. Hyperbaric oxygen has been tried without success.

(5) Pain relief. The pain of crisis is severe and requires appropriate analgesics, which you should not under any circumstances withhold. Opiates (morphine 10 mg or diamorphine 5 mg i.m. are now preferred to pethidine) are often necessary. For lesser degrees of pain, first try simpler analgesics, such as aspirin (or one of the more recently developed non-steroidal anti-inflammatories) and paracetamol. Patient-controlled analgesic regimes are being used in some places, and we encourage this initiative, as there are still all too frequent reports of inadequate pain control in patients with sickle crisis.

(6) Correction of anaemia. As mentioned above, 'sicklers' usually live with an Hb of around 9.0 g/100 ml. Unless there is profound anaemia (Hb<6.0 g/100 ml) transfusion is unnecessary to raise the haemoglobin. However, partial exchange transfusions to replace some of the sickle cell haemoglobin have been suggested as a mode of treatment. There is no convincing evidence for its efficacy, but in desperate circumstances it is worth trying.

(7) The acute chest syndrome. This is a particularly serious complication of sickle disease, due to a combination of pulmonary infarction and infection. It is, at least in Jamaica, the commonest cause of death in sicklers.[6] In the face of pronounced hypoxia, you may need to ventilate these patients. Urgent exchange transfusion is very important, and should be undertaken as soon as possible.

(8) Specific anti-sickling drugs as therapeutic agents. Advances in understanding of the theoretical basis of sickling have made possible several specific therapeutic approaches. So far none

has been proven effective. However, as many of these treatments had been advocated, we feel that a brief survey of the mechanism and agents used is warranted, if only to warn against undue optimism. Agents tried so far are:

(i)   compounds that prevent sickling by inhibiting intracellular gelation (gelation inhibitors), such as urea, dichloromethane gas, dimethyladipimidate and piracetam;

(ii) compounds which inhibit sickling independently of gelation—oral zinc cyanates; cysteamine therapy is said to be beneficial in the prevention of painful crisis. We do not think that there is presently enough evidence to justify the use of any of these compounds.

(9) Pregnancy. A recent trial has shown no difference in perinatal outcome in a group of women sicklers given exchange transfusions through pregnancy.[4]

REFERENCES

1   Alavi J. B. (1984) Sickle cell anaemia—pathology and treatment. *Med. Clin. North Am.* **68:** 545.

2   Davies S. (1991) The vaso-occlusive crisis of sickle cell disease. *Br. Med. J.* **302:** 1551.

3   Onwubalili J. K. (1983) Sickle-cell anaemia: an explanation for the ancient myth of reincarnation in Nigeria. *Lancet* **ii:** 503.

4   Platt O. (1988) Is there treatment for sickle cell anaemia? *N. Engl. J. Med.* **319:** 1479.

5   Serjeant G. R. *et al.* (1981) Outbreak of aplastic crisis in sickle cell anaemia associated with parvovirus like agents. *Lancet* **ii:** 595.

6   Thomas A. (1982) Causes of death in sickle-cell disease in Jamaica. *Br. Med. J.* **285:** 633.

The overdose

The overdose: general management[1,4,6]

DIAGNOSIS

(1) The majority of patients attending the accident and emergency department following an episode of self poisoning are sufficiently coherent to tell you what the problem is, and indeed what they have taken. In an unconscious or uncooperative patient, the diagnosis usually rests on circumstantial or third party evidence. It is therefore important to interview relatives, ambulance men or other patient advocates, and to contact the patient's family doctor as soon as possible.

(2) Overdose must be considered in any comatose patient.

(3) The effects may include:

(i) impairment of consciousness;
(ii) respiratory and cardiovascular depression;
(iii) dehydration;
(iv) hypothermia;
(v) convulsions.
(vi) cardiac arrhythmias.

MANAGEMENT

Management does not depend at the onset on the precise identification of the drugs involved. Measures in order of priority are as follows.

(1) Clear and maintain an airway. Remove teeth, food, secretions etc., and, if necessary, insert an airway.

(2) Maintain respiration. The immediate need for assisted ventilation has to be assessed clinically but the efficiency of ventilation can only be gauged by measuring the blood gases. Retention of carbon dioxide—$Paco_2 > 6$ kPa (45 mm/Hg)—and hypoxia—$Pao_2 < 9.3$ kPa (70 mmHg)—despite oxygen being given by an MC face mask, are indications for artificial ventilation. It is unusual for a patient with a minute volume of >4l measured with a Wright spirometer to require ventila-

tion. Remember that ventilatory function may fluctuate and can deteriorate suddenly. Always remember too that your patient may have inhaled stomach contents if his or her protective airways reflexes have been lost (see p. 101).

(3) Maintenance of arterial pressure. Hypotension in the context of acute poisoning is defined as a systolic pressure of below 85 mmHg in patients under the age of 40, and below 90 mmHg in those above 40. If hypotension so defined, or adequate tissue perfusion, is not maintained:

  (i) Put up a central venous pressure line and infuse plasma expanders and normal saline in the usual way (see p. 338) until the CVP is in the upper range of normal. If this does not restore tissue perfusion, raise the systolic arterial pressure to above 90 mmHg by:

  (ii) Dopamine and/or dobutamine, or failing these, isoprenaline (see p. 340 for dosage of both these, and the section on the hypotensive patient for a more detailed account of the pathogenesis and management of shock in overdose patients).

(4) Treat arrhythmias as necessary. Serious arrhythmias are uncommon in acute poisoning. Conduction defects only require pacemaker insertion if they are compromising the circulation; likewise, other arrhythmias only need treatment if they are compromising the circulation (see p. 26).

(5) Correct hypothermia (see p. 289).

(6) Convulsions may complicate poisoning with a wide variety of substances, either through a direct toxic effect, or hypoxia. The most important of these are tricyclic antidepressants, mefanamic acid, dextropropoxyphene, propranolol and theophylline. Unless the fits are protracted, or recurrent, it is probably best not to treat them. Treatment, when required, should be along conventional lines (see p. 224).

(7) General nursing care of the unconscious patient (see p. 361).

(8) Take blood and store this for subsequent drug analysis. There are only a few circumstances where urgent blood levels are helpful: paracetamol, a level of which should be taken in all patients with impaired consciousness following acute poisoning; iron; salicylates; lithium; barbiturates and other hypnotics; paraquat; methanol and ethylene glycol (see section on specific substances for further details).

(9) When all this has been instituted consider measures designed to remove the substance from the body.

   (i)   A stomach washout seems a logical measure in any patient who has taken a potentially toxic dose of poison. However, it is unproductive if performed more than 4 h after the tablets have been taken, except in poisoning due to salicylates, tricyclic antidepressants, carbamazepine and barbiturates, when it is worth doing up to 12 h after the overdose. If the patient is conscious, consent for this procedure must be obtained and if he or she persists in withholding consent, so be it. It is dangerous to perform a stomach washout on the unconscious patient without having a cuffed endotracheal tube in place. Put the patient in the head-down position and pass a well lubricated 30–40 French gauge orogastric tube into the stomach (it is virtually impossible to pass a large bore tube directly into the trachea). Aspirate the stomach contents and introduce 250 ml of luke-warm water. Leave 2–3 min and then re-aspirate. Repeat this procedure until 2 litres have been used, or until the lavage fluid is clear. If laryngeal spasm occurs during gastric lavage, some inhalation of stomach contents has probably occurred. In this case aspirate the remainder of the stomach contents and withdraw the tube. If serious inhalation of stomach contents occurs, institute suction, give hydrocortisone 200 mg i.v., oxygen as necessary, broad spectrum antibiotics, including one effective against anaerobes (see p. 102) and arrange for physiotherapy. Treat wheezing as for asthma (see p. 81). Gastric lavage should not be undertaken in any patient who has taken petroleum distillates, for fear of aspiration with subsequent pneumonitis. In patients who have taken corrosives, lavage should only be used if there is a serious danger of systemic effects developing, as in the case of formic acid and paraquat. Nasogastric aspiration may be safer in these circumstances.

   (ii)   Emesis. Some authorities now favour inducing emesis as an alternative to gastric lavage. Syrup of ipecacuanha certainly induces emesis, but there is no evidence that it helps,[7] and we do not use it, or any other emetic.

   (iii)   Activated charcoal is able to adsorb a wide variety of drugs and toxins. A single dose of 25–100 g will prevent the absorbtion of toxic material present in the gut at the time of its administration. Although it is not known whether it is helpful to combine it with gastric lavage, a common practice is to insert the charcoal into the stomach through the nasogastric tube with which you have just performed the lavage. Charcoal is most effective when given within 4 h of the episode of poisoning, except for tricyclics and aspirin, when it can be used up to 12 h after ingestion. Toxins which are poorly adsorbed by charcoal are:

(a) acids and alkalis;
(b) ethanol and methanol;
(c) ethylene glycol;
(d) iron and lithium;
and so it's not worth using where these are known to have been the only toxin ingested.

(iv) Repeated doses of activated charcoal, 50 g 4-hourly, given until your patient has recovered, probably aids elimination in patients severely poisoned with

    (a) aspirin,
    (b) carbamazepine,
    (c) cyclosporin,
    (d) dapsone,
    (e) digoxin,
    (f) meprobamate,
    (g) phenytoin,
    (h) piroxicam,
    (i) phenobarbitone
    (j) theophylline,
    (k) some sustained release preparations, such as tricyclics, and should be used in such patients in the hope that it will obviate the need for other more invasive treatment.[2]

Activated charcoal is a very safe treatment provided that your patient does not inhale any. Therefore make sure that the airway is protected before you give it.[5]

(10) As a general rule the above measures are all that is required in the management of overdoses. However, there are a few

specific occasions when something further can be done (no more than 5% of poisoning cases); these are discussed below and in ensuing sections (q.v.).

(11) Further ways of speeding elimination are:

(i) Forced diuresis, which may be worth doing in cases of poisoning due to the following:

(a) long-acting barbiturates, e.g. barbitone and phenobarbitone (see below);
(b) salicylates (see below);
(c) amphetamines and fenfluramine and phencyclidine, the excretion of which are promoted by an acid diuresis (although we have never seen this used in practice).

(ii) Haemoperfusion,[8] using a column containing activated charcoal or a resin is an efficient and safe method of removing short- and long-acting barbiturates, glutethimide, salicylates, and some other drugs from the body. It was formerly the treatment of choice for severely intoxicated patients who failed to respond to supportive measures, but now that repeat doses of activated charcoal have proved to be so effective, it is seldom used. The levels at which the procedure may be considered are:

(a) Phenobarbitone >100 mg/l
(b) Barbitone >100 mg/l
(c) Other barbiturates>50 mg/l
(d) Ethchlorvynol >150 mg/l
(e) Glutethimide >40 mg/l
(f) Methaquolone >40 mg/l
(g) Theophylline >60 mg/l
(h) Trichlorethanol derivatives >50 mg/l
(i) Salicylates >100 mg/l

(iii) Haemodialysis—this only removes substances which are water-soluble and which the kidney can likewise excrete. Effective forced diuresis is as efficient as haemodialysis which should therefore only be used if there is renal failure, if charcoal haemoperfusion or resin is not available, or in cases of lithium, ethylene glycol or methyl alcohol poisoning. In methyl alcohol poisoning you should use haemodialysis if there is a metabolic acidosis, neurological symptoms or signs, a blood concentration of >0.5 g/l, or proved ingestion of more than 30 g of methanol.

(iv) But, as we have mentioned above, there is increasing evidence that repeat doses of activated charcoal may be more effective than any of these manoeuvres and this treatment has in effect superseded them.[2]

(12) Naloxone.[3] This is a specific antidote for morphine and morphine-like compounds. It acts immediately (within 5 min) and its effect will be dramatic if your patient has taken an opiate or opiate derivative (including codeine, dextropropoxyphene and pentazocine). It will not do any harm if your patient turns out to have taken some other substance. Thus if there is uncertainty as to which drug has been taken in any overdose with poor perfusion and poor respiration, naloxone (1.2 mg–2.4 mg i.v. over 3 min) should be used both as a diagnostic and therapeutic agent. There may be an incomplete response to naloxone with some opiods, and in for instance pentazocine poisoning, large doses may be required. Also remember that most opiods have a longer duration of effect than naloxone, and so beware of a possible recurrence of coma and respiratory depression if only a single dose of naloxone has been given. Indeed you may need to give naloxone by continuous infusion. Make up 2 mg in 500 ml of saline (a concentration of 4 μg/ml), and titrate the dose you require according to the response of your patient.

(13) Flumazenil.[9] This is an effective benzodiazipine antagonist, when given in incremental doses of 0.5–1.0 mg. However, it is not presently licensed for use in overdoses, and given the lack of serious problems associated with benzodiazipine overdose, its use in these circumstances is, in our view, not justified.

Information as to the constituents of compounds and advice as to the management of their ingestion may be had from the following Poisons Information Centres:

Belfast:	Royal Victoria Hospital	Tel:0232 240503
Birmingham:	Dudley Road Hospital	Tel:021 554 3801
Cardiff:	Llandough Hospital	Tel:0222 709901
Dublin:	Beaumont Hospital	Tel:0103531 379966

Edinburgh:	Royal Infirmary	Tel:031 229 2477
Leeds:	General Infirmary	Tel:0532 430715
London:	New Cross Hospital	Tel:071 635 9191
Newcastle:	Royal Victoria Infirmary	Tel:091 232 1525

All these measures, complicated as they are, only constitute first aid and are relatively simple compared to the patient's problems on regaining consciousness.

REFERENCES

1   Henry J., Volans G. (1984) *ABC of Poisoning*. (A series of articles from *Br. Med. J.* published in book form.)
2   Leader (1987) Repeated oral activated charcoal in acute poisoning. *Lancet* **i**: 101.
3   Leader (1975) Naloxone. *Lancet* **i**: 734.
4   Mathew H. (1971) Acute poisoning: some myths and misconceptions. *Br. Med. J.* **1**: 519.
5   Menzies D. *et al.* (1988) Fatal pulmonary aspiration of oral activated charcoal. *Br. Med. J.* **297**: 459.
6   Prescott L. (1983) New approaches in managing drug overdosage and poisoning. *Br. Med. J.* **287**: 274.
7   Vale J. *et al.* (1986) Syrup of ipecacuanha: is it really useful? *Br. Med. J.* **293**: 1321.
8   Vale J. A., Rees A. J., Widdop B. *et al.* (1975) The use of charcoal haemoperfusion in the management of severely poisoned patients. *Br. Med. J.* **1**: 5.
9   Whitwam J. (1988) Flumanezil: a benzodiazepine antagonist. *Br. Med. J.* **297**: 999.

Salicylates[1]

The fatal dose in adults is 25 g but death can occur from the ingestion of lesser doses when there are other complicating factors, such as pre-existing disease. One aspirin tablet (BP) contains 300 mg of acetyl salicylic acid, but you should check the exact quantities in any tablet with a poisons information centre.

DIAGNOSIS

The patient is confused, restless, flushed, sweating, hyperventilating and complains of tinnitus. Coma is unusual unless a really massive and frequently fatal overdose has been absorbed. The following metabolic changes may be present.

(1) A hypokalaemic alkalosis caused by vomiting.
(2) A respiratory alkalosis (low $Paco_2$, high bicarbonate) caused by hyperventilation.
(3) A metabolic acidosis possibly caused by absorption of acid, dehydration and disturbed carbohydrate, lipid and protein metabolism.
(4) Dehydration, caused by hyperventilation, sweating, vomiting, reduced fluid intake, and an osmotic diuresis.
(5) Hypo- or hyperglycaemia.
(6) Pulmonary oedema—a hypersensitivity phenomenon which thus gives rise to the shock lung syndrome (see p. 97).

In young children (<12 years) the acidosis is likely to predominate; adults are nearly always alkalotic when first seen. The clinical state is due to combination of the direct effect of salicylates, dehydration and altered acid–base status.

MANAGEMENT

In salicylate poisoning, early measurement of blood levels is very useful. Some patients with high blood levels show little clinical evidence of it and yet are in great danger. Symptoms occur at about 1.9 mmol (300 mg)/l. Intoxication is reckoned as severe if the level is more than 3.1 mmol (500 mg)/l and a forced alkaline diuresis may then be indicated, although now that repeated doses of activated charcoal, a regime which is simple, safe and effective, is the treatment of choice, you will rarely have to use any other form of treatment (see p. 256). Charcoal haemoperfusion or, failing that, haemodialysis may be indicated if the level is more than 6.2 mmol (1000 mg)/l, or if more than 4.3 mmol (700 mg)/l and the level is rising rapidly, or if the patient is in coma, or if there is impairment of renal function. One value does not necessarily act as a guide to management. Far more useful are levels taken at regular intervals, e.g. every 6 h. Finally, do not rely on blood levels alone. The most important guide to the severity of the poisoning is the patient's condition. If it is bad and deteriorating despite the activated charcoal regime then further measures should be instituted whatever the salicylate level.

(1) Take blood for serum salicylate, haemoglobin and PCV, electrolytes and urea, arterial pH and $Paco_2$. Of these results, the arterial pH is needed first.

(2) A forced alkaline diuresis should be started if:

   (i)   the clinical condition is poor, i.e. the signs above are marked;

   (ii) the salicylate level is more than 1.9 mmol (300 mg)/l in children and more than 4.6 mmol (750 mg)/l in adults; or 3.1 mmol (500 mgm)/l in the presence of a metabolic acidosis;

   (iii) there is a history of ingestion of more than 50 tablets.

(3) Alkalinisation is unnecessary if the urine pH is already more than 8.5 and is dangerous if the arterial pH is more than 7.5. In either of these situations merely start a forced diuresis (see below). If the urine pH remains acid in the face of an apparent arterial alkalosis, there is usually intracellular potassium depletion. Until this is corrected by potassium supplements, it is difficult to achieve production of an alkaline urine.

(4) If the indications for forced diuresis are absent, simply observe the patient closely and encourage oral fluids.

(5) If pulmonary oedema occurs, manage as for shock lung (see p. 98).

FORCED DIURESIS—ALKALINE AND ACID

(1) Catheterise the bladder and keep the urine.

(2) Set up a central venous pressure line (see p. 381) and when it

reads within the normal range (you may have to give i.v. saline and dextrose to achieve this) assess the rate of urine flow.

(3) If the rate of urine flow is above 4 ml/min with the patient adequately perfused, you may start the forced diuresis; if the urine flow is less than this, give frusemide 20 mg i.v. If the frusemide produced a urine flow of greater than 4 ml/min it is safe to start the diuresis. If after the frusemide the urine flow is less than 4 ml/min, it is likely that renal insufficiency is present, and the diuresis should not be undertaken. If you consider it safe to carry out the diuresis, proceed in rotation with the following infusions:

1.26% NaHCO$_3$	—500 ml (90 mmol NaHCO$_3$)
5% dextrose	—500 ml
5% dextrose	—500 ml
0.9% N saline	—500 ml

Do not give the bicarbonate until the arterial pH is known. Give 1 litre of this regime each hour for 6 h, and 500 ml/h thereafter. Provided the patient was adequately perfused prior to starting the diuresis (which, as pointed out in (2) above, may require an initial infusion of up to 5 litres of N saline and 5% dextrose), urine output should approximate fluid input. If this is not the case, give i.v. frusemide, 20 mg as needed to keep up the urine output. If, after frusemide, the urinary output does not increase, or if the patient develops fluid overload, it is probable that a degree of renal impairment is present (but check that the urinary catheter is not blocked!). The diuresis should therefore be stopped, and charcoal haemoperfusion or haemodialysis considered. For a forced diuresis, rather than a forced alkaline diuresis, merely substitute 0.45 N saline for the 1.2% NaHCO$_3$ and proceed as above. To induce an acid diuresis, you should give 10 g of arginine or lysine hydrochloride i.v. over 30 min, and then give oral ammonium chloride 4 g 2-hourly as necessary to keep the urine pH between 5.5 and 6.5.

(4) Give K$^+$ 40 mmol with each litre of fluid to start with.
(5) Measure and chart:

    (i)   the total fluid input and the fluid output with a cumulative total every hour;

    (ii)   the central venous pressure every 30 min;

    (iii) the urine pH hourly (if possible on a pH meter, which is more accurate than the universal indicator strip)—

remember the achievement of an alkaline urine is more important than the high urine output, and you must act on the regular pH readings;

(iv) the urinary and blood electrolytes and urea, and the arterial pH and Paco$_2$ every 4 h;

(v) The serum salicylate every 6 h while the patient's condition is critical.

(6) Intensive monitoring is necessary because salicylate intoxication is one of the most complex metabolic states you will have to treat, and because a necessary forced diuresis, if not carefully watched, can be extremely dangerous. It follows therefore that the patient should be transferred to a centre where this is possible.

These measurements will allow for the following adjustments.

(i) Fluid (see above).

(ii) As soon as the urine pH is above 8, substitute 0.5 N saline for the bicarbonate.

(iii) If hyponatraemia develops, substitute N saline for one of the bottles of 5% dextrose.

(iv) Replace the measured potassium loss in the urine over 4 h at the end of which time re-measure and repeat the process.

(7) Continue this regime, repeating the serum salicylate level, urinary and serum electrolytes and urea every 6 h. Similarly, the arterial pH and Paco$_2$ should be measured 6-hourly until the serum salicylate level is less than 3.1 mmol/l (50 mg%).

(8) If the diuresis continues for more than 6 h, give 10 ml of 10% calcium gluconate 6-hourly. This will protect your patient against hypocalcaemic tetany, an occasional complication of prolonged alkaline diuresis.

(9) Remember that forced alkaline diuresis is hazardous; before embarking on it, ask yourself if you and your patient could do as well with activated charcoal.

REFERENCE

1 Proudfoot A. T. (1983) Toxicity of salicylates. *Am. J. Med.* **75** (Suppl.): 99.

Digoxin[1,3]

Acute overdosage due to this widely prescribed drug is uncommon, but toxicity may readily arise from its therapeutic use. The maximal therapeutic dose is about 60% of the minimal toxic dose and toxicity is especially likely to occur:

(1) if diuretics are given without potassium supplements;
(2) after a bout of diarrhoea or vomiting (both of which may cause K^+ depletion);
(3) if the patient is old and/or small;
(4) if the patient had renal impairment;
(5) if other drugs, e.g. verapamil, quinidine, nifedipine or amiodarone, are being given.
(6) in a patient with coexisting hypothyroidism.

DIAGNOSIS

The patient may complain of the following.

(1) Vomiting and diarrhoea (which may exacerbate pre-existing hypokalaemia).
(2) Central nervous system problems, which may range from restlessness to frank delirium. Visual disturbances (blurring, flashes and, more specifically, problems with colour vision) occur early. Indeed, bedside testing of colour vision may be helpful in the diagnosis of toxicity.
(3) Cardiac arrhythmias, the commonest being A-V block, supraventricular tachycardia, ventricular etopics and ventricular tachycardia. Worsening heart failure may also occur.
(4) Clinically, digoxin toxicity may be difficult to distinguish from the underlying heart disorder for which it was prescribed. Blood levels may be helpful, provided the blood sample is taken 6 h after the last oral dose, the normal therapeutic range being 1.0–2.0 ng/ml, with a level of above 3 ng/ml generally associated with toxic symptoms and signs. Toxicity may, however, occur at a lower level, particularly in patients above 60 years, with serum creatinine >150 μmol/l, and K^+ <5.0 mmol/l.

MANAGEMENT

(1) In all cases of toxicity, the drug should be stopped.

(2) If the patient is nauseated and is having occasional ventricular ectopics, it is usually sufficient to discontinue the drug for a day or two. The effect of digoxin can be partially reversed by potassium, and 20–40 mmol of KCl per day orally should be given.

(3) If the situation is more urgent (e.g. the patient has persistent vomiting, is in heart failure, heart block or has an arrhythmia compromising output), the following measures should be instituted.

    (i) Intravenous K^+ should be given: 40 mmol K^+ in 5% dextrose should be infused over 1 h, with continuous ECG monitoring. The drip should be stopped immediately if sinus rhythm returns or if peaking of T waves (evidence of hyperkalaemia) occurs. Up to 120 mmol K^+ may have to be given. If the initial serum K^+ was normal, it is wise to infuse the K^+ in 250 ml of 20% dextrose with 30 units of soluble insulin added.

    (ii) Magnesium also counteracts the toxic effects of digoxin on the myocardium. Therefore, as well as giving K^+, give 2 ml of 50% $MgSO_4$ diluted to 50 ml over the course of 1 h, and repeat as necessary.

    (iii) Repeated doses of activated charcoal should be given (see p. 255).

(4) If the above therapy is unsuccessful, DSFab treatment is probably warranted (see below). If this is not available, or considered inappropriate, try:

    (i) propranolol 1–2 mg i.v. slowly for digoxin-induced ectopics and tachycardias; or

    (ii) phenytoin 3.5–5.0 mg/kg by slow i.v. injection to a maximum of 50 mg in 1 min is an alternative;

    (iii) atropine 0.6 mg i.v. may counteract digoxin-induced bradycardias.

    (iv) Transvenous pacing may be required for persistent heart block, or a widening PR interval despite K^+ therapy.

(5) In patients with digoxin-induced arrhythmias, DC cardioversion may provoke either heart block or, rarely, resistant ventricular tachycardia. So cardioversion should not be used

lightly in such patients, who will probably require DSFab (see below). However, in the face of a persistent life-threatening arrhythmia, DC reversion (see p. 28) should be undertaken. Very low energies, e.g. 10 J, should be used to start with. Since heart block may occur, transvenous pacing should be readily available.

(6) Digoxin specific fab (DSFab), antidigoxin antibodies, are now the definitive treatment for severe digoxin overdose.' Response to therapy usually occurs within 30 min and is complete in 3–4 h. The dose is calculated in one of two ways.

    (i)   If you know the ingested dose, multiply this by 60, and give that amount of DSFab. For instance for 10 mg of digoxin give 600 mg of DSFab.

    (ii)   If you do not know the ingested dose, the body load of cardiac glycoside is estimated by multiplying the serum drug concentration by body weight and a factor reflecting the particular glycoside's distribution. An example for digoxin itself would be that a 70 kg patient with a level of 20 ng/ml (25 nmol/l) would require 480 mg of DSFab.

(7) Digoxin undergoes an enterohepatic circulation, and cholestyramine can bind it in the gut. This provides a possible, but as yet untested, way of getting rid of digoxin.

REFERENCES

1   Aronson J. K. (1983) Digitalis intoxication. *Clin. Sci.* **64:** 253.
2   Hewick D. (1989) Antibodies and the reversal of drug toxicity. *Hospital Update* January, p. 11.
3   Smith T. (1988) Digitalis—mechanism of action and clinical use. *N. Engl. J. Med.* **318:** 358.

Iron[1]

Some iron tablets look like Smarties, and sometimes small children unwittingly take handfuls of them. A toxic dose of elemental iron is 30 mg/kg, a lethal dose 150 mg/kg (a 200 mg tablet of ferrous sulphate contains 60 mg and a 300 mg tablet of ferrous gluconate contains 36 mg of elemental iron). The features of iron poisoning are as follows.

Diagnosis

(1) Acute gastroenteritis, which may be haemorrhagic, up to 6 h after ingestion (but may be further delayed after overdose of a sustained release preparation). There may be a recurrence after an interval of apparent recovery.
(2) Acute encephalopathy may occur early (within 24 h) or after an interval of apparent recovery.
(3) Hypotension, shock and metabolic acidosis may occur early or late.
(4) Occasionally acute hepatic or renal failure occurs.
(5) Following recovery from these reactions there may be subsequent cicatricial strictures of the gut.

MANAGEMENT

If treatment is started as soon as possible, the complications outlined above may be avoided.

(1) Give desferrioxamine 2 g i.m.
(2) Wash out the stomach and leave behind desferrioxamine 5–10 g in 50 ml of fluid.
(3) Take an abdominal x-ray after lavage, to ensure that there is not still a tablet mass left in the stomach.
(4) Take blood for haemoglobin and PCV electrolytes, and urea and serum iron.
(5) If a history of ingestion of considerable quantities is obtained or vomiting or bloody diarrhoea occurs, or serum iron is

      above 90 μmol/l (500 μg%), give desferrioxamine 15 mg/kg/h
      i.v. to a maximum of 80 mg/kg/24 h. This, if necessary, may
      be infused added to blood.

(6) Continue giving desferrioxamine 2 g i.m. 12-hourly until the
      serum iron is less than 90 μmol/l (500 μg%) and the clinical
      state is satisfactory. This will have to be continued for 24 h as
      iron which is initially taken up by the reticuloendothelial
      system is released 12 h later.

(7) Blood may need to be given if haemorrhage has been severe.

(8) If diarrhoea has been severe, 0.9% N saline, 5% dextrose and
      potassium supplements may need to be given.

REFERENCE

1   Lavender S., Bell J. A. (1970) Iron intoxication in an adult.
     Br. Med. J. **2:** 406.

Barbiturates

DIAGNOSIS

Barbiturate overdose leads to an impaired level of consciousness, hypoventilation, hypotension, hypothermia and peripheral dilatation, and occasionally, a blistering rash. As patients are often deeply comatose on admission, other causes of coma must be considered (see p. 355). A simple method for assessing blood barbiturate levels should be available to you through your biochemical laboratory.

MANAGEMENT

(1) very few patients with barbiturate poisoning need more than supportive management. The mortality in those seriously affected is often due to irreversible changes, e.g. cerebral anoxic damage, sustained before starting treatment. It can also be due to overenergetic treatment.

(2) Charcoal haemoperfusion was the treatment of choice for all severe barbiturate overdoses (see p. 257), but there is now increasing evidence that repeated doses of activated charcoal are just as good, and this should be your first intervention. (see p. 255).

(3) Given these newer and safer treatments, forced alkaline diuresis (see p. 261), which does help in the elimination of phenobarbitone and barbitone, should rarely be required. For all other barbiturates, it is of no avail.

(4) You may wish to supplement your treatment of repeated dose activated charcoal with either charcoal haemoperfusion or a forced diuresis, at least until the role of the activated charcoal is established more firmly. The decision to use either charcoal haemoperfusion or alkaline diuresis is primarily a clinical one. The indications are as follows.

   (i) A history of considerable ingestion coupled with a rapidly deteriorating patient.

(ii) A patient who is sufficiently unconscious that there is no response to pain (as produced by rubbing the knuckles over the patient's sternum). The pupillary and tendon reflexes are very variable and frequently lead one to suppose that the patient is more severely poisoned than is the case. Inadequacy of the patient's spontaneous respiratory efforts and hypotension occurring in the absence of hypovolaemia are sinister signs.

(iii) If the patient's clinical state deteriorates markedly in the face of rising or constant blood barbiturate levels (see below).

Provided that reliable laboratory techniques are available, the blood barbiturate level must be assessed, as a high level may act as a warning of the seriousness of the situation, i.e. over 0.21 mmol (5 mg)/100 ml for short- and medium-acting barbiturates and 0.43 mmol (10 mg)/100 ml for phenobarbitone.

(5) There is no place for the use of bemegride, at one time thought to be a specific barbiturate antagonist. In fact, its use has been associated with increased mortality.

Tricyclic and tetracyclic anti-depressants[2]

Today, drugs of this group are amongst those most commonly taken in overdose.

DIAGNOSIS

Clinical features include depression of consciousness, which is seldom severe, dilated and sometimes unequal pupils responding poorly to light, increased muscle tone which may be accompanied by tremor or frank convulsions, pronounced tendon reflexes and urinary retention. Additionally, cardiac dysrhythmia and respiratory depression are important features of overdose in this group of drugs. In the early stages patients may also be agitated and aggressive. Metabolic acidosis and hypokalaemia may occur.

MANAGEMENT

(1) The management is essentially supportive care as outlined on p. 263, as there is no known way of accelerating elimination of these drugs, apart from gastric lavage, and activated charcoal, of which you should give repeated doses (see p. 255).

(2) Ensure prompt and adequate correction of any acidosis by giving appropriate doses of bicarbonate intravenously, together with supplements as necessary.[1]

(3) Monitor ECG. Prolonged inter- and intraventricular conduction times lead to the appearance of bizarre complexes on the ECG, often simulating ventricular and supraventricular tachycardia with aberrant conduction. These arrhythmias do not have the same prognostic significance as when following mycoardial infarction or in ischaemic heart disease. Since the majority of conventional antiarrhythmic agents are in fact toxic, the use of antiarrhythmic agents should be avoided if at all possible, particularly if the cardiac output is maintained. If you have to give an antiarrhythmic, give phenytoin (see

p. 224). If necessary, volume repletion and an ionotropic agent, such as dobutamine 5–40 $\mu g/kg/l$ by i.v. infusion may be used to maintain the arterial pressure.

(4) Convulsions, if they are recurrent or long-lived, should be controlled without delay by conventional means (see p. 224), but hypoxia should first be excluded as the primary cause.

REFERENCES

1   Leader (1976) Sodium bicarbonate and tricyclic antidepressant poisoning. *Lancet* **2:** 838.
2   Meredith T. J., Vale J. A. (1988) Poisoning due to psychotropic agents. *Adverse Drug Reactions and Acute Poisoning Reviews.* **4:** 83.

Paracetamol[1]

An overdose of this drug may give rise to no more than nausea as an initial symptom, but doses of 25 g or more may later cause acute hepatic necrosis and failure. Approximate blood levels, after which hepatic necrosis is likely, are given in Fig. 22. If these blood levels are exceeded, treatment with a specific protecting agent should be considered. About 10% of patients consume sufficient paracetamol to cause liver damage. Without treatment, one in five of these would die of liver failure. In this group, the liver function tests are maximally abnormal at 3 days after the overdose; a prothrombin time of >25 s 48 h post-poisoning is prognostically ominous (see below).

(1) If the patient is at risk of hepatic damage, as determined by the paracetamol level, and presents within 10–12 h of the overdose, methionine may be given orally.[4] Give 2.5 g as the intial dose, followed by three more doses, each of 2.5 g at 4-hourly intervals. If your patient is vomiting, or oral methionine is not available, use N-acetylcysteine (see below).

(2) Alternatively, give N-acetylcysteine by the intravenous route at an initial dose of 150 mg/kg in 200 ml 5% dextrose over 15 min, followed over the next 4 h by a second dose of 50 mg/kg in 0.5 l of 5% dextrose and finally over 16 h, a dose of 100 mg/kg in 1 litre of 5% dextrose.[2] We now recognise that

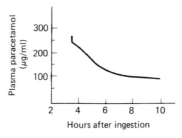

Fig. 22 Plasma paracetamol concentration after overdosage. Treatment is indicated in patients with concentrations exceeding those shown in the graph. (Reproduced with permission from L. F. Prescott *et al.* and the editors of the *Lancet.*)

administration of N-acetylcysteine should be continued until the prothrombin time is less than 20 s. It should also be given to those who present late with a paracetamol overdose, and who have an abnormal prothrombin time. Preliminary evidence suggests that oral N-acetylcysteine 140 mg/kg body weight initially, then 70 mg/kg each 4 hours for 17 more doses, is equally good at preventing liver damage if given early, and may be better when started after 10 h.[3]

(3) It is often sensible to start the antidote before you get the plasma paracetamol levels, and then to make a decision to continue or to stop treatment based on these results.

(4) Gastric lavage within 4 h of ingestion, and activated charcoal, should be given (see p. 255). (Activated charcoal should not be given if you are using oral methionine, as the methionine will be adsorbed by the charcoal.)

(5) Liver damage. The prothrombin time is the most sensitive indicator of the degree of liver damage, and if, because the above treatment has not been successful, acute liver necrosis occurs, liver transplantation may be life-saving. The following are the indications for transplantation:

  (i) Acidosis—ph <7.3;
  (ii) plus all three of the following—PT >100 s, creatinine >300 $\mu g/l$, Grade 3 or worse encephalopathy (see p. 141).

(6) But you should clearly consult your local transplant centre before your patient has got to this stage. We suggest acting on the prothrombin time, as outlined below:

  (i) If the PT at 24 h from the time of ingestion is >20 s, or >40 s at 48 h, consult the local transplant unit.
  (ii) If the PT is between 20 s and 40 s at 48 h, check it again, and if it is still above 20 s at 72 h, consult the transplant unit.

REFERENCES

1 Mitchell J. (1988) Acetominophen toxicity. *N. Engl. J. Med.* **319:** 1601.

2 Prescott L. F., Illingworth R. N., Critchley J. A. J. H. *et al.* (1979) Intravenous N-acetylcysteine: the treatment of choice for paracetamol poisoning. *Br. Med. J.* **2:** 1097.

3 Smilkstein M. (1988) Efficacy of oral N-acetylcysteine in the treatment of acetaminophen overdose. *N. Engl. J. Med.* **319:** 1557.

4 Vale J. A., Meredith T. J., Goulding R. (1981) Treatment of acetaminophen poisoning—the use of oral methionine. *Arch. Intern. Med.* **141:** 394.

Distalgesic (coproxamol)[1,2]

This analgesic is still frequently prescribed, despite the fact that there is little evidence that it is in any way superior to other simple analgesics. Each tablet contains 32.5 mg dextropropoxyphene and 325 mg paracetamol. The patient presents with respiratory depression and coma; 10% may have epileptic attacks. The finding of constricted pupils on examination is highly discriminating, as unless the patient is deeply unconscious, poisonings other than with opiates are associated with dilated pupils.

MANAGEMENT

(1) Dextropropoxyphene is closely related to methadone, and thus any cardiorespiratory depressant effects are reversible with naloxone (see p. 258). Remember that the metabolites of dextropropoxyphene have long half-lives, and there is a tendency for late and unpredictable deterioration to occur. As the duration of action of naloxone is relatively short, repeated doses may be necessary.
(2) Gastric lavage and activated charcoal should be used (see p. 255).
(3) The paracetamol level should be measured, and appropriate therapy started as necessary (see p. 273).

REFERENCES

1   Proudfoot A. T. (1984) Clinical features and management of distalgesic overdose. *Hum. Toxicol* **3:** 853.
2   Young J. B. (1983) Dextropropoxyphene overdose. *Drugs* **26:** 70.

Beta blockers[1]

(1) Beta blockers may produce hypotension, bradycardia, coma, convulsions and myocardial depression leading to cardiogenic shock. Conventional advice is to give atropine 0.6–1.2 mg i.v. while you perform a gastric lavage, and instill activated charcoal (see p. 255). The atropine is to prevent vaso-vagal cardiovascular collapse during the procedure.

(2) In the face of severe hypotension, glucagon, which acts to stimulate the heart by bypassing the beta receptors, is the drug of choice. Give glucagon 5–10 mg i.v. by bolus injection followed by an infusion, in 5% dextrose, sufficient to maintain an adequate cardiac output, usually 1–5 mg/h. Hyperglycaemia, a further effect of glucagon, does not seem to be a problem, but you should monitor the blood sugar. (The Lilly product of Glucagon contains a phenolic preservative, and should not be used for continuous infusions. The Novo product should therefore be used in these circumstances.)

REFERENCE

1   Prescott L. F. (1983) New approaches in managing drug overdosage and poisoning. *Br. Med. J.* **87:** 276.

Methanol[1]

Toxic effects may be delayed from 8 to 36 h, as toxicity is due to a metabolite. The patient presents with confusion, ataxia, epigastric pain and vomiting and blurring of vision. A metabolic acidosis with a large anion gap (see p. 180) and coma may supervene. You should measure the level as soon as possible, as this will guide you as to the need for invasive treatment (see below).

TREATMENT

(1) Correct the acidosis with $NaHCO_3$ (see p. 342).
(2) Ethyl alcohol. This inhibits the oxidation of methanol to aldehydes. Give ethyl alcohol 50 g orally or i.v. initially, followed by an infusion of 10–12 g/h, to maintain plasma ethanol levels of 1–2 g/l.
(3) Haemodialysis or haemoperfusion should be undertaken if your patient is known to have ingested more than 30 g of methanol, or has a level of 0.5 g/l. If either of these is used, you will need to increase the infusion rate of ethyl alcohol to 17–22 g/h.
(4) Folate therapy, which is said to promote the metabolism of formate, may be helpful. Give 1 mg/kg (up to a maximum of 50 mg) every 4 h for 6 doses.

REFERENCE

1   Leader (1983) Methanol poisoning. *Lancet* **1:** 910.

Ethylene glycol (anti-freeze)[2]

(1) Ingestion of this is an infrequent, but important cause of acute renal failure. Patients present with vomiting, polyuria and drowsiness, and are found to have hypocalcaemia, a low bicarbonate and high anion gap (see p. 180). It is said that the ingestion of 100 ml of ethylene glycol, if untreated, will be fatal.

(2) Traditional therapy is as for methanol; i.v. ethyl alcohol and haemodialysis if the level of ethylene glycol is above 25 mg/100 ml.

(3) The toxic effects of ethylene glycol are due to its conversion by alcohol dehydrogenase into glycolic acid, and recent experience with 4-methyl pyrazole, an inhibitor of alcohol dehydrogenase, suggests that this could be a specific and highly effective treatment.[1] If you have access to this (and it is still available in the UK), give a loading dose of 9.5 mg/kg i.v, followed at 12 h by a dose of 7.0 mg/l, at 24 h 3.6 mg/l, 36 h 1.2 mg/l and finally 48 h 0.6 mg/l. Such treatment might, in the future, obviate the need for haemodialysis.

REFERENCES

1　Baud F. (1988) Treatment of ethylene glycol poisoning with intravenous 4-methylpyrazole. *N. Engl. J. Med.* **319:** 97.
2　Porter G. (1988) The treatment of ethylene glycol poisoning simplified. *N. Engl. J. Med.* **319:** 109.

Theophylline[1]

(1) Acute theophylline overdose presents with severe nausea and vomiting, accompanied by abdominal pain and diarrhoea. Restlessness, hyperventilation, irritability, tremulousness and headache are also common, as are supraventricular and ventricular tachycardias. These are best treated with short-acting beta blockers, such as atenolol 5 mg i.v. at 5-min intervals to a maximum of 20 mg.
(2) Convulsions are common, occurring in 10% of patients with theophylline levels above 50 mg/l, and 90% of patients with levels above 100 mg/l. They may be controlled with diazepam 5–10 mg i.v., repeated as necessary.
(3) Marked hypokalaemia, due to a shift of potassium into the cells, is common, and contributes to the arrhythmias. Measure and monitor the K^+ regularly—you may require to give up to 60 mmol of K^+/l of infused fluid.
(4) There is often an associated metabolic acidosis, which does not however usually require any specific therapy.
(5) The gastrointestinal onslaught may give rise to GI haemorrhage. If you need to use a H_2 antagonist, use ranitidine, as cimetidine inhibits the metabolism of theophylline.

OTHER ASPECTS OF MANAGEMENT

(1) Take blood for electrolytes and urea, blood gases and theophylline levels, which you should ask for as a matter of urgency, as levels help you monitor the success, or otherwise, of your therapy.
(2) Gastric lavage should be undertaken.
(3) Activated charcoal, given in repeated doses (see p. 255) is presently the most effective way of reducing the absorbtion of theophylline as well as increasing its elimination. This has superseded haemoperfusion, which used to be recommended for patients with theophylline levels above 60 mg/l 4 hours after the overdose.

REFERENCES

1   Leader (1985) Self poisoning with theophylline. *Lancet* **i:** 146.

Carbon monoxide

(1) Carbon monoxide causes 1000 deaths from poisoning in the UK each year, about one-third of the total annual deaths from self poisoning.

(2) Acute heavy exposure results in coma, convulsions and then death. Pallor of the skin is more common than the classic cherry red colour, but venous blood frequently looks arterial. Early skin necrosis at pressure points can be a helpful sign.

(3) Carbon monoxide causes these problems because it has an affinity for haemoglobin 250 times that of oxygen, and also inhibits cellular respiration.

(4) Therapy is based on the fact that the half-life of elimination of CO is 250 min in a patient breathing room air, but 50 min when 100% oxygen is inspired at sea level. Hyperbaric oxygen at 250 kPa further reduces the elimination half-life to 22 min, and also increases the amount of oxygen dissolved in plasma.

(5) So the first essential is to deliver 100% oxygen, either by a tightly fitting face mask (commonly used plastic masks deliver only 60% oxygen, even at high flow rates), or by mechanical ventilation with 100% oxygen.

(6) An unresolved issue is whether hyperbaric oxygen is ever helpful.[1] As suggested above, there is a good physiological reason why it should be, but one preliminary assessment does not confirm this. However, we feel that if your patient:

   (i)   is, or has been, unconscious, or has neurological symptoms or signs more significant than a headache;
   (ii)   has any cardiac complications;
   (iii) has a carboxyhaemoglobin (COHb) level of above 40% (some would even suggest 20%) regardless of symptoms;
   (iv) has any symptoms and is pregnant, as the fetus is highly susceptible to CO;

you should consider hyperbaric oxygen.

In the UK you can find out the whereabouts of a suitable chamber by ringing Portsmouth (0705) 822351, and asking for the duty diving or staff officer, or by ringing a poisons unit (see p. 258).

(7) Treatment, by whatever means, should be continued until the COHb level is below 5%.

REFERENCE

1   Raphael J. (1989) Trial of normobaric and hyperbaric oxygen for acute carbon monoxide intoxication. *Lancet* **ii:** 414.

Organophosphate poisoning[1]

The organophosphates are commonly used as insecticides, particularly in developing countries, and sheep dips in the developed ones. Overdose, either intentional or accidental, is common. They are also, of course, used as nerve gases.

These compounds irreversibly bind to the cholinesterases in the body. The cholinesterases normally inactivate acetylcholine, so when they are not working, acetylcholine levels rise; the effect of organophosphate intoxication is due to an increase in the levels of acetylcholine.

Exposure to these organophosphate compounds is either through the skin or by inhalation (usually accidental in farm workers) or ingestion (usually intentional). They vary in toxicity, malathion being of low toxicity, parathion being of high toxicity. The time of onset after acute exposure varies from a few minutes with nerve gases to between a few and 24 h.

DIAGNOSIS

The overactivity of acetylcholine, most pronounced at autonomic postganglionic fibres, gives rise to the following symptoms:

(1) Bradycardia and hypotension.
(2) Miosis and blurred vision.
(3) Vomiting, abdominal colic and diarrhoea. Urinary and faecal incontinence.
(4) Dyspnoea due to airways obstruction and respiratory muscle dysfunction.
(5) Bronchial hypersecretion, excessive salivation and sweating.
(6) Fasciculation and convulsions.
(7) Weakness and headache.
(8) Disorientation, progressing to coma and death.

The setting and clinical findings are usually sufficient to make the diagnosis. This can, however, be confirmed by measuring the blood pseudocholinesterase level which is reduced, commonly to very low levels. The breath may also smell of garlic.

It is important to remember that serum pseudocholinesterase

levels are neither a good marker of the severity of poisoning, nor a good predictor of recovery. Red cell cholinesterase levels, reflecting tissue cholinesterases, are considerably more helpful in this regard. Even so, these levels can be depressed to 60% of normal without clinical signs, especially if the patient has been handling organophosphates previously.

MANAGEMENT

Non-Specific

(1) The most common immediate cause of death is respiratory failure. Check the vital capacity hourly, which will give you a lead on the progression of the illness, and blood gases. Respiratory failure, as defined by abnormal Pao_2 and $Paco_2$ (see p. 71), requires ventilatory support. Remember that sudden deterioration in the respiratory status is common; hence the need to measure vital capacity, peak flow and blood gases regularly.

(2) Remove contaminated clothing.

(3) Wash your patient—organophosphates are excreted in sweat and may be resorbed through the skin. Some authorities recommend hourly bathing.

(4) Your patient may be hypovolaemic due to excessive fluid loss through diarrhoea, sweating and salivation. Appropriate circulatory support monitored using a CVP line, should be given. Remember that the lungs may appear 'wet': this is not due to fluid overload, but due to excessive bronchial secretions which you hope to control with atropine (q.v.). You will also need to suction the copious oropharyngeal excretions.

Specific

(1) Atropine is the mainstay of treatment. The questions are, how much and for how long?

    (i)   *How much?* You should start with 1.2 mg–2.0 mg i.v stat. and then at 10-min intervals. You will almost certainly have to use this order of dose for the first 24 h (the range of atropine required varies between 40 mg and 500 mg/day). After the first day you may be able to reduce it. Monitoring is on the basis of the development of atropinic side-effects. None is absolutely reliable, but a dry mouth, a pulse rate above 100 beats per minute, and decreasing secretions in the lungs indicate satisfactory atropinisation. When these features appear, you can reduce the dose to 0.6–1.0 mg and increase the interval between doses to 20–30 min. An alternative is to give atropine by continuous infusion, at a dose of 0.02–0.08 mg/kg/h, monitoring the requirement in the same way.

(ii) *For how long?* You may need to continue atropine for up to 2 weeks. After each 6–12 h period, provided there is adequate atropinisation, further increase the dose intervals to 1 and then 2 h. You can then give atropine orally 4-hourly, and so titrate the amount downward gradually over a 2 week period.

(iii) You should not start atropine before correcting hypoxia, as otherwise you may induce ventricular tachycardia.

(2) Atropine, while blocking the effects of acetylcholine at postganglionic nerve endings, does not affect brain cholinesterase. This has two main consequences:

(i) If your patient is seen within 12 h of the overdose, give an oxime which does have an effect on brain cholinesterase. Oximes act by deconjugating the organophosphate from the cholinesterase enzymes, a process which becomes more difficult once more than 12 h have elapsed after the overdose, but you should consult with a poisons unit, as for some organophosphates, oxime therapy is effective much later than 12 h. Use either of the following.

(a) Toxigonin (obidoxime), which is not readily available in the UK, is the most potent preparation available and it crosses the blood–brain barrier. Give 3–6 mg/kg body weight i.v. repeated 4-hourly for 12—24 h, depending on the response.

(b) Pralidoxime is an acceptable alternative. Give 30–60 mg/kg body weight i.m. 4-hourly, or i.v. 4-hourly (do not exceed 500 mg/min) for 12–24 h, depending on response.

(ii) Atropine does not have a predictable effect on the disorientation and confusion induced by organophosphates. As an excess of atropine may also cause confusion, you may be faced with a confused, disorientated and sometimes violent patient, and not know whether this is due to an excess of atropine. Our experience is that such symptoms occurring within the first 3 days are due to the effects of the organophosphate overdose and not the atropine. Therefore, in these circumstances, be very wary before reducing atropine.

(3) Diazepam 5–10 mg i.v. may be given for muscle cramps and twitching. It has been shown to act synergistically with pralidoxime to reduce the severity of CNS symptoms.

(4) Remember that many of the accidental overdoses are due to inadequate safety precautions. Enquire about the working environment and take appropriate steps if this is deemed dangerous.

REFERENCES

1   Tafuri J. (1987) Organophosphate poisoning *Ann. Emerg. Med.* **16:** 193.

Hypothermia

Hypothermia[2,3,4]

Hypothermia has been defined as a central (usually rectal) temperature of less than 35°C (95°F).

DIAGNOSIS

(1) Hypothermia can only be diagnosed using a low-reading rectal thermometer. A recording of 33°C should arouse suspicion that the true temperature may be lower as this is the lowest reading on an ordinary thermometer.

(2) Hypothermia may be the sole cause of coma in anyone exposed to a low environmental temperature.

(3) Alternatively it may complicate coma from other causes—especially hypoglycaemia, strokes, alcohol and self poisoning with various drugs, such as barbiturates, benzodiazepines, phenothiazines and tricyclics. It may either precipitate or be caused by myxoedema (see p. 188) and hypopituitary coma (see p. 175).

(4) Below about 31°C (88°F) shivering gives way to muscular rigidity accompanied by a slow pulse and respiration and hypotension. Acidosis, caused by hypoventilation and excessive lactic acid production, may be present. The ECG shows J (junctional) waves (Fig. 23). Ventricular fibrillation can occur at any temperature below 30°C (86°F) as a central (usually rectal) temperature of less than 35°C (95°F).

MANAGEMENT

(1) Take blood for full blood count, electrolytes and urea, serum amylase, blood glucose, blood gases, thyroid function and cortisols. Measure the rectal temperature half-hourly. Further measures are:

    (i) The general care of the unconscious patient (see p. 361).
    (ii) Treatment of the hypothermia and its complications.

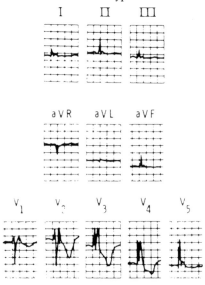

Fig. 23 The ECG in hypothermia. (Reproduced with permission from Drs D. Emslie-Smith, G. E. Sladden and G. Stirling and the publishers of the *British Heart Journal*.)

(2) Rewarming. The Biblical method, whereby the beautiful Shunamite, Abishag, was laid beside the freezing David, should seldom be used. If hypothermia occurs in a young patient as an acute episode after, for example, immersion in cold water, put the patient in a bath at 45°C and then, when the core temperature has risen to 33°C, into a bed with warm blankets. In other circumstances controversy over the rate of rewarming still exists. Traditionally, slow warming (0.8°C per hour) has been advocated. This is achieved by nursing the patient covered with blankets in a room at 26–29°C. However, the morbidity from hypothermia is directly related to the time spent hypothermic. Therefore, more rapid warming at a rate of about 1.5°C per hour may be advisable. The problem here is that the vasodilatation and consequent relative hypovolaemia which occurs on rewarming will be more marked with rapid rewarming. However, as you should anyway nurse your patient in the ITU and monitor the cardiovascular system

closely, this should not constitute a problem for you. Therefore, we opt for fast rewarming, as this seems more logical to us. This can be achieved by a combination of electric blankets, warm air fans and the warming of inspired gases and i.v. fluids. In addition to rewarming your patient, correct those factors which can complicate hypothermia (see below).

(3) Hypothermia may be complicated by:

(i) Hypotension. This may be caused by:

(a) Steroid insufficiency. Take blood for a cortisol level and then give 200 mg of hydrocortisone i.v. followed by 50 mg i.v. 4-hourly if there is an initial response.

(b) Relative circulatory insufficiency produced by peripheral vasodilatation as rewarming proceeds (see above). Insert an arterial and CVP line, and infuse plasma in the usual way (see p. 382) until the CVP is normal. In severe hypothermia—core temperature below 30°C—a Swan–Ganz catheter to measure PCWP is useful in helping you to assess fluid replacement (see p. 387). Avoid using catecholamines in this condition if possible—they are especially likely to cause ventricular arrhythmias.

(ii) Hypoventilation. This may need treatment (indicated as always by measurement of the arterial blood gases). Hypothermia may lead to dependence on hypoxic drive (as in some patients with chronic respiratory failure) and artificial ventilation may be necessary.

(iii) Acidosis, which may be severe. Calculate the base deficit (see p. 342) and restore with the appropriate amount of sodium bicarbonate in the usual way.

(iv) Ventricular fibrillation. As the oxygen demand of tissues is reduced by about 7% per °C fall in temperature, it may be worth while continuing cardiac massage for longer than usual in hypothermic patients. If ordinary methods of DC cardioversion do not cause a return to sinus rhythm, it has been suggested that a thoracotomy should be performed and the pericardium irrigated with warm saline—internal defibrillation then being attempted.

(v) Pulmonary oedema. This is an occasional complication of rewarming, due to leaky capillaries, and is thus really

a form of 'shock lung' (see p. 97). Intermittent positive
pressure ventilation, with PEEP, may be necessary.

(vi) Infection. A broad spectrum antibiotic should be given
i.v. as pneumonia usually develops.

(vii) Acute pancreatitis—although the incidence is over-
estimated.

(ix) Blood glucose concentration. This is often abnormal in
hypothermia; it may be either high or low, and should
be treated accordingly.

REFERENCES

1   Emslie-Smith D., Sladden G. E., Stirling G. R. (1959) The
significance of changes in the ECG in hypothermia. *Br. J.
Hosp. Med.* **21:** 343.

2   Exton-Smith A. M., (1973) Accidental hypothermia. *Br.
Med. J.* (1973) **4:** 727.

3   Leader (1978) Treating accidental hypothermia. *Br. Med. J.*
2: 1383.

4   Paton B. C. (1983) Accidental hypothermia. *Pharmacol.
Ther.* **22:** 331.

Acute febrile illness

The acutely febrile patient

Thermoregulatory neurons in the hypothalamus, sensitive to endogenous pyrogen (see below), control body temperature. In a healthy person there is a diurnal variation around the normal temperature of 37.0°C (98.6°F), the evening temperature being 0.5–1.0°C higher than in the morning.

Endogenous pyrogen is a small molecular weight protein released by monocytes and many of the fixed phagocytic cells of the body, such as Kuppfer cells. The release of endogenous pyrogen is activated by:

(i) many infective agents;
(ii) lymphokines formed by antigenic stimulation of lymphocytes;
(iii) soluble complexes;
(iv) some tumours produce endogenous pyrogen-like proteins.

The sudden onset of a fever below 40.5°C (105°F) is not of itself harmful, may be helpful in man,[3] and certainly is in lizards.[2] It only requires lowering if it:

(1) Produces a tachycardia sufficient to cause cardiac embarrassment (usually only in patients with pre-existing cardiac disease).
(2) Produces febrile convulsions (usually in children).
(3) Makes your patient extremely uncomfortable.

So your main concern with a fever of this level is diagnostic; an approach to this problem is outlined in the Diagnosis section below.

A fever above 41.1°C (106°F) may, of itself, cause an encephalopathy, and therefore requires treatment. This extreme hyperpyrexia is usually caused by:

(1) Heat stroke, which is defined as a rapid rise in temperature to above 40°C following exposure to intense heat. Your patient's skin is hot and dry, as there is generalized anhydrosis, and initial confusion may progress to coma. It is thought to be due to a control failure of the sweating mechanism.[1]

(2) Primary neurological lesion of the pons or hypothalamus involving the thermoregulatory centre.

(3) Is only rarely caused by infection. Falciparum malaria is the most important of these, and should always be excluded in hyperpyrexial patients.

Each 1°C rise in fever increases the pulse rate by about 10–15 beats/min and the respiratory rate by about 3–5/min.

MANAGEMENT OF FEVER

(1) If the temperature is below 40.5°C (105°F) and you deem treatment necessary (see above) you should:

    (i)   Commence tepid sponging, cooling with a fan and, if available, use cooling blankets.

    (ii) Give aspirin 300–600 mg 4-hourly (but not to anyone under 14 years old). Alternatively, paracetamol, 500–1000 mg 4–6-hourly (max. 4 g in 24 h) may be used.

(2) If the oral temperature is above 41.1°C (106°F), this constitutes a medical emergency in its own right (see above).[1] Your aim is to reduce the oral temperature to 38.3°C (101°F) within an hour. You should:

    (i)   Immerse your patient in a bath containing cool water and ice chips.

    (ii) Take the temperature at 5 min intervals.

    (iii) When it has dropped to 38.3°C, nurse your patient on a bed in a cool room.

    (iv) The temperature usually then continues to fall to around 37°C.

    (v) If after the initial rapid cooling, the temperature starts to rise again, it can usually be controlled by the methods outlined in (1) above.

    (vi) Where restlessness is a problem, chlorpromazine 25–50 mg i.v. can be used in addition to the physical methods of treatment.

    (vii) If, during cooling, your patient becomes shocked, you should institute measures as outlined on p. 338.

    (viii) Convulsions should be treated with 10 mg of i.v. diazepam, or phenytoin (see p. 224).

DIAGNOSIS OF FEVERS

(1) Worldwide, viral illnesses are the commonest cause of acute pyrexial illness. These give rise to pyrexia alone, or accompanied by non-specific symptoms of headache, abdominal pain, vomiting, sore throat and nasal discharge. Such viral illnesses are self-limiting, usually settling within 3–4 days, and are not at present amenable to specific therapy.

(2) Fever may also be the initial symptom of other more serious infections and if associated with rigors, bacteraemia or parasitaemia is likely. The range and diversity of these varies considerably from one geographical location to another, and doctors should apprise themselves of the local circumstances. Trypanosomiasis causing sleeping sickness in central Africa, various of the haemorrhagic fevers which are specific to certain localities, are examples of locally relevant pyrexial illnesses.

(3) Notwithstanding particular local circumstances, acute febrile illnesses of consequence (temperature >39.5°C (102°F) and often rigors) frequently have associated clinical features which allow you to make an informed decision about diagnosis and treatment.

   (i) The clinical features may point to a specific system involved with the infection:

   (a) Headache, photophobia, stiff neck and positive Kernig's sign suggest meningitis or meningo-encephalitis (see p. 376).

   (b) Pleuritic pain, cough and disproportionate dyspnoea suggest pneumonia (see p. 104).

   (c) An acutely painful joint suggests a bacterial arthritis (see p. 372).

   (d) Lower abdominal tenderness, associated with an offensive vaginal discharge in a sexually active woman, or sexually abused girl, suggests pelvic inflammatory disease.[7] The gonococcus (a gram-negative coccus) must be excluded, but multiple organisms, including anaerobes, *chlamydia trachomatis* and *ureaplasma urealyticum* may be involved. Therapy should include metronidazole, a broad spectrum antibiotic active against *chlamydia*, and an antibiotic active against the prevailing gonococcus. Septic abortion has a similar presentation, with the addition of an enlarged tender uterus and dilated os. The likely organisms are again multiple, and include anaerobes. These patients are best treated with a penicillin, metronidazole and a broad spectrum antibiotic such as gentamicin or chloramphenicol.

(e) A sore throat, with enlarged exudative tonsils, enlarged lymph nodes, difficulty in swallowing and prostration suggests a bacterial tonsillitis (usually a β-haemolytic streptococcus, and therefore sensitive to penicillin). An associated erythematous rash, especially on the face and flexor surfaces of the arms and legs, which desquamates after fading, is characteristic of scarlet fever. Diphtheria is now uncommon.

(f) If difficulty in breathing is associated with a sore throat, consider acute epiglottitis. If you confirm this, and in adults indirect laryngoscopy does not precipitate an airway crisis, a critical issue is whether to establish an artificial airway. The best advice is to treat these patients in a high dependency unit, and if there is progressive respiratory distress (approx. 10% of patients) proceed to intubation or emergency tracheostomy. Acute epiglottitis is usually caused by the gram-negative rod *Haemophilus influenzae* and responds to chloramphenicol.

(g) Local skin sepsis, either a cellulitis most commonly due to a β-haemolytic streptococcus, or a boil most commonly due to *Staphylococcus aureus*, may progress to septicaemia. Penicillin will be active against the streptococcus, but the staphylococcus may be penicillinase-producing, and, if you suspect this, you should use flucloxacillin as well.

(h) Acute tenderness over a bone, with associated local swelling, suggests osteomyelitis, the treatment of which is initial drainage and flucloxacillin, on the assumption that the causal organism is *Staphylococcus aureus*, and may produce penicillinase.

(i) Bloody diarrhoea associated with a high fever is often infective, and implies not only local invasion of the colon but also bloodstream invasion by the organism. In these circumstances a broad spectrum antibiotic active against the likely pathogens—the shigellas (ampicillin 50 mg/kg/d in four divided doses), campylobacter (erythromycin 500 mg q.d.s), less commonly the non-typhoid salmonellas (ampicillin as above)—should be started. Chloramphenicol 1 g 6-hourly orally or i.v. is effective against all the above as in ciprofloxacin 500 mg b.d. orally. *Entamoeba histolytica* should first be excluded by examining a fresh stool—if present, metronidazole 400 mg t.d.s. should be started.

(j) Pain in the loin, frequency and dysuria suggests a urinary tract infection. If this is community-acquired, the infecting organism is likely to be an *Escherichia coli* (a Gram-negative rod) sensitive to trimethoprin or ampicillin 500 mg.

(k) A painful enlarged liver, usually without jaundice but with signs at the base of the right chest, suggests a liver abscess which may be amoebic. Amoebic abscesses respond well to metronidazole 800 mg t.d.s. and aspiration is now considered to be unnecessary. There is not always a history of preceding diarrhoea. In 50% of bacterial liver abscesses there is no obvious primary site; there are usually a number of different bacteria involved, some of which are anaerobes. Bacterial abscesses should be aspirated, and metronidazole and ampicillin given pending the results of culture.

(l) Jaundice. Apart from yellow fever, viral hepatitis is unlikely to cause significant pyrexia. Malaria, leptospirosis, Q fever are specific infections which are commonly associated with jaundice. Septicaemias may also cause a non-specific toxic hepatitis.

(m) Abdominal pain. The acute infective diarrhoeas often cause pain, as may cholecystitis and diverticulitis, where there will also be localised tenderness and often a mass.

(n) Earache, a red drum or a discharging ear, suggests an acute otitis media, usually caused in adults by the Gram-positive diplococcus *Streptococcus pneumoniae*, and therefore responsive to penicillin.

(o) A herpes simplex eruption is commonly associated with malaria, bacterial meningitis, pneumococcal pneumonia, leptospirosis and severe viral infections. It is uncommon in other acute febrile illnesses.

(ii) In addition, the clinical features may suggest a possible cause through association:

(a) Contact with animals, either recreational, occupational or inadvertent, should be asked for.

● *Anthrax*, caused by *Bacillus anthracis* a Gram-positive rod, is common amongst the cattle rearing peoples of East and Central Africa, and in those intimately involved in the handling of hides. There may be a characteristic malignant pustule and surrounding oedema, but the respiratory variety occurs without the pustule. Penicillin 4 megaunits 6-hourly is the treatment of choice.

● *Brucellosis*, a septicaemic illness caused by a gram negative rod conveyed to man through intimate contact with infected goats and cows, or through consuming infected milk or cheese, responds to tetracycline or chloramphenicol. A leucopenia is characteristic.

● *Leptospirosis*. The leptospira, finely coiled motile spirochaetes, are concentrated in the urine of rodents. Man, when in contact with infected non-salt water is at danger, and so the disease particularly affects sewer workers, farmers, swimmers, fishermen and canoeists, as well as those who work in abattoirs. Penicillin 4–10 million units a day may be helpful.

● *Psittacosis*, caused by the obligate intracellular organism *Chlamydia psittaci*, and usually transmitted to man by the otherwise inoffensive parrot family, gives rise to an atypical pneumonia responsive to tetracycline 500 mg q.d.s.

● *Q fever* is an illness caused by the Rickettsial organism *Coxiella burnetti*. Man is infected by inhalation or ingestion of the organism after exposure to infected goats, cattle or sheep. Farmers and those involved in animal husbandry are at risk. Unpasteurised milk, though often contaminated with *Coxiella burnetti*, does not seem to transmit the disease. Q fever responds to tetracycline 500 mg q.d.s.

● *Lyme disease* is caused by *Borrelia burgdorferi*, a spirochaete which inhabits a tick of the *Ixodes* species, and is spread to man through contact with wild animals, particularly deer. The initial symptom is an erythematous rash, occurring within a few days of the tick bite; many other systems can be involved—arthritis occurs in 60%, aseptic meningitis in 15% and cardiac problems in 8%. The organism is highly sensitive to tetracyline.[8]

- *Lassa fever*, an arenavirus infection endemic to West Africa, and fatal to 50% of those who contract it, gives rise to initial non-specific symptoms, and progresses to prostration with multiple petechiae. Its importance lies in the fact that high dose i.v. ribavarin is effective therapy for life-threatening disease.[5]

(b) If there is evidence that your patient is from an overcrowded, unhygienic, deprived community, particularly one recently overtaken by any social calamity, you should think of the following pyrexial illnesses:

- *Yersinia pestis* is the gram-negative bacillus causing plague. Here the disease is transmitted to man when there is close cohabitation between infected fleas, rats, man and his domestic animals. The septicaemic illness is associated with swollen tender and sometimes discharging local lymph node (the bubo). The disease responds briskly to tetracycline 500 mg q.d.s. and streptomycin.

- *Epidemic louse borne typhus* is caused by body lice infected with *Rickettsia prowakezi* living in intimate contact with man. Here the initial septicaemic illness is followed by a diffuse purpuric rash; tetracycline 500 mg q.d.s. is the most effective drug.

- *Tick typhus and scrub typhus*.[6] A group of Rickettsial diseases transmitted to man by the bite of an infected tick or mite, so this may afflict hunters as well as the underprivileged. Some varieties produce an initial eschar at the site of the bite, and all are then followed by a headache, fever and petechial rash. They respond briskly to tetracycline 500 mg q.d.s.

(c) Recent travel may be relevant, particularly if it has been to recognised infectious areas (see Lassa fever above).

(d) Your patient may be aware of recent exposure to infection, or a close contact may have a similar illness, which may even have been diagnosed.

(e) Prior surgery or trauma should alert you to the possibility of associated infection.

(f) A menstruating woman using tampons may have the toxic shock syndrome caused by a staphylococcal exotoxin (see p. 347). Antibiotics do not appear to help, but it is reasonable to give flucloxacillin.

(g) Diarrhoea, sometimes bloody, following a course of antibiotics suggests *Clostridium difficile* infection (see p. 130). Sigmoidoscopic appearances are characteristic.

(h) Previous immunisation may be of relevance, if only to exclude those illnesses from which your patient ought to have been protected.

(4) You may however be faced with a patient with a severe pyrexial illness without any clear localising or associated features. Worldwide, the two problems here are malaria (see p. 316) and typhoid (see p. 134), which should be considered in every seriously ill pyrexial patient.

Virally induced influenza-like syndromes can simulate these two diseases, but viraemias do not usually give rise to rigors, or the same degree of prostration as these more serious conditions.

Many of the conditions mentioned in (3) above can give a septicaemic picture, but the presence of discriminatory symptoms and signs should help you decide between the various causes.

(5) There are non-infective causes of acute pyrexia. Some have already been mentioned and are easily excluded (see (5) p. 299). In addition:

(i) Adverse reactions to drugs can produce a fever; again the circumstances usually indicate the diagnosis.

(ii) Tumours, immunological disorders, chronic infections such as tuberculosis and infective endocarditis, can produce fever. These conditions do not usually present acutely, assuming major importance only in the investigation of pyrexia of unknown origin.[4]

(6) Increasingly, acute pyrexial illness occurs in association with the HIV-1 infection or AIDS. You should always consider this possibility (see p. 315).

INVESTIGATIONS

Your aim is to identify the specific causal organism as soon as possible; only in this way will you be able to offer rational therapy.

(1) Take a specimen of urine, stool, sputum, pus or a swab from any relevant sites, for culture before you begin an antibiotic. Immediate Gram staining of this material should be carried out. This will often give you a vivid demonstration of the correctness of your diagnosis.

(2) Take blood cultures; three from different sites is reasonable. Anaerobic cultures should be set up, and you should ask your bacteriologist to let you have a preliminary result in 12–24 h.

(3) Examine the urine for cells, blood and protein, the presence of which will suggest a urinary tract infection.

(4) Take a chest x-ray.

(5) Do a full blood count and stain a blood film, which may show the following:

    (i) Malarial parasites or trypanosomes.

    (ii) A lymphocytosis with abnormal mononuclear cells, suggestive of mononucleosis.

    (iii) An absolute neutrophilia, suggestive of bacterial infection. Typhoid and brucella are the exceptions, as both are associated with a low white blood count ($<5 \times 10^9/mm^3$). Viral infections do not raise the white count.

    (iv) A normochromic, normocytic anaemia may suggest haemolysis, common in malaria, in which there is frequently a low platelet count as well. Alternatively, this may suggest that you are dealing with a more chronic disease.

(6) If there is any suggestion of meningism, perform a lumbar puncture (see p. 367).

(7) Liver function tests are seldom immediately helpful. If you suspect focal intra abdominal pathology, an abdominal ultrasound is helpful; it is anyway a very useful investigation in seeking the cause of occult sepsis.

(8) Take blood for serological investigations. These only assume importance retrospectively, as you have to demonstrate a fourfold rise in titre to confirm a particular infection.

TREATMENT OF ACUTE PYREXIAL ILLNESS

(1) Your clinical history and examination, and preliminary investigations, will nearly always suggest the most likely diagnosis, which can then be treated appropriately.

(2) Difficulty arises when, despite your best endeavours, you do not have a clear idea of the cause of the pyrexia. You have several options.

    (i)   Treat with broad spectrum antibiotics, as for bacterial shock (see p. 349). This is the right course of action if your patient is poorly perfused, is very toxic with rigors, or has evidence of organ failure.

    (ii)   In anyone who has been to a malarious area, especially if there is doubt about the validity of your blood smear, give chloroquine or quinine (see p. 317).

    (iii)   If neither of the two above situations pertains, adopt a wait-and-see policy, examine your patient frequently, and be guided by clinical developments and the results of your investigations.

REFERENCES

1   Anderson R. (1983) Heatstroke. *Adv. Int. Med.* 115.

2   Atkins E. (1983) Fever—new perspective on an old phenomenon. *N. Engl. J. Med.* **308:** 958.

3   Dixon B. Sweating it out. *Br. Med. J.* **299:** 866.

4   Jacoby G. *et al.* (1973) Fever of undetermined origin. *N. Engl. J. Med.* **289:** 1407.

5   Johnson K. (1990) Imported Lassa fever—re-examining the algorithms. *N. Engl. J. Med.* **323:** 1139.

6   Leader (1988) Scrub typhus pneumonia. *Lancet* **ii:** 1062.

7   Pearce J. (1990) Pelvic inflammatory disease. *Br. Med. J.* **300:** 1090.

8   Steere A. (1989) Lyme disease. *N. Engl. J. Med.* **321:** 586.

Infections associated with acquired immunodeficiency syndrome (AIDS)[5]

(1) The human immunodeficiency virus (HIV-1) causes a progressive, time-dependent destruction of the CD4-positive (T4) lymphocyte cell population. The CD4+ve lymphocyte is central to the integrity of host cell mediated immunity. Approximately 50% of HIV-1 infected individuals progress to AIDS over a 7 year period.

(2) Infections against which cell mediated mechanisms play an important defensive role therefore commonly occur in patients with late stage HIV-1 infection, i.e. AIDS. AIDS is arbitrarily defined by the development of certain opportunistic infections or malignancies or a CD4+ve lymphocyte count of <350 cells/mm³. (See Centers of Disease Control, Atlanta, USA, definition of AIDS.)

(3) These infections may present acutely in a patient in whom the diagnosis of HIV-1 infection has not previously been established, but more commonly in the UK, occur in people who are known to harbour the virus.

(4) Infections in patients harbouring HIV-1 are usually caused by endogenous reactivation of previous infectious agents. Therefore the clinical spectrum of disease will reflect local circumstances. For instance, *Pneumocystis carinii*, common in the UK, is very rare in Uganda, where tuberculosis causes most of the respiratory disease.

(5) Fungal, parasitic and viral organisms are commonly involved, and when occurring in association with long term immunodeficiency, as in HIV-1 infection/AIDS, are rarely completely curable. At best they can be controlled during an acute episode, and usually thereafter require long-term suppressive therapy.

(6) You should remember that infections in patients who harbour HIV-1 (or have AIDS) are often multiple.

(7) Pneumonia, acute neurological syndromes such as meningitis, transverse myelitis, encephalitis, gastrointestinal and dermatological problems are the common ways in which HIV-1 infection (AIDS) can present acutely. These will be dealt with each in turn.

(8) HIV-1 related illness produces such a wide variety of problems that you should consider it as a possibility in anybody presenting with an acute illness. Remember too that as heterosexual transmission becomes increasingly important, so HIV-1 transmission and infection is not restricted to the previously so called 'high risk groups'.

DIAGNOSIS AND MANAGEMENT—General

There is a great deal of sensitivity and anxiety in all sections of our society over HIV-1 infection (AIDS). So, before you embark on excluding an HIV-1-related infection, you must be clear about the implications of the diagnosis, and the need for explicit informed consent and counselling prior to doing an HIV-1 antibody test.

(1) In taking your history, you need to have a sensitive awareness of the modes of transmission of HIV-1 infection[3] namely:

    (i)   Inoculation of blood:

        (a) Transfusion of blood and blood products, although as all blood presently donated for transfusion in the UK is now tested for HIV-1, this should no longer be a significant problem.

        (b) Needle sharing amongst i.v drug abusers.

        (c) Needle stick, open wound and mucous membrane exposure in health care workers.

        (d) Injection with unsterilised needles.

    (ii) Sexual:

        (a) Homosexual—between men.

        (b) Heterosexual, from men to women and women to men.

    (iii) Perinatal:

        (a) Intrauterine.

        (b) Peripartum.

(2) Routes investigated and not shown to be involved in transmission are:

    (i)   Close personal contact.

    (ii) Household contacts.

(iii) Health workers without exposure to blood or blood products, provided of course that none of the factors in (1) is applicable.

(iv) Biting insects.

(3) Non-specific symptoms of malaise, lethargy, weight loss, night sweats, diarrhoea and fevers have often been present for a long time prior to the evolution of a more specific acute illness. Similarly, your patient may have had oral candidiasis causing painful swallowing, a variety of skin rashes including sebhorroeic dermatitis, and generalised lymphadenopathy all unrelated to any acute illness.

(4) The non-specific laboratory findings are:

(i) Normochromic anaemia—frequently 8–9.0 g/dl.

(ii) markedly raised ESR.

(iii) Reduced total lymphocyte and absolute CD4+ve cell count.

(iv) Neutropenia and thrombocytopenia may also be found.

(5) So the acute illness usually occurs within the above frame-work.

DIAGNOSIS AND MANAGEMENT—Specific Syndromes

Respiratory infections and HIV-1 infections/AIDS.[7]

(1) In the UK, HIV-1-related pneumonia is caused by the following pathogens.

(i) *Pneumocystis carinii* pneumonia (PCP). In the UK, 80–85% of acute respiratory illness in HIV-1 infected patients is related to pneumocystis. In 15–20% of patients there may be a co-pathogen (see below).

Typical symptoms are of dry coughs (sometimes lasting months, difficulty taking deep breaths, increasing breathlessness, in a patient who is found to be pyrexial, in whom there may be fine crackles in the chest and often has some of the general stigmata of HIV-1 infection. These symptoms may however also occur in the other common HIV-1-related respiratory infection, tuberculosis. The characteristic chest x-ray abnormality in PCP is perihilar shadowing classically with a ground glass interstitial infiltrate, but appearances varying from normal to local cavitating lesions or pleural involvement have been reported. Focal abnormalities are, however, more suggestive of tuberculosis or a bacterial pneumonia.

(ii) The other 15% of cases of acute respiratory illness are due to:

   (a) *Mycobacterium tuberculosis*—this is the key differential diagnosis.[1]

   (b) *Pneumococcus, Legionella* and *Haemophilus influenzae*, all of which are commoner in HIV-1 infected patients than in the normal population, but tend to present clinically in a similar fashion.

   (c) Cytomegalovirus and *mycobacterium avium intracellulare*, which are not uncommonly present in the sputum, but whose pathogenicity is in doubt, and the treatment of which does not seem to have major benefit using present therapies.

(iii) Investigations are directed at differentiating between the above possibilities, and assessing the severity of the illness. In approaching a patient with HIV-1-related pneumonia we suggest you follow a flow diagram as outlined in Figure 24.

   (a) Sputum and induced sputum. Routine sputum examination for bacteria, including mycobacteria, is essential. Pneumocystis is rarely found in routine sputum. Inducing sputum by asking your patient to inhale 5ml of nebulised saline via a tightly fitting face mask is more productive. If no pathogens are found, assume you are dealing with PCP.

   (b) Arterial blood gases (ABG). Hypoxia is a sensitive indicator of the severity and progression of the disease. Improvement in the Alveolar–arterial (A–a) gradient after 4–5 days means that you have introduced the correct treatment.

   (c) If your patient is getting worse, fibreoptic bronchoscopy (FOB), broncho-alveolar lavage (BAL) and transbronchial biopsy should be undertaken. This

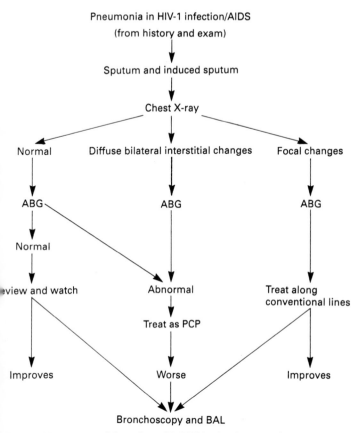

Fig. 24 Management of the patient with HIV-1 related pneumonia.

will determine the presence of other pathogens, or non-infectious lung problems, such as Kaposi's sarcoma or lipoid interstitial pneumonia, and allow you to alter your therapy appropriately.

(d) Serum LDH is often raised in PCP and may be used as a non-specific marker for diagnosis, but its decline can be followed as an indicator of response.

Treatment of PCP[8]

(1) Oxygen therapy—give oxygen via an MC mask. If despite this, the Pao[2] is falling you will need to consider intensive care therapy, with continuous positive airway pressure (CPAP) or intermittent positive pressure ventilation (IPPV). The survival from ventilation in a first attack of respiratory failure in AIDS is reasonable, and we believe such therapy should be offered.[2] Mortality in subsequent attacks is very high, and so we would not routinely ventilate such patients. It is, however, vital to discuss these issues openly with your patient, so that the patient's views can guide your decision-making.

(2) Co-trimoxazole—this should be given i.v. (20 mg/kg/day of the trimethoprim component) for at least 2 weeks and preferably orally for a third week. Nausea and skin rashes are the major toxicities, and you should give prophylactic anti-emetics, such as metoclopramide. Folinic acid 15 mg daily should also be given if the WBC is less than $2.0 \times 10^9/l$, or the platelet count below $50\ 000 \times 10^9/l$.

(3) Pentamidine, 4 mg/kg/day given i.v or i.m, is just as effective. The main side-effects are skin rashes, and hepato- and nephrotoxicity, but immediate hypotension and hypoglycaemia may also occur.

(4) Whichever of these two you start with, in 20–30% of treatments you may have to change to the alternative treatment because of intolerable side-effects. This does not affect the prognosis.

(5) Alternative oral therapies that have been shown to be effective in mild to moderate disease are dapsone—trimethoprim (100–120 mg/kg/day) and combined clindamycin 900 mg t.d.s for 10 days; clindamycin 450 mg q.d.s for 11 days with primaquine 30 mg/day.

(6) Corticosteriods. The early use of prednisolone 60 mg/day, with a rapidly tapering dosage regime over several days, in patients with even moderately severe PCP (Pao[2] at rest of <10 kPa, i.e. <80 mmHg) reduces the requirement for ventilation and improves the outcome from the acute attack.[4]

Central Nervous System Involvement[6]

Forty per cent of patients with AIDS get neurological involvement, and in the majority of these cases this is due to an infectious agent. The common pathogens are *Toxoplasma gondii*, the human DNA papovirus, designated the JC virus which causes progressive multifocal leucoencephalopathy (PML), and *Cryptococcus neoformans*. While toxoplasmosis and PML usually present with focal neurological lesions, cryptococcus and herpes simplex encephalitis usually present as a diffuse meningo-encephalitis. The features of these two modes of presentation are as follows.

(1) *Focal cerebral lesions*. Symptoms usually evolve over 2–3 weeks, and consist of hemiparesis, aphasia, ataxia, and movement disorders. It is important to remember that 40% of patients have headache, fever, lethargy and confusion, but only 5% have seizures or neck stiffness. A specific focal lesion is acute cytomegalovirus retinitis, which causes increasing loss of visual acuity and ultimately blindness, over the course of a few weeks.

(2) *Diffuse cerebral lesions* Symptoms usually evolve over a few weeks. Headache, fever and malaise are found in up to 70% of patients and may progress to meningism, although this is only found in about 30% of patients. Focal lesions may then supervene (approximately 15% of patients).

These features, however, are not sufficiently reliable to be diagnostic.

As always in HIV-1 infected patients, you must be aware that non-infectious causes, such as primary intracerebral lymphoma, and the direct effect of the human immunodeficiency virus itself, may cause similar cerebral symptoms. However, as these are essentially untreatable, whereas the infective pathogens are not, you must always assume infection until proved otherwise.

Diagnosis

(3) Because of the possibility of focal lesions in any patient with neurological complications of HIV-1 infection, you should do either a CT or MRI scan with delayed contrast injection, prior to performing a lumbar puncture. If there are multiple mass lesions, established practice is now to treat for toxoplasmosis. If only a single lesion is seen, you should consider stereotactic biopsy. If this is not feasible, treat as toxoplasmosis, or otherwise await the definitive biopsy diagnosis. If no mass lesion is seen, you should consider the possibility of herpes simplex encephalitis, with the typical temporal lobe changes on CT or on radioisotope brain scan. You should also perform a lumbar puncture, and examine the cerebrospinal fluid for cryptococcus, *M. tuberculosis* and *Treponema pallidum* (neurosyphilis) as well as for 'conventional' organisms.

Treatment

(1) Tuberculosis, neurosyphilis and other bacterial meningitides are treated in the conventional fashion (see p. 368).

(2) Toxoplasmosis is treated with a combination of oral pyrimethamine, 100 mg on day one, and 50 mg/day thereafter; sulphadimidine 6–8 mg/day and folinic acid 10–20 mg/day. Toxicity occurs in 40–70% of patients on this regime. Alternative therapies are clindamycin 900–1200 mg twice daily with pyrimethamine as above. In the event of non response within 14 days, a biopsy of the mass lesion should be considered. Should this turn out to be refractory toxoplasmosis the new macrolide antibiotics clarithromycin or azithromycin may be effective alternatives alone or combined with pyrimethamine.

(3) Cryptococcal meningitis is treated with amphotericin B (0.5–0.8 mg/kg/day up to a maximum of 20 mg/kg in total, and flucytosine (maximum 100 mg/kg/d) as for non HIV-1 infected/AIDS patients (see p. 352). In HIV-1 positive patients fluconazole (400 mg on day 1 then 200 mg/day oral or i.v.) has also been shown to be effective as an alternative or adjunctive to amphotericin B therapy.

(4) Herpes simplex encephalitis: see p. 370.

(5) Cytomegalovirus retinitis: ganciclovir (dihydroxy-phenylguanosine) 5 mg/kg i.v twice daily (but concomitant AZT must be discontinued due to the combined severe bone marrow suppression) has now been superseded by the more effective regime of foscarnet (trisodium fosphonoformate) 60 mg/kg i.v three times a day (AZT can be continued with this therapy).

(6) Short-term therapy with corticosteroids should be given to unconscious patients for their mass reducing effect.

HIV–1 infection AIDS and the gastrointestinal tract[9]

(1) *Oropharyngeal and oesophageal lesions*. These give rise to pain in the mouth and swallowing. The commonest cause is *Candida albicans*, which is diagnosed from the typical appearance of white plaques on an erythematous base. The treatment is with amphotericin B lozenges, or nystatin. If oesophageal candidiasis is severe, systemic therapy with amphotericin B or fluconazole may be required. Cytomegalovirus and herpes simplex infection can also cause a painful oesophagitis, which

if severe, may require therapy with foscarnet or ganciclovir (see p. 312 for dose regimes).

(2) *Small bowel*. Torrential diarrhoea with malabsorption and weight loss occurs at some time in between 30% and 80% of HIV-1 infected patients. It is usually due to infection with cryptosporidium or *Isospora belli*. Neither is amenable to specific treatment, but fortunately often settles spontaneously, if only for a short time. Octreotide (Sandostatin), an octapeptide with somatostatin-like activity when given either intravenously or subcutaneously (in doses ranging from 100 to 300 μg thrice daily) has been found to be effective in the amelioration of intractable diarrhoea due to cryptosporidiosis. You must, however, exclude other pathogens by culturing the stool, as giardiasis, campylobacter, salmonella, *M. avium intracellulare*, cytomegalovirus and herpes simplex may occasionally be the cause of the symptoms.

(3) *Hepatobiliary disease*. Fever, malaise and right upper quandrant pain with abnormal liver function tests, a relatively common symptom complex in HIV-1 infected patients, may be caused by:

(i) Any of the many causes of viral hepatitis, for which there is no acutely effective therapy.

(ii) A granulomatous hepatitis. This may be drug-induced—many of the drugs used in HIV-1-related therapy are hepatotoxic (e.g. isoniazid, co-trimoxazole, pentamidine, sulfonamides) but you need to exclude. *M. tuberculosis* and *M. avium intracellulare*, and cryptococcus, histoplasmosis and herpes simplex virus infection.

(iii) Biliary tract disease; acalculous cholecystitis is usually due to cytomegalovirus (CMV) or cryptosporidial infection. Presently there is no effective therapy for cryptosporidium and no evidence that treating such CMV infections is beneficial.

HIV-1 infection/AIDS and the skin

(1) *Staphylococcus aureus* (presenting as impetigo, furuncles, folliculitis, carbuncles and cellulitis) is the most common bacterial skin pathogen in HIV-1 individuals. Therapy with standard anti-staphylococcal agents is usually adequate.

(2) The commonest viruses producing skin lesions in HIV-1

infected patients are the herpes virus family. Herpes simplex
virus (HSV) 1 and 2 cause chronic painful genital, rectal or
orofacial ulcers. As the stage of HIV-1 disease advances
reinfections with HSV become more common and refractory.
Outbreaks of HSV infection early in HIV-1 disease often
respond to topical acyclovir; if this fails 200 mg of acyclovir
orally five times a day or alternatively intravenously 5–10 mg/
kg three times a day may be needed. Ulcerative skin lesions
failing to respond to acyclovir should be re-evaluated for
the presence of acyclovir-resistant herpes virus. Vidarabine
10 mg/kg/day or foscarnet 50–70 mg/kg i.v. given three times
a day could be used as alternatives.

(3) Herpes zoster infections in HIV-1 infected individuals are
usually unidermatomal. Acyclovir 800 mg, orally, five times a
day for 7–10 days is the treatment of choice and corticosteroids
are contraindicated.

(4) Epstein–Barr virus causes oral hairy leukoplakia which can
resemble candida. Generally this is asymptomatic, but will
disappear with treatment with azidothymidine, acyclovir, ganciclovir or foscarnet.

(5) Human papillomavirus causes condylomata acuminata in
HIV-1 infected patients. These lesions are likely to recur after
CO_2 laser therapy. Isoretinoin and interferon therapy is worth
considering if these lesions are troublesome in patients with
advanced HIV-1 disease.

(6) Adverse skin reactions associated with HIV-1 disease. The
incidence of cutaneous eruptions to a variety of drugs
especially antibiotics in HIV-1 infected individuals, is higher
than in the normal population. The most common causative
agents are sulfonamides and amoxycillin/clavulanate. Some
50–60% of patients with PCP develop a rash 8–10 days after
starting therapy with co-trimoxazole, in approximately one
third of whom this will require discontinuation of therapy.
The treatment is to stop the drug and if the skin reaction is
severe (e.g. Stevens–Johnson syndrome) corticosteroids may
be required.

REFERENCES

1   Barnes P. *et al.* (1991) Tuberculosis in patients with human
     immunodeficiency virus infection. *N. Engl. J. Med.* **324:** 1644

2   Efferen L.S. *et al.* (1989) Survival following mechanical ventilation for *Pneumocystis carinii* pneumonia in AIDS. A different perspective. *Am. J. Med.* **87:** 401.

3   Friedland G. *et al.* (1987) Transmission of the human immunodeficiency virus. *N. Engl. J. Med.* **317:** 1125.

4   Gagnon S. *et al.* (1990) Corticosteroids as adjunctive therapy for severe *Pneumocystis carinii* pneumonia in AIDS. *N. Engl. J. Med.* **323:** 1444.

5   Glatt A. *et al.* (1988) Treatment of infections associated with human immunodeficiency virus *N. Engl. J. Med.* **318:** 1439.

6   Manji H. *et al.* AIDS and the central nervous system. *Hospital Update* December, p. 965; and January 1992, p. 28.

7   Millar A.B. (1988) Respiratory manifestations of AIDS. *Br. J. Hosp. Med.* March; p. 205.

8   O'Doherty M.J. (1991) Prophylaxis and treatment of *Pneumocystis carinii* pneumonia. *Br. J. Hosp. Med.* **45:** 277.

9   Smith P. (1992) Gastrointestinal infections in AIDS. *Ann. Intern. Med.* **116:** 63.

Malaria[1,4]

Malaria due to any of the *Plasmodium* species is, world wide, one of the commonest causes of an acute pyrexial illness. It often administers the coup de grace to an individual already primarily debilitated and anaemic from a combination of previous infections and malnutrition. Moreover, *Plasmodium falciparum* can give rise to dire complications in previously healthy individuals as follows.

(1) Cerebral malaria. Definitions vary, but this is usually taken to mean a severe encephalopathy with or without focal neurological signs in the patient with acute falciparum infection. The pathogenesis is probably a clogging of small intracerebral blood vessels by parasitised and haemolysed blood cells.

(2) Massive intravascular haemolysis leading to jaundice and/or acute renal failure—'blackwater (haemoglobinuria) fever'. Again the pathogenesis is obscure—it may occur in the absence of parasitaemia, and is so presumed to be an immunological response to the parasite.

(3) Diagnosis of malarial infection depends primarily on seeing parasites in a blood smear. Because the intensity of parasitaemia can vary from hour to hour, several serial blood smears should be examined before abandoning the search. But it is uncommon for a second smear to be positive if no parasites are seen in the initial one.

(4) There is usually a normochromic normocytic anaemia, normal or low white blood count and the platelet count is frequently reduced to around $100 \times 10^9/l$. This last is presumably due to platelet consumption, but a full blown disseminated intravascular coagulation (DIC—see p. 342) is very uncommon.

(5) Hypoglycaemia may contribute to the coma of malaria, particularly in those treated with quinine. This should always be looked for, and treated with intravenous 10% dextrose infusions (see below). It may, however, be that this hypoglycaemia is merely a manifestation of the parlous state of many of the patients who get malaria, as it also occurs in other serious illnesses.[3]

(6) Malaria can be confused with many other acute pyrexial illnesses. An approach to this problem is outlined on p. 297.

TREATMENT

(1) The mainstay has been oral chloroquine 0.6 g given immediately followed by 0.3 g 6 hours later and 0.3 g daily for 2 days. The intramuscular route, 3.5–5.0 mg/kg 6-hourly, or intravenous route, a continuous infusion of 1.25 mg/kg/h for 8 h, and then 0.62 mg/kg/h over 24 h, to a total dose of 25 mg/kg, are suitable alternatives for a patient who is persistently vomiting, or fails to tolerate a nasogastric tube. Clearly, oral therapy should be started as soon as possible.

(2) However, the emergence of chloroquine-resistant strains has, in a variety of localities, forced an alternative regime with quinine. Quinine dihydrochloride is given first with a loading infusion of 20 mg/kg in 500 ml of 5% dextrose infused over 4 h. This is followed by 10 mg/kg doses every 8 h given as infusions of 250 ml of 5% dextrose over 4 h. Quinine is just as effective if, where i.v. infusion is not possible, the same dose is given i.m.[8]

Quinidine may be used, as an alternative, and indeed seems to be more effective against *Plasmodium falciparum* than quinine. It is given as a loading dose of 10 mg base/kg infused over 2 h, followed by a continuous infusion of 0.02 mg/kg/min, for a maximum of 72 h. The infusions may be discontinued when the patient can take by mouth. A side-effect of both drugs is hypoglycaemia secondary to induced insulin release. This should be looked for regularly—if necessary being controlled by the use of 10% dextrose rather than 5%.

(3) Some authorities give pyrimethamine 25 mg b.d. for 3 days plus a sulphonamide such as sulphadiazine 2 g initially followed by 0.5 g 6-hourly for 5 days in conjunction with quinine. We do not.

(4) Resistance to quinine, and therefore presumably quinidine, is emerging.

    (i) Qinghaosu, an artemisinine used for many years in China, is highly effective in severe falciparum malaria, with little toxicity, and we hope that it will become more easily available in the West soon. It seems to be most effective when given orally, at a dose of 1.0 g initially, and repeated at 24 h, but an intramuscular preparation is available.[2]

    (ii) Mefloquine, in a single oral dose of 1.0–1.5 g, has also been used in these circumstances.

(5) Anaemia should be treated on its merits by blood transfusion. In desperately ill patients with over 10% of red blood cells parasitised exchange transfusion should be considered, and continued until the parasitaemia is below 2%.[5,6]

(6) As mentioned above, the pathogenesis of cerebral malaria is obscure. However, cerebral oedema does not play a signficant part. Dexamethasone seems to prolong coma in survivors as well as exposing them to the risks of steroid therapy. It has no beneficial effect on mortality.[7]

(7) Convulsions in cerebral malaria. Their frequency can be much reduced by a single i.m. dose of phenobarbitone, 3.5 mg/kg, which should therefore be given as soon as the diagnosis is confirmed.[9]

(8) Having given anti-malarials the treatment of cerebral malaria is as for the unconscious patient (see p. 355).

(9) Renal failure in blackwater fever is treated along the usual lines (see p. 152).

(10) Pulmonary oedema, due to leaky capillaries (the ARDS, see p. 97) occurs in a few patients with severe falciparum malaria. You must be alert to this possibility. Management is as for other causes of the ARDS (see p. 98).

REFERENCES

1   Cook G. (1988) Prevention and treatment of malaria. *Lancet* **i:** 32.

2   Jiang J. *et al*. (1982) Antimalarial activity of mefloquine and qinghaosu. *Lancet* **ii:** 285.

3   Kawo N. *et al*. (1990) Specificity of hypoglycaemia for cerebral malaria in children. *Lancet* **336:** 454.

4   Krogstadt D. (1988) Chemoprophylaxis and treatment of malaria. *N. Engl. J. Med.* **319:** 1538.

5   Miller K. *et al*. (1989) Treatment of severe malaria in the USA with a continuous infusion of quinidine gluconate and exchange transfusion. *N. Engl. J. Med.* **321:** 65.

6   Leader (1990) Exchange transfusions in falciparum malaria. *Lancet* **335:** 324.

7   Warrell D.A., Looareesuwan S. *et al*. (1982) Dexamethasone proves deleterious in cerebral malaria. *N. Engl. J. Med.* **306:** 313.

8   Wattanagoon Y. *et al.* (1986) Intramuscular loading dose of quinine for falciparum malaria: pharmacokinetics and toxicity. *Br. Med. J.* **293:** 11.

9   White N. *et al.* (1988) Single dose phenobarbitone prevents convulsions in cerebral malaria. *Lancet* **ii:** 66.

Typhoid[1,2,4]

PRESENTATION AND DIAGNOSIS

(1) Typhoid, due in 95% of cases to infection with the Gram-negative motile rod *Salmonella typhi*, is a leading cause of acute pyrexial illness in underdeveloped countries. The initial symptoms (first phase of the disease) are non-specific and 'flu' like, viz: stepwise increase in fever, headache, malaise, anorexia, cough, sore throat and musculoskeletal aches; 10% of patients have associated gastroenteritis. At this stage 90% of patients will have positive blood cultures. Positive stool cultures (in 80%) and urine cultures (in 25%) occur during the second phase of the illness. The bacillus may also usefully be cultured from bone marrow.

(2) The second phase, that of the established disease, begins 2–3 weeks after ingestion of the organism. It is here that the widely known but seldom seen rose red spots occur; more reliably these patients have bronchitis, lymphadenopathy, splenomegaly, occasionally hepatomegaly, a relative bradycardia, constipation and typhoid stupor. Stupor describes the characteristic mental anergy which may progress to frank confusion and coma which is the hallmark of the toxic encephalopathy related to typhoid. Ileal perforation can occur in this phase of the disease.

(3) Occasionally patients present with the late complications of the disease, either metastatic spread to any site, or immune complex deposition responsible for the glomerulonephritis and probably myocarditis.

(4) So typhoid usually presents as an acute febrile illness. It may present as an emergency in one of three guises:

    (i) Deteriorating consciousness progressing to coma.

    (ii) Intestinal perforation. Pain in the right lower quadrant is the commonest initial sign followed by signs of localised or generalised peritonitis. Abdominal x-ray should reveal free air.

    (iii) Intestinal haemorrhage. Macroscopic bleeding occurs not infrequently—massive haemorrhage is fortunately rare signalled by a sudden fall in arterial pressure and temperature.

(5) Most but not all patients will achieve at least a fourfold rise in antibodies to O antigen (the Widal test), but this is an unreliable diagnostic pointer, particularly in communities in which salmonella infections are endemic.[3]

(6) Ninety per cent of patients have a normal or low white blood count, and most have a normochromic normocytic anaemia. Jaundice is uncommon, but mild abnormalities of liver enzymes are present in 40% of patients.

(7) In the early stages, typhoid may be confused with many other acute pyrexial illnesses. An approach to the differential diagnosis is outlined on p. 297.

INVESTIGATIONS

Take blood for full blood count, electrolytes and urea and liver function tests. Take three blood cultures and send urine and faecal specimens for bacteriology. Consider a bone marrow culture.

MANAGEMENT

If the diagnosis is suspected the patient should be isolated and barrier nursed.

(1) The drug of choice is chloramphenicol. Give 50 mg/kg/day in divided doses 6-hourly orally if possible, intravenously if not, for 2 weeks.

(2) Coma in typhoid has been assumed to be due to a combination of toxaemia, inanition and fluid and electrolyte derangement. Treatment therefore depends not only on chemotherapy, but also ensuring appropriate volume replacement.

(3) Steroids. High dose intravenous dexamethasone—3 mg/kg stat., followed by 8 doses of 1 mg/kg 6-hourly each given by i.v infusion over 30 min, may improve the prognosis in the most severely ill patients who are comatosed or shocked.

(4) If a large perforation is suspected a laparotomy should be carried out. These patients are obviously not ideal surgical candidates. Careful attention to volume replacement with a CVP line will maximise their chances (p. 382).

(5) Intestinal haemorrhage is treated with blood replacement in the usual way (p. 113).

(6) Remember that typhoid is a notifiable disease in the UK. You will anyway have to get hold of your local public health physician to help trace the source of the infection.

REFERENCES

1   Hoffman T.A. *et al.* (1975) Waterborne typhoid fever in Dade county, Florida. Clinical and therapeutic evaluation of 105 bacteraemic patients. *Am. J. Med.* **59:** 481.

2   Hook E.W. (1984) Typhoid fever today. *N. Engl. J. Med.* **310:** 116.

3   Reynolds D.W. *et al.* (1970) Diagnostic specificity of Widal's reaction for typhoid fever. *J. Am. Med. Assoc.* **214:** 2197.

4   Rubin H. (1983) Enteric fever (case report). *N. Engl. J. Med.* **309:** 600.

General clinical problems

Acute confusional states—delirium[1,2]

(1) Delirium, defined as an acute organic disorder involving a reduced awareness of, and inability to maintain, appropriate sustained attention toward the environment, is characterised by:

   (i)   A global disorder of thinking, memory and perception. Perceptual disturbances usually consist of paranoid misinterpretation of the environment, coupled with visual hallucinations.
   (ii) Inability to sustain attention and respond appropriately to stimuli.
   (iii) A reduced level of consciousness, with disorientation in time, place and person.
   (iv) An abnormally increased or decreased psychomotor pattern, with restlessness and agitation sometimes merging into apathy.
   (v)   A disturbed sleep/wake pattern, with drowsiness during the day, and night sleep characteristically shortened and fragmented.

(2) Its onset is acute, and it fluctuates in intensity, usually being worse at night. A delirious person may express the whole gamut of emotions, ranging from apathy to fear and rage, which gives the syndrome its colour, and creates both diagnostic and therapeutic problems. Handling delirium constitutes one of the severest tests of your clinical skills.

(3) It must be distinguished from acute functional psychosis; the crucial difference is that in a psychosis, orientation in time, place and person is intact, and the course over 24 h is stable.

DIAGNOSIS

The widespread reduction in cerebral metabolism and disturbance of neurotransmission underlying delirium may be caused by a wide range of problems, many of which are easily reversible. Four major groups of such causal factors can be distinguished:

Primary intracerebral disorders

(1) An intracranial space-occupying lesion, e.g. tumour, abscess or haematoma—either extradural, subdural or intracerebral.
(2) Meningitis and encephalitis, (see p. 367).
(3) Ictal or post-ictal states.
(4) Stroke (see p. 201).

Exogenous toxic agents

(1) Drugs—the following most frequently:

    (i)   Tranquillisers and hypnotics, such as barbiturates, benzodiazepines and phenothiazines.
    (ii)   Anticholinergics, such as atropine, antiparkinsonians and tricyclic antidepressants.
    (iii) Dopamine agonists, such as levodopa, bromocriptine and amantadine.
    (iv) The opiates
    (v)   Cardiotherapeutics, such as digoxin, diuretics and beta blockers.
    (vi) Non-steroidals and cimetidine.
    (vii) Drugs of abuse, such as amphetamines, LSD, cocaine, Ecstasy and NMDA (metholene dioximetamphetamine).

Almost every drug has been implicated in provoking delirium, and you should be meticulous in identifying all the drugs that your patient is taking. Polypharmacy and its consequences is probably the commonest cause of delirium.

Systemic disease secondarily affecting the brain

(1) Cerebral hypoxia (poor perfusion, or poor oxygenation).
(2) Any infection, especially of the urinary tract and lungs.
(3) Any pain or discomfort (commonly urinary retention) in a patient already seriously ill.
(4) Hypoglycaemia or more rarely, hyperglycaemia.
(5) Endocrine disorders, such as myxoedema (see p. 188), thyrotoxicosis (see p. 191).
(6) Electrolyte or fluid disturbance, commonly

    (i)   hypo- or hypernatraemia;
    (ii)   hypokalaemia.
    (iii) hypercalcaemia.

(7) Deficiency of thiamine, (Wernicke/Korsakoff syndrome—external ophthalmoplegia, ataxia and confusion), nicotinamide and vitamin B_{12}.

(8) Cardiac, hepatic or renal failure.

(9) Collagen vascular diseases, such as SLE.

(10) Acute porphyria.

(11) Hypertensive encephalopathy (see p. 48).

(12) Surgery. It is said that up to 15% of elderly people become delirious following surgery.

Withdrawal from substances of abuse

This applies particularly to alcohol (see p. 331) and sedative hypnotic agents.

Two or more of these may occur together. Any may be exacerbated by anaemia, hypotension or pre-existing chronic dementia.

MANAGEMENT

(1) Management involves a careful and complete history and examination to exclude the above possibilities. This will nearly always suggest the correct cause, which must then be treated on its merits. The following investigations may either corroborate your diagnosis, or clarify the situation if uncertainty remains. So you must ask for:

    (i) Haemoglobin and PCV;

    (ii) electrolytes and urea;

    (iii) blood sugar;

    (iv) blood calcium;

    (v) blood gases;

    (vi) liver function tests, including a prothrombin time;

    (vii) cultures of blood, urine or other relevant sites;

    (viii) consider a lumbar puncture; and take a careful drug history.

    (ix) A CT scan may be required to exclude or confirm intracranial pathology.

(2) Confusion is always worse at night. Disorientation may be helped by an easily visible clock, a familiar nurse and a light.

(3) (i) Never attempt to sedate an uncontrolled patient without due consideration of the cause, it may make the situation

worse and it may be fatal. If sedation is vital or is deemed unharmful give chlorpromazine (50–100 mg i.m.) initially or diazepam 10 mg i.v.

(ii)   If the above are ineffective give either

(a) chlormethiazole (see p. 225); or

(b) Haloperidol. This is effective orally, i.m. or i.v. in doses ranging from 0.5 mg to 10 mg. The problem with haloperidol is that extrapyramidal side-effects are common, and you should be on the look out for these.

(c) Never give paraldehyde to a confused but conscious patient as the pain provides considerable force and direction for the structure of his delusions.

It goes without saying that your verbal or pharmacological attempts to calm the patient must not be attended by any hint of aggression. It not only betrays lack of insight on your part, it may also be the only facet of your relationship to be grasped by the patient—and is therefore disastrous.

REFERENCES

1   Davidson K. (1989) Acute organic brain syndromes. *Br. J. Hosp. Med.* **41:** 89.

2   Lipowski Z. (1989) Delirium in the elderly patient. *N. Engl. J. Med.* **320:** 578.

Acute psychoses

DIAGNOSIS

The clinical picture may at first sight be similar to that of delirium, and as in delirium, psychoses may also be provoked by sudden medical or surgical illness. There may be a history of previous mental illness. A helpful point of distinction between an acute psychosis and a confusional state is that in acute psychoses, the sensorium is clear and the patient orientated in time, place and person although the content of thought is disordered. In addition, the hallucinations of psychoses when they occur are usually auditory, rather than visual. Consider:

(1) Substance abuse—for example, amphetamines, cocaine, including crack, and LSD.
(2) Puerperal psychosis.
(3) Acute schizophrenia. This usually presents a characteristic mixture of disorders of thinking and feeling, with hallucinations and disorders of conduct. This closely resembles the picture of amphetamine psychosis.
(4) Acute depression. Delusions and hallucinations are usually of a self-deprecatory nature. Hypochondriasis, suicidal ruminations and a tendency to depersonalisation may be evident.
(5) Acute mania. Elation combines characteristically with easily provoked irritability. The patient talks rapidly, jumping from one subject to another.
(6) Acute hysterical episodes. Overtones of acting and self-dramatisation may be apparent. Even when at his most violent, the patient rarely injures himself.

MANAGEMENT

The management of these cases involves the following actions.

(1) Achieving, if at all possible, some kind of contact with the patient, if only to establish yourself as a harmless and possibly helpful comrade.

(2) Excluding any underlying medical or surgical illness, as for delirium (see p. 326).

(3) Initiating the treatment of specific psychiatric syndromes. If more urgent therapy is required, treat as for delirium (see p. 328).

(4) Seeking psychiatric consultation as soon as possible. If possible, discuss this before giving medication since if sectioning is to be considered, the psychiatrist really needs to evaluate the unsedated patient.

Toxic confusional state due to acute alcohol withdrawal—delirium tremens[2]

Acute withdrawal from alcohol causes a characteristic toxic confusional state, which, if uncontrolled, may be fatal.

DIAGNOSIS

(1) The risk of problems from alcohol withdrawal begins at alcohol consumptions of about 10 units/day (80 g of alcohol) and becomes appreciable in patients who drink upwards of 15 units/day. The alcohol withdrawal syndrome usually starts about 8 h after a substantial fall in the blood alcohol level in a susceptible patient and then progresses over the next 48 h. It can, however, start up to 2 weeks after withdrawal. About 10% of patients will evolve to the most severe stage, delirium tremens.[4]

(2) Recognition of the possibility of alcohol withdrawal depends on taking an accurate history of alcohol consumption. Recognising the early symptoms of tremor, sweaty palms, tension and sleep disturbance in a predisposed person may allow you to give appropriate sedation in anticipation, and thereby forestall progression to DTs. A suitable regime is: chlormethiazole, 1.5 g q.d.s. for 2 days, then 1.00 g q.d.s. for 3 days and finally 500 mg q.d.s. for 4 days.

(3) The characteristic symptoms of DTs are tremulousness, apprehension, disorientation in time and place and visual, tactile and auditory hallucinations. In addition, insomnia, nausea and vomiting and motor incoordination may be present.

(4) Excessive intake of alcohol may also give rise to cirrhosis, cardiomyopathy and various neurological syndromes such as peripheral neuropathy due to vitamin deficiency, chronic cerebellar disease and Wernicke's encephalopathy. Thus, DTs may be superimposed on an already debilitated patient.

(5) There is a substantial and rather unpredictable variability in the severity of the symptoms of withdrawal. About 80% of

patients get mild symptoms, 14% moderate trouble and 6% progress to full-blown DTs.

MANAGEMENT

Non-specific

(1) It is very important to establish contact with the patient, who is frightened, disorientated and frequently aggressive.

(2) Thiamine 50 mg i.v. and 50 mg. i.m. should always be given before starting a dextrose infusion thereby avoiding the possibility of precipitating Wernicke's encephalopathy in a susceptible patient.

Specific

(1) The aim of treatment is the induction of light sleep sufficient to control symptoms, while leaving vital functions unimpaired. Drugs to achieve this end are best given orally, but may have to be given i.v.

(2) Chlormethiazole (Heminevrin) is the drug of choice.[2] The dose required to achieve light sleep ranges between 4.0 and 10.0 g/day. It requires being reviewed daily, the highest dose generally being needed 24–48 h after alcohol withdrawal. Patients generally do not need this drug after the seventh day. If oral administration is impossible, i.v. chlormethiazole may be given. Give a loading dose of 30–50 ml of a 0.8% solution over 3–5 min to induce sleep, and continue an infusion of this concentration at 0.5–1.0 ml/min, adjusting the rate to the minimum dose required to keep the patient just sleeping lightly. Usually 500–1000 ml are needed in the first 6–12 h. If it is used in this way for a maximum of 12–18 h, chlormethiazole is a safe drug, but none the less your patient should be observed in a high dependency unit, or an ITU. Side-effects, which are dose-related, are respiratory depression, hypotension and supraventricular tachycardia culminating in respiratory arrest. As the drug accumulates with long-term use, you should not continue the infusion for longer than 18 h without first measuring chlormethiazole levels.

(3) Chlordiazepoxide, either orally or i.v., in sufficient dosage necessary to induce light sleep may be used as an alternative

to chlormethiazole. Start with 40 mg 4-hourly and increase to 100 mg 2-hourly if necessary.

(4) Ethanol. An initial i.v. loading dose of 30 ml, followed by 10 ml hourly in 5% dextrose, is a perfectly reasonable alternative.[1]

(5) Although the tremulousness, fever, tachycardia and hallucinations subside over 3–4 days, there may be an interval of over 1–2 weeks before full return to the patient's previous mental state. This interval is characterised by a lack of concentration and intermittent disorientation and agitated confusion. The latter is best treated with haloperidol 10 mg i.m. or i.v. 1 hourly as necessary (with a maximum of 60 mg/24 h). This may precipitate dystonic reactions which may be relieved by benztropine 1–2 mg i.m. or procyclidine 5 mg i.m. or i.v.

(6) Promazine derivatives should not be used, because of their hepatoxic effect, and opiates should be avoided as they may cause respiratory depression in persons with liver damage.

(7) The possibility of cirrhosis, heart failure and neurological disease induced by alcohol should be considered during examination of the patient, as these may need treating also. To this end, the following investigations should be done as soon as possible: chest x-ray, ECG, liver function tests and serum proteins, full blood picture and ESR, serum folate, electrolytes and blood urea.

(8) Beta blockers. Atenolol, 50 mg/day if the pulse rate is consistently between 50 and 80/min, and 100 mg/day if the pulse rate is higher, has been shown to be of symptomatic benefit in those with mild to moderate withdrawal.[3]

Remember all this is only first aid, and your psychiatric colleagues should be involved as early as possible.

REFERENCES

1   Chick J. (1989) Delirium tremens. *Br. Med. J.* **298:** 3.
2   Hollister L.E. *et al.* (1972) Treatment of acute alcohol withdrawal with chlormethiazole. *Dis. Nerv. Sys.* **33:** 247.
3   Kraus M. *et al.* (1985) Randomized clinical trial of atenolol in patients with alcohol withdrawal. *N. Engl. J. Med.* **313:** 905.
4   Lerner W.D., Fallon H.J. (1985) The alcohol withdrawal syndrome. *N. Engl. J. Med.* **313:** 951.

The poorly perfused patient[2,3,6]

DIAGNOSIS

A persistently low arterial pressure (systolic <70mmHg) is of itself life-threatening, but a lesser degree of hypotension does not in itself matter unless there is also evidence of inadequate tissue perfusion, when it should always be regarded as a medical emergency. This combination also provides a working definition of shock. In physiological terms, shock may be defined as a state of inadequate tissue oxygenation leading to vital organ dysfunction. We increasingly use blood lactate levels as a proxy measure of tissue oxygenation, and hence the severity of shock (see p. 343 below).

An alternative, perhaps more apposite definition of shock is the sensation experienced by the house officer after he or she has been looking after a deteriorating patient for 3 h.

Poor tissue perfusion is most easily seen when it affects:

(1) The brain—mental confusion.
(2) The extremities (including the nose)—which are cold, pale, moist and mottled with peripheral cyanosis and collapsed veins.
(3) The kidneys—the minimal acceptable urine flow rate is 0.5 ml/kg/h. If it is less than this, renal hypoperfusion is likely to be present. If the temperature of the extremities falls much below that of the central temperature (as measured on a rectal thermometer) this implies poor tissue perfusion and a fall in the glomerular filtration rate is also likely.
(4) The coronary arteries—this may be the cause of arrhythmias and also of impaired myocardial contractility.

The shock syndrome can arise from four basic causes.

(1) Cardiogenic (more accurately—primary pump failure). The main causes here are:

    (i) Myocardial infarction (see p. 11) and/or heart failure from any cause.
    (ii) Cardiac arrhythmias—particularly Stokes–Adams attacks and ventricular tachycardias (see p. 26).

(2) Decreased circulating volume leading to hypovolaemia.[1] The main causes here are:

   (i)   Salt and water depletion as in severe diarrhoea and vomiting, heat exhaustion and diabetic and Addisonian crisis.
   (ii) Haemorrhage (see p. 112).
   (iii) Anaphylaxis (see p. 345).

(3) Decreased vascular resistance, leading to abnormalities of distribution. Here there is a mis-match between the vascular bed and the circulating blood volume from the outset. The main causes here are:

   (i)   Septic shock (see p. 347).
   (ii) Barbiturate and other overdoses.

(4) Obstructive. Here the venous return to the right or left atrium is compromised. The main causes here are:

   (i)   Cardiac tamponade (see p. 65).
   (ii) Mediastinal shift. This is usually due to massive pulmonary collapse (see p. 90), a large pleural effusion (see p. 95), over-hasty relief of a large pleural effusion (see p. 95), or a pneumothorax.
   (iii) Pulmonary embolism (see p. 52).
   (iv) Dissecting aneurysm (see p. 63).

(5) Any of the above causes, if sufficiently prolonged or severe, may cause a reduced cardiac output and high peripheral resistance. The ensuing poor tissue perfusion causes a profound acidosis which dilates the precapillary arterioles, but not the post capillary venules. This causes stagnation of blood within the capillaries which both exacerbates cellular hypoxia, and because of damage to the capillary walls, causes leakage of crystalloid and colloid from the vascular compartment. Further, in shock the entire capillary bed is involved, so that the capacitance of the vascular compartment is increased. Thus, the initiating sequence of events in shock is compounded by:

   (i)   stasis of blood within the capillaries;
   (ii) extravasation of crystalloid and colloid from damaged capillaries.
   (iii) increase in capacitance of the circulatory system. The

result of all this is a serious mis-match between the effective blood volume (much reduced) and the capacitance of the vascular compartment (increased). This mis-match is reflected clinically in the poor tissue perfusion, hypotension, tachycardia and lowered CVP which characterises shock. Prompt treatment is intended to reverse the above outlined sequence thereby preventing the inexorable progression which will otherwise ensue.

An understanding of the pathogenesis of shock is essential to its proper management, which is further outlined below.

MANAGEMENT

Monitoring and Investigations

Patients with shock in whom aggressive therapy is warranted, need to be looked after in an intensive care unit. Basic monitoring should include the following.

(1) Arterial pressure. Measured ideally by an intra-arterial catheter which will not only give you a continous read out, but can be used to get arterial blood for blood gas measurements.
(2) Pulse and respiratory rate.
(3) Temperature. You need to measure core (rectal) and toe temperature. Moderate pyrexia is a valuable asset in combating infection (most obviously in the lizard, which, when ill, seeks a warm niche in which to induce a temperature), and is also, of course, a frequent pointer to infection. In addition skin temperature is a reflection of the peripheral blood flow. Normally the gradient between core and periphery is 3°C, whereas in shock, the peripheral temperature (most conveniently measured on the big toe) is often only 2°C above the ambient temperature. A closing of the core–peripheral temperature gap is valuable evidence of improvement.
(4) Central venous pressure (CVP) and pulmonary capillary wedge pressure (PCWP). These measure the right- and left-sided filling pressures respectively, and so can be used to guide your fluid replacement. (see p. 382).
(5) A continuous ECG recording should be established.
(6) Urinary output. As mentioned above, this is an important indicator of tissue perfusion. You may also need to test the

urinary osmolality (see p. 149) to assess whether renal function is adequate.

(7) Investigations. You will need to do a haemoglobin, white cell count, platelet count and clotting studies if there is any evidence of bleeding (see section below). Take arterial blood for gases and pH, and venous blood for electrolytes including Ca^{2+}, Mg^{2+} PO_4^{2-}, LFTs and urea. You should measure lactate (see below). Blood cultures, and cultures from any other relevant site, should be taken so that you can prescribe antibiotics intelligently (see p. 349).

(8) Colloid osmotic pressure (COP). Traditionally, we have equated serum albumin with COP. We now realise that this is not a very satisfactory equation. However, it is now possible to measure COP directly, the norm being 25mmHg. In accordance with Starling's law, raising the intravascular COP will increase the amount of fluid in the intravascular compartment, and so will be useful in assessing how much of which fluid, particularly colloid, you should give. As this is one of the major unresolved problems in the treatment of shock (see below), you should strive to get access to COP measurements. While awaiting this technological advance, it is better to use the total protein rather than the albumin, as an indirect measure of COP.

(9) Daily chest X-rays are desirable, if only to make sure you have not produced a pneumothorax inserting your central lines!

(10) Transcutaneous O_2 and CO_2 monitoring is emerging as a continous guide to tissue perfusion and oxygenation, and may be available to you.

Specific Treatment

Specific treatment is directed towards removing the cause, which is usually apparent from the history and examination. This is, however, not usually sufficient, further measures being required to correct tissue perfusion.

Non-specific treatment

(1) You must ensure that your patient has a clear airway. If there is doubt in your mind, or if the airway is at risk, intubate the patient.

(2) Restoring the circulating volume. Effective restoration of the circulating volume is the single most important measure in reversing shock, and should be undertaken as quickly as possible. The questions to be answered are how much will be required and of which fluids?

    (i)   *How much?* As outlined above, many factors contribute to the hypovolaemia of shock. Thus the volume of fluid required to restore perfusion is always greater than any fluid loss (which is, anyway, difficult to measure). Improving tissue perfusion is evidenced by a warming of the extremities, increasing renal flow and disappearance of mental confusion. The amount of fluid to achieve this is best assessed by serial central venous pressure and pulmonary wedge readings (see p. 382).

           A central venous pressure line is thus mandatory in the proper treatment of shock, but of course fluid replacement should begin immediately, and not wait on the placement of the line, which may be difficult. Insertion of a pulmonary artery flotation catheter (see p. 388), enabling you to record pulmonary wedge pressure and cardiac output, can also be very helpful in assessing fluid requirements, and is being used more frequently in the monitoring of shock patients.

    (ii)   *Which fluids?* Irrespective of the cause of shock, both crystalloids and colloids are lost, and both require replacement. The circumstances in which shock occurs will obviously determine the ratio of colloid to crystalloid used, but as a general rule, one-half to three-quarters of the necessary volume should be as crystalloid, and the rest as colloid, although controversy over the exact ratio abounds.[10]

    (iii)   Crystalloids. These should be given initially as normal saline, as salt replacement has first priority. However, in overall terms there is usually more water than salt lost, thus it is reasonable to give one-third of the overall crystalloid replacement as 5% dextrose.

    (iv)   Colloids. Colloid replacement can be given as:

          (a) Albumin,[7] plasma or fresh frozen plasma. FFP should not, however, be given unless there is evidence of bleeding due to coagulation deficiencies, as in DIC.[4]

(b) One of the artificial plasma expanders, such as dextran or Haemaccel. Dextran is cheap, readily available and free from the risk of hepatitis, and has, as an additional bonus, an anti-thrombotic property. However it does tend to block the reticuloendothelial system, an undesirable property. Dextran 70 in saline in a dose of no more than 1000 ml/ 24 h is still regarded by some as the colloid of choice. Dextran 40, while having the theoretical advantage of reducing viscosity, can cause renal failure; we do not use it. If colloid additional to the dextrans proves to be necessary, plasma may be used. In cardiogenic shock if there is associated hypovolaemia, or in any other circumstances where saline infusion is undesirable, dextran made up in dextrose can be used. As dextrans cause rouleaux formation, blood must be taken for cross-matching before they are infused. Haemaccel, a colloid made from degraded gelatine, does not have anti-thrombotic properties. It does not cause cross-matching difficulties, and is said to have renal protective effects, so we use it in preference to dextran. We do not use more than 2000 ml in any single shock episode.

(3) The purpose of giving colloid is to raise the intravascular oncotic pressure, and so entrain fluid into the vascular compartment. Normal colloid osmotic pressure is 25 mmHg, and research is under way to assess which colloid solution is best at raising the intravascular osmotic pressure. This will mean that in the near future we should be able to advance a more rational colloid replacement policy.

(4) In haemorrhagic shock, blood will be required in addition to the above fluids. It is probably desirable to transfuse the patient to a haemoglobin of around 11 g/100 ml. Higher than this does not materially alter oxygen delivery, but does have the disadvantage of increasing viscosity. The blood that you give may obviate the need for any other colloid.

(5) The perflurochemicals, oxygen-carrying substances, are being evaluated as substitutes for blood. Their role is not yet defined.[8]

(6) Reversing hypoxia. The importance of ensuring a clear airway has already been stressed. Use of high (40–60%) concentra-

tions of oxygen will improve the Pao_2 and ensure maximal saturation of haemoglobin. This may prevent some cell damage. This oxygen concentration can be achieved by most commercially available face masks using oxygen flow rates of about 10 1/min. Assisted ventilation may be required particularly if shock lung occurs (see p. 97).

(7) Reducing arteriolar constriction. Arteriolar constriction should reverse when the cardiac output and arterial pressure are restored to normal with your fluid replacement. If, however, fluid replacement alone is not sufficient, you should use either:

(i) Beta-adrenergic agents, such as dopamine and dobutamine.

(a) Dopamine. At low infusion rates (<5 μg/kg/min) dopamine induces selective vasodilatation of the renal, cerebral, coronary and mesenteric circulation. At slightly higher doses (5–20 μg/kg/min, it increases the force, but not the rate of myocardial contraction (i.e. it is inotropic not chronotropic). It also acts as a vasoconstrictor at doses above 10 μg/kg/min. Its maximal effect is said to triple the heart force. It is thus the agent of choice in shock, once you are satisfied that volume repletion is adequate (see p. 382).

(b) Dobutamine (2.5–10 μg/kg/min) is more strongly inotropic than dopamine, but does not have dopamine's vasodilator properties. Using the two together makes good sense, as we have outlined in the section on cardiogenic shock (p. 17).

(c) If these are not available, or do not work, use isoprenaline. Put 2 mg of isoprenaline in 500 ml of 5% dextrose and give the infusion sufficiently fast to raise the systolic arterial pressure to about 95 mmHg. If this is ineffective or leads to a large volume of fluids being infused, double or treble the concentration.

(d) All these are preferable to metaraminol (aramine), which has both alpha-mimetic and beta-mimetic properties and may increase the arterial pressure at some expense to tissue perfusion.

(e) Noradrenaline and methoxamine should not be

used. They constrict arterioles and further decrease tissue perfusion. Their use is therefore illogical, and in practice is rarely successful.

or:

(ii) Alpha-adrenergic blocking agents the use of which has been largely superseded by dopamine and dobutamine. These reduce arteriolar constriction. The agents most commonly used are phenoxybenzamine, phentolamine, chlorpromazine and nitroprusside. They can cause a disastrous fall in arterial pressure unless the expanded circulatory volume is taken up by infusing fluid preferably blood, plasma, dextran 70 or Haemaccel. It is essential for the central venous pressure and/or the pulmonary capillary wedge pressure (PCWP) to be at the upper limit of the normal range before these drugs are given.

   (a) Infuse phenoxybenzamine 10–15 mg in 100 ml of 5% dextrose over 2 h, or phentolamine at a rate of 0.5–1 mg/min; or
   (b) chlorpromazine 5 mg i.v. every 15 min to a maximum of 20 mg; or
   (c) give nitroprusside.

As any of these drugs are given, the central venous pressure will probably fall together with the PCWP and arterial pressure. The central venous pressure and or PCWP must be maintained within the upper half of the normal range by further infusions of fluid. This ensures an adequate venous return, and cardiac output.

(8) Glucocorticoids. There is no role for high dose steroids in shock (except for their use in the wheezing accompanying anaphylactic shock, see p. 345). However, adrenal insufficiency may be provoked in shocked patients, and it is perfectly reasonable to give hydrocortisone 100 mg to a patient who has persistent hypotension for which there is no other obvious cause.

(9) Increasing myocardial contractility. The reason for myocardial depression in shock is not clear, although certain products of cell necrosis have been implicated. You should attempt to reverse this depression with adrenergic agents, with the correction of the acidosis, and by ensuring that your patient has

correct levels of all the other electrolytes, including K^+, Mg^{2+}, Ca^{2+} and PO_4^{2-}. It may also be of benefit to digitalise the patient (see p. 18).

(10) Reversing acidosis. As acidosis has a well-recognised negative inotropic effect; its correction is important, and is usually achieved by restoring tissue perfusion. However, if the pH is below 7.1 it is reasonable to give small quantities of bicarbonate. Theoretically the bicarbonate deficit (mmol) is given by [body weight (kg) × 3/5 × 25-serum HCO_3 mmol/l]. Give half this amount and repeat the arterial pH before deciding whether to give more.

(11) Disseminated intravascular coagulation (DIC).

   (i) This often occurs in the setting of poorly perfused patients, particularly in association with sepsis. Enzymes released from damaged cells convert fibrinogen to fibrin. In its turn this activates plasminogen, and the resulting plasmin dissolves both unwanted and haemostatic fibrin. The resultant cascade creates the paradoxical state of simultaneous thrombosis and haemmorhage which characterises DIC. The most obvious clinical manifestation is usually haemorrhagic rather than thrombosis, but either may further impair perfusion.

   (ii) The evidence for DIC is a bleeding tendency with low platelets, raised prothrombin time (PT) and kaolin cephalin time (KCT), low fibrinogen titres and raised fibrin degradation products. There may be fragmented red cells on the blood film. A reasonable bedside test for the presence of DIC is as follows. Take blood into a plain tube and keep this at 37°C by holding it in your hand or putting it in your pocket. Invert it at 30 s intervals. Normal blood should clot within 2–3 min. Failure to do this is good evidence for DIC.

   (iii) These abnormalities are often reversed when the underlying cause of shock is corrected: there is no good evidence that the use of heparin increases survival.

   (iv) If, after the underlying disorder is corrected, bleeding persists with a low plasma fibrinogen level (<1.0 g/l) and a low platelet count (<40 × 10⁹/1), fresh frozen plasma, which supplies all the major clotting factors, fibrinogen concentrate and fresh platelet concentrates may be required.

(12) Stress ulceration. Patients who are shocked frequently develop superficial gastric erosions which may bleed profusely (see section on ARDS, p. 97 for risk factors). Enteral feeding helps prevent this complication as does sucralfate, which you should start as soon as possible in a dose of 1–2 g t.d.s.[5]

(13) Lactate. Lactate levels go up if either oxygen delivery to the tissues, or consumption by the tissues is inadequate, and so is a good measure of tissue perfusion. The level is usually above 5 mmol/l in shock. The change in level over time may give you an insight into how well you and, more importantly, your patient are doing.

(14) Selective decontamination of the digestive tract, while undoubtedly reducing the number of nosocomial infections in very ill patients, has not reduced overall mortality. We do not practise it.[9]

REFERENCES

1   Baskett P. (1990) Management of hypovolaemic shock. *Br. Med. J.* **300:** 1453.

2   Davies J.M. (1982) Cardiovascular problems. *Hospital Update* November, p. 1359.

3   Houston M.C. (1984) Shock. Diagnosis and management. *Arch. Intern. Med.* **144:** 1433.

4   Jones J. (1987) Abuse of fresh frozen plasma. *Br. Med. J.* **295:** 287.

5   Leader (1989) Stress ulcer prophylaxis in critically ill patients. *Lancet* **ii:** 1255.

6   Ledingham I. McA. *et al.* (1982) Prognosis in severe shock. *Br. Med. J.* **284:** 443.

7   McClelland D. (1990) Human albumin solutions *Br. Med. J.* **300:** 35.

8   Odling-Smee W. (1990) Red cell substitutes. *Br. Med. J.* **300:** 599.

9   Vandenbroucke-Grauls C. *et al.* (1991) Effect of selective decontamination of the digestive tract on respiratory tract infections and mortality in the ITU. *Lancet* **338:** 859.

10 Yates D. (1987) Volume replacement: the choice of fluid. *Hospital Update* April, p. 297.

Blood transfusion reactions

A mild reaction following blood transfusion consisting of flushing, itching, urticaria and pyrexia is quite common, especially in those with a history of allergic reactions. Their incidence may be reduced by antihistamines, e.g. diphenhydramine (Benadryl) 50 mg orally 1 h before transfusion and 50 mg during it. If wheezing starts to occur or hypotension (which is not due to haemorrhage) develops, the blood should be stopped at once and saved for retesting. Give hydrocortisone 200 mg i.v. or adrenaline 1:1000 0.5 ml i.m. immediately. Also give an i.v. antihistamine such as diphenhydramine 20 mg i.v.

Acute renal failure as a complication of blood transfusion has been dealt with elsewhere (see p. 150).

Anaphylactic shock[1,2]

(1) Never give any drug or vaccine to a patient who says she or he is allergic to it, even if the evidence is unconvincing. Do not attempt to obtain the evidence by skin testing. This may be misleading and may occasionally be fatal.

(2) Warning signs of an allergic response are flushing, itching and urticaria. However, they may be absent. The symptoms of a more severe attack are wheezing, a feeling of chest constriction and impending doom, abdominal pain, nausea and vomiting. Laryngeal oedema may be experienced as a lump in the throat, hoarseness or stridor. Circulatory collapse and death may follow. Symptoms usually occur within seconds to minutes of exposure, either i.v. or occasionally orally, to the triggering agent. It is important to remember, however, that reactions can be delayed for up to several hours.

MANAGEMENT

(1) Give adrenaline 500–1000 μg (0.5–1.0 ml of 1:1000) i.m. This is the most important immediate treatment, and will tend to reverse bronchospasm, laryngeal oedema, urticaria and angio-oedema. This dose should be repeated at 15 min intervals until improvement occurs. If your patient is profoundly hypotensive (systolic arterial pressure <80 mmHg), 3–5 ml of 1:10 000 solution may be given slowly i.v., at a rate of 0.5–5.0 μg/min.

(2) Give diphenhydramine hydrochloride (Benadryl) 20 mg slowly i.v. to counteract the excessive histamine release.

(3) Give hydrocortisone 200 mg i.v. to suppress any further allergic reaction.

(4) Give aminophylline 250–350 mg i.v. over 15 min if there is evidence of continuing airways obstruction. Salbutamol 250 μg i.v. over 5 min is an alternative. Do not forget dyspnoea may also be due to acute laryngeal oedema (see above and p. 92).

(5) Give high concentration of oxygen.

(6) If hypotension persists after this immediate treatment, establish a CVP line and infuse plasma, Haemaccel or alternating

bottles of N saline and 5% dextrose to maintain a CVP in the upper half of the normal range. This is usually sufficient to restore the arterial pressure. If, however, it remains low, it may be necessary to give isoprenaline or dopamine (see p. 340).

(7) If there is increasing shortness of breath, consider elective intubation, as this can be very difficult once florid laryngeal oedema has developed.

REFERENCES

(1) Bochner B. *et al.* (1991) Anaphylaxis. *N. Engl. J. Med.* **324:** 1785.

(2) Brueton M. *et al.* (1991) Management of anaphylaxis. *Hospital Update* May, p. 386.

Bacterial Shock

DIAGNOSIS

(1) Bacterial shock occurs when large numbers of either Gram-positive or Gram-negative bacteria get into the bloodstream. The common organisms and surrounding circumstances are detailed below.

  (i) Gram-negative bacteraemia quite often follows surgery to the bowel or instrumentation of the lower urinary tract. The infecting organisms are commonly *Escherichia coli* or other coliforms; less commonly anaerobes or *Pseudomonas aeruginosa*.

  (ii) Gram-positive bacteraemias.

   (a) Staphylococcal infections are often secondary to joint or chest sepsis or drug abuse, but the source is not always found.

   (b) Streptococcal infection is found in association with cellulitis, puerperal infection and septic abortion. In septic abortion, the streptococcus is often accompanied by *Clostridium welchii* and other *anaerobes*, as well as coliforms.

  (iii) A further important sub group to consider is focal, often trivial staphylococcal infection causing toxic shock encephalopathy. In this group circulating exotoxins cause multi-organ damage. A significant proportion of cases have been associated with the use of tampons during menstruation. Toxic shock encephalopathy may be distinguished clinically. A characteristic macular erythroderma is followed by desquamation, including the palms and soles, within 2 weeks of onset. Mucous membrane changes, oropharyngeal oedema, ulceration and conjunctivitis develop soon after the fever. Fits may occur. Hypotension is often profound.

(2) Additional factors which predispose toward sepsis are:

  (i) Pre-existing disease, such as diabetes, alcoholism, malnutrition, uraemia and liver disease.

(ii) Drug therapy, such as steroids, chemotherapeutic agents, previous courses of antibiotics.

(iii) Invasive procedures, such as instrumentation of the urinary tract, arterial and venous lines, nasotracheal tubes and enteral feeding.

(3) The onset of septic shock is usually marked by rigors associated with nausea, vomiting and diarrhoea.

(i) Initially the patient is peripherally vasodilated, flushed, pyrexial and hypotensive. Cardiac output is at this stage increased, but as much of the blood is being shunted through arteriovenous communications, the Pao_2 is low and tissue oxygen utilisation is deficient. The situation is peculiar to bacteraemic shock, and accounts for the paradox of an apparently well-perfused patient who is, none the less, confused and oliguric. The mortality of this group is about 25%.

(ii) This state gives way to the classical shock picture of a confused or comatose patient with cold, clammy peripheries, acidosis and a fall in urinary and cardiac output with or without pyrexia. The mortality of this group is at least 60%. Early recognition and energetic treatment of the former state may forestall the appearance of the latter with consequent saving of life.

MANAGEMENT

In about half the patients the interval between onset of shock and death is 48 h, and a successful outcome is partially dependent upon the speed with which the following measures are carried out.

(1) Laboratory investigations. Take blood for blood cultures, full blood count, electrolytes, urea, and creatinine, group and cross-match and arterial blood gases. If possible take three blood cultures, each from a different site, within ½ h. Take swabs from throat and rectum. Microscope and plate out a clean specimen of urine.

(2) Antibiotics.

(i) Start initial treatment as soon as possible after (**NEVER** before!) culture specimens have been taken.

Table 4   Table of sensitivity of common organisms to various antibotics

	1	2	3	4	5	6	7	8	9	10
					Organism					
Azlocillin/piperacillin	R	S	SS	S	S	SS	HS	SS	S	S
Ceftazidine	S	S	S	SS	S	R	S	S	S	R
Chloramphenicol	S	S	R	S	SS	S	S	S	S	S
Aminoglycosides (gentamicin)	HS	HS	S	S	S	R	R	S	R	R
Benzyl penicillin/ erythromycin	R	HS	R	R	R	R	HS	R	HS	S
Metronidazole	R	R	R	R		S	S	R	R	R
Cloxacillin	S	S	R	R	R	R	?	R	S	R
Vancomycin	S	HS	R	R	R	R		R	HS	HS
Ciprofloxacin	S	HS	S	HS	R	SS		HS	S	SS

HS, highly sensitive; S, sensitive; SS, slightly sensitive; R, resistant; ?, data poorly established.

1. Hospital-acquired *Staphylococcus aureus*.
2. Non-hospital-acquired *Staphylococcus aureus* (gram +ve coccus).
3. *Pseudomonas aeruginosa* (gram −ve rod).
4. *Escherichia coli* (gram −ve rod).
5. *Proteus* sp. (gram −ve rod).
6. *Bacteroides* sp. (gram −ve rod).
7. *Clostridium welchii* (gram +ve coccus).
8. *Klebsiella aerobacter* sp. (gram −ve rod).
9. *Streptococcus pyogenes* (gram +ve coccus).
10. *Streptococcus faecalis* (gram +ve coccus).

Clearly antibiotics to which organisms are either highly sensitive or sensitive should be used wherever possible.

(ii)   Use a combination of a penicillin plus an aminoglycoside plus metronidazole (see (iii), (iv) and (v) below).

(iii)   Choice of penicillin.

(a)   Benzyl penicillin, in combination with an aminoglycoside, is effective against virtually all Gram-positive organisms (penicillinase-producing staphylococci will be dealt with by the aminoglycosides). A suitable penicillin dose for severe infections is 2 megaunits i.v. every 6 h.

(b)   If the patient is allergic to penicillin, substitute erythromycin 500–1000 mg i.v. 6-hourly.

(c)   If pseudomonas infection or other resistant gram-negative infection is considered likely, substitute piperacillin (200–300 mg/kg i.v. daily in four divided doses) or azlocillin 5 g 8-hourly i.v. for the penicillin.[3]

(d) Azlocillin is synergistic with gentamicin but must be given in separate infusions, as they react chemically, inactivating each other. This reaction is only of serious consequence in the bloodstream when renal function is seriously impaired.

(e) Remember that 15 g of azlocillin contains 33 mmol of Na^+, and so Na^+ administration should be adjusted accordingly.

(f) If your patient is allergic to penicillin, use ceftazidime 1–6 g i.v. daily in three divided doses in place of piperacillin or azlocillin.

(iv) Choice of aminoglycoside.

(a) Aminoglycosides are highly active against nearly all Gram-negative organisms. Gentamicin, given as an initial loading dose of 120 mg i.v, and then 5 mg/kg/day in three divided doses (normally 80 mg 8-hourly) is the aminoglycoside of first choice, unless the patient is known to have poor renal function. If you do use gentamicin when renal function is impaired, the interval between doses must be modified as outlined in Table 5 below. An alternative way of calculating the dose interval is: serum creatinine (μmol) divided by 15 = approximate dosage interval (h). In every case serum gentamicin levels should be measured daily. You should aim for peak levels (1 h after i.v. or i.m. administration) of 7–12 μg/ml, and trough levels (just before the next dose) of less than 2 μg/ml, and you will have to alter your dose as necessary to achieve this.

(b) Netilmicin is safer in renal impairment, as it is less oto- and nephrotoxic. The usual adult dose is 150 mg b.d. (4–7 mg/kg/d in two divided doses). You should aim at peak levels of 5–12 μg/ml, and troughs of less than 3 μg/ml.

(c) Amikacin. This very expensive aminoglycoside should only be used if organisms resistant to gentamicin and netilmicin have been identified. The usual dose is 15 mg/kg/d in two divided doses).

(d) The interval between doses of both the above will have to be modified along the same lines as gentamicin if your patient has renal impairment.

Table 5 Modification of gentamicin dosage in patients with renal impairment

Blood urea (mmol/l)	Dose (mg) and frequency of administration (for a 70 kg patient)	
7	*80	8-hourly
7–18	*80	12-hourly
18–36	*80	24-hourly
36	*80	48-hourly

*60 mg if patient is below 60 kg weight.

(v) Metronidazole.[4] This is the agent of choice against anaerobes. As mentioned above, we use it routinely in septic shock, as anaerobic organisms are frequently present. The dose is 500 mg in 100 ml infused over ½ h, 8-hourly or 400 mg orally or 1 g rectally 8-hourly.

(vi) Fucidic acid. If severe staphylococcal infection is strongly suspected, give 500 mg fucidic acid dissolved in 250 ml of N saline and infused over 4 h four times a day. Vancomycin in a dose of 1 g b.d. i.v. is an alternative.

(vii) Chloramphenicol. This is a highly effective antibiotic whose role has been somewhat eclipsed by the aminoglyosides, and its undoubted, though rare, propensity to cause an idiosyncratic irreversible aplastic anaemia. More common is the dose-related, reversible marrow suppression. Neither should stop you using it, in a dose of 50–100 mg/kg body weight i.v. 6-hourly, if the newer antibiotics are not available to you. A usual adult dose would be 1 g 6-hourly.

(viii) The quinolones, such as ciprofloxacin, may acquire a role in serious sepsis[8]. However, we see no need to change from the well-tested regimes detailed above.

(3) Systemic fungal infections in association with seriously ill patients.[2,6]

(i) These occur commonly in immunocompromised patients, 80% of infections occurring in this group (see p. 305). The others occur in patients who are already seriously ill, often with bacterial sepsis, and therefore usually in the ITU.

(ii) The three fungi most commonly involved are *Candida,* aspergillosis and *Cryptococcus neoformans.* Cryptococcal infection occurs almost exclusively in patients with T lymphocyte deficiency, such as AIDS, whereas systemic (as opposed to mucocutaneous) infections with *Candida* and *Aspergillus* are more common in neutropenic or otherwise seriously ill patients.

(iii) *Candida.*[5] If you have a positive blood culture for *Candida* in a patient who is seriously ill, you should start treatment with:

(a) Amphotericin B i.v. Give a test dose of 5.0 mg, and then, if there is no adverse reaction, give 0.3 mg/kg in a 5% dextrose infusion over 2–4 h on the first day, and 0.6–1.0 mg/kg/d thereafter. Amphotericin may cause hypokalaemia and renal impairment, and you should temporarily stop the drug if the creatinine rises to above 200 μmol/l.

(b) If there is intraocular or CSF involvement, add flucytosine—in a dose of 37.5 mg/kg/6 h orally if renal function is normal. If the creatinine clearance is between 20 and 40 ml/min, reduce the dose interval to 12-hourly, and if it is 10–20 ml/min to 37.5 mg/kg each 24 h.

(c) A promising, but as yet not fully evaluated new treatment is with fluconazole, 400–600 mg/day.

(iv) Aspergillosis. The lung is the commonest site of involvement, and while isolating *Aspergillus* from a likely patient is helpful in making the diagnosis, lung biopsy may be necessary to confirm it. Treatment is with amphotericin.

(v) *Cryptococcus*. The diagnosis is made by demonstrating the organism, using the traditional indian ink stain. The treatment is as for *Candida*.

(4) The restoration of tissue perfusion and correction of metabolic abnormalities are as detailed on p. 338. But—

(5) These patients are particularly prone to hypoxia, and frequently require assisted ventilation to maintain the Pao_2. This should be undertaken in conjunction with you anaesthetic colleagues. Even despite ventilatory assistance respiratory failure is a frequent mode of death. The lung capillaries appear to become leaky, giving an x-ray appearance of

widespread consolidation. This respiratory complication is rather unsatisfactorily labelled shock lung or the adult respiratory distress syndrome (ARDS) (see p. 97).

(6) Endotoxin antibody (HA–1A–centoxin).[1,7] The lipopolysaccharide in the outer membrane of Gram-negative bacteria is not affected by antibiotics, and is thought to be a major factor in the pathogenesis of bacteraemic shock. A recent trial using human monoclonal IgM antibody to this lipopolysaccharide showed a greatly increased survival in patients with proved Gram-negative sepsis, although there is still some disquiet about the validity of these findings[10]. Until the situation is clarified, we suggest using Centoxin, in a dose of 100 mg, in the following circumstances:

(i) You must be certain that there is evidence of systemic response to infection, with associated hypotension (systolic blood pressure <90mmHg), or two of the following signs of organ system dysfunction or peripheral hypoperfusion:

(a) unexplained metabolic acidosis—cH >50nmol/l or an elevated lactate level (see p. 179).
(b) arterial hypoxaemia—Pao_2 <10 kPa;
(c) oliguria—urinary output <0.5 ml kg^{-1} h^{-1};
(d) elevated PT or PTT, or reduction in platelet count to <100 000 mm^3;
(e) sudden decrease in mental acuity;
(f) cardiac output of >4.0 $l/min/m^2$.

(ii) There should be a high likelihood that the infection is caused by a Gram-negative organism i.e.:

(a) peritonitis due to bowel perforation or complicating abdominal surgery;
(b) nosocomial pneumonia;
(c) pyelonephritis;
(d) wound or soft tissue infection complicating abdominal surgery;
(e) septic shock without evidence of the source of infection.

(7) Naloxone. Its use has not been associated with improved survival, and we do not use it.

(8) Steroids. There is now good evidence that these do not help.[9]

REFERENCES

1   Colman R. (1989) The role of plasma protease in septic shock. *N. Engl. J. Med.* **320:** 1207.

2   Davey P. (1990) New antiviral and antifungal drugs. *Br. Med. J.* **300:** 793.

3   Donowitz G. (1988) Beta-lactam antibiotics. *N. Engl. J. Med.* **318:** 419.

4   Goldman P. (1980) Metronidazole. *N. Engl. J. Med.* **303:** 1212.

5   Edwards J. (1991) Invasive candida infections. *N. Engl. J. Med.* **324:** 1063.

6   Hay R. (1991) Systemic fungal infections. *Prescribers Journal* 160.

7   Leader (1991) Endoxin bound and gagged. *Lancet* **337:** 588.

8   Neu H. (1987) Clinical use of the quinolones. *Lancet* **ii:** 1319.

9   Veteran Administration Study Group (1987). Effect of high dose steroids therapy on mortality in patients with clinical signs of systemic sepsis. *N. Engl. J. Med.* **317:** 659.

10   Wenzel R. (1992) Anti-endotoxin monoclonal antibodies—a second look. *N. Engl. J. Med.* **326:** 1151.

The unconscious patient—coma[1-5]

DIAGNOSIS

Coma is an unrousable lack of awareness. It is better defined as a rating on the Glasgow coma scale of less than 8 (see p. 216). Consciousness depends on activity in neurons of the ascending reticular formation of the brain stem, which pass through the diencaphalon and ramify with neurons thoughout the cerebral cortex. Therefore a depression of consciousness leading to coma can be due to either:

(1) Bilateral and widespread dysfunction of both cerebral hemispheres.
(2) Damage to, or compression of, the activating centres of the brainstem and diencephalon. (These structural causes constitute around 33% of cases in most series of coma.)
(3) Metabolic disturbance involving either of the above regions, accounting for a further 65% of cases.

Coma needs to be distinguished from:

(4) Psychogenic unresponsiveness, which, because it is initially diagnosed as coma, accounts for the residual 2% of cases.
(5) Brain death (see p. 242).

The exact nature and evolution of the neurological abnormality provides information about not only the localisation of the lesion causing coma, but also its likely aetiology. Since both these are crucial to management, a careful history from relatives (or other witnesses, including the family practitioner or ambulance driver as necessary) and examination are mandatory.

When examining a comatose patient, you aim to find out:

(1) The depth of coma. A convenient way to do this is to use the Glasgow coma scale (see p. 216). The depth of coma should be charted at frequent (15–30 min) intervals in the acute stages, and any deterioration should call for immediate re-assessment of your patient, if necessary by a more experienced colleague.
(2) The presence of focal lesions. Asymmetrical motor responses

are the easiest to identify, and these should already have been detected while the depth of coma was being assessed. Asymmetry of the brainstem reflexes is also important in this respect (see Part B below and Table 6). The presence of persistent focal lesions implies structural, rather than metabolic, causes for coma.

(3) The anatomical level of involvement of the neuraxis. Here you must be guided by the patterns of involvement of the brainstem reflexes, the type and rate of respiration, and the pulse rate, as detailed in Part B below in Table 6.

(4) Knowledge of these three aspects of coma will help you arrive at a differential diagnosis, as discussed below. In Parts A and B, we give an account of the diagnosis and progression of structural lesions causing coma, and in Parts C and D of metabolic and psychogenic causes of coma. In Part E we present a flow diagram illustrating our approach to the management of coma.

MANAGEMENT

Part A: Structural coma due to widespread dysfunction of both cerebral hemispheres

(1) Post-ictal stupor may, if history is lacking, cause diagnostic confusion, which fortunately is temporary since the patient will usually rouse within 6 h.

Other causes are more serious and essentially are limited to:

(2) Catastrophic intracerebral or intraventricular haemorrhage (see p. 202).

(3) Closed head injury with contusion and/or intracerebral haemorrhage (see p. 215).

(4) Encephalitis and meningo-encephalitis (see p. 367).

The picture of neurological disability in all the above will depend upon the site of maximal cortical involvement. In addition, the primary cerebral damage will give rise to secondary vasomotor paralysis with congestion and oedema of the brain. This will produce a downward displacement of the cerebral hemispheres leading to diencephalic and brainstem compression, which we describe in Part B below.

Table 6 Localisation of brainstem involvement (see text for full explanation)

	Diencephalic		Midbrain and upper pons	Lower pons and upper medulla	Lower medulla
	Upper	Lower			
Response to pain	Appropriately directed	Abnormal flexor	Abnormal extensor	Nil	Nil
Pupils	Small with intact light reflex	Small with intact light reflex	3–5 mm irregular	3–5 mm and unresponsive	Dilated and unresponsive
Eye movements	Full (roving)	Full	Hard to elicit internuclear ophthalmoplegia	Absent	Absent
Respirations	Eupnoeic Cheyne–Stokes	Eupnoeic	Tachypnoeic	Shallow 20–40/min	Slow and irregular
Other	Grasp reflexes	—	Diabetes insipidus	—	Falling arterial pressure
Ocular vestibular (ice-water calorics)	Deviation of both eyes to side of lesion		Adducting eye fails to move across the midline	Absent	Absent
Oculocephalic (doll's head manoeuvre)	Normal	Normal (see text)	Adducting eye fails to move across the midline	Absent	Absent

Part B: Structural coma due to involvement of diencephalic and brainstem activating centres

The diencephalon and brainstem may be effected:

(1) As a result of brainstem compression. This gives an orderly progression of rostral to caudal brainstem dysfunction.

   (i)   At first reactive small pupils and Cheyne-Stokes respiration are present, and the subject may be roused by painful stimuli. As only the upper brainstem is involved, the eye reflexes elicited as described below, are intact.

      (a)   When the eye reflexes are intact, there may be spontaneously rolling eye movements and there will be an appropriate response to doll's head manoeuvre or ice-water calorics (see below).

      (b)   The doll's head manoeuvre is carried out by observing the effect on eye movements of briskly and fully rotating the head on the neck and trunk (if necessary while the patient is temporarily disconnected from the ventilator). In normal people the eyes will stay looking forward while the head is moved. The abnormal response is when the eyes move in the same axis as the head.

      (c)   The ice-water caloric test is carried out as follows. First, inspect the external auditory canal to ensure the tympanic membrane is intact and, if necessary, remove wax. Lift the head if possible to 30° to the horizontal. Using a thin catheter inserted into the external auditory canal, slowly instil up to 50 ml of ice-cold water while observing the eye movements. In a conscious patient this is extremely uncomfortable, for it induces severe vertigo, nausea and vomiting, together with nystagmus of which the fast component is away from the irrigated ear. In the unconscious patient with an intact brainstem, the response obtained is of tonic conjugate deviation of the eyes towards the irrigated ear. Having tested one side, 5 min should elapse before testing the other in order to allow the currents induced in the semicircular canals to subside.

   (ii)   With involvement of the mid-brain, decerebrate rigidity (here the arms are extended and internally rotated, the wrists and fingers flexed, the legs extended adducted and internally rotated with the feet plantar flexed and inverted, and the trunk extended, with the head retracted) dysconjugate eye movements, (see Table 6) and fixed medium sized pupils are present. The patient often becomes tachypnoeic.

(iii) Finally, as the lower brainstem is involved, the pupils dilate, no eye movements can be elicited, and the patient is totally unresponsive to pain arising from stimulation in the trigeminal area.

(2) The brainstem can also be involved as a result of direct injury, when there will be localising eye signs and bilateral limb signs from the onset of the coma. The localising signs depend on the level of the brainstem involved. Thus:

(i) Midbrain lesions, if centrally placed, interrupt the light reflex and oculomotor interconnections. Thus, pupils are mid position and fixed with either nuclear or internuclear opthalmoplegia. There may also be bilateral, frequently asymmetrical, corticospinal tract signs.

(ii) Upper and mid pontine involvement are marked by small reactive pupils, a gaze palsy to the side of the lesion and sometimes evidence of fifth (absent corneal) or seventh (lower motor neuron facial symmetry) nerve involvement.

(iii) Lower pons lesions similarly have small reactive pupils with lateral eye movements absent, but vertical eye movements spared (vertical doll's head manoeuvre). There may be flaccid quadriplegia, or alternatively abnormal extensor posturing. The respiratory rhythm is shallow and irregular.

(iv) If cerebellar and brainstem signs are elicited, the possibility of cerebellar haemorrhage (p. 205) must not be forgotten. Cerebellar infarcts accompanied by developing oedema may also behave like an expanding mass lesion and are similarly susceptible to potentially life-saving neurosurgical decompression.

Part C: Metabolic encephalopathy

There are a number of features which distinguish metabolic encephalopathy from the previously discussed structural causes of coma.

(1) Coma is nearly always preceded by an interval of decreased awareness, impaired cognitive function and personality disturbance.

(2) Even when other brainstem functions are lost with depression of consciousness, absent ice-water caloric reflexes and abnormal extensor posturing, the pupillary light reflex is usually preserved. This simultaneous involvement of many levels of the neuraxis with relative sparing of some functions at the same levels is typical of metabolic encephalopathy. Progressive rostrocaudal deterioration does not occur.

(3) Abnormal movements typical of metabolic encephalopathy include a fine tremor at 8–10 Hz, flapping tremor of the hands (frequently found in, but not confined to, hepatic encephalopathy) and multi-focal myoclonic jerks.

(4) Sustained focal neurological deficits are usually absent. There are two exceptions to this rule, which can be a trap, however:

    (i)   Hypoglycaemic hemiplegias which may completely resolve with prompt and adequate treatment (p. 183). Similar findings have been reported in hepatic coma, uraemia and hypernatraemia.

    (ii) Although lateral conjugate deviation of the eyes strongly suggests a structural lesion, downward conjugate deviation may be caused by metabolic disturbance—particularly certain drug overdoses.

(5) There are a number of categories of metabolic coma, knowledge of which will help you direct your examination and investigations more effectively.

    (i)   Hypoxic-ischaemic, as after cardiac arrest, and now the commonest cause of metabolic coma.

    (ii) Self-poisoning, including carbon monoxide (see p. 281).

    (iii) Alcohol intoxication.

    (iv) Organ failure—the commonest is hepatic encephalopathy, but coma can occur in association with respiratory, renal or cardiac failure.

    (v) Endocrine—of which hypoglycaemia or hyperglycaemia are the commonest. Myxoedema may also cause coma.

    (vi) Electrolyte disturbances—particularly hyponatraemia and hypercalcaemia.

    (vii) In association with diffuse intracranial or systemic infection; particularly meningitis, encephalitis and cerebral malaria.

Your comprehensive examination should therefore include smelling the breath (diabetic ketoacidosis, uraemic fetor, fetor hepaticus and alcohol) and testing for neck stiffness (meningitis, subarachnoid haemorrhage and tonsilar herniation). You will also need to undertake the relevant investigations to confirm or exclude the above (see (6) below).

Part D: Psychogenic unresponsiveness

There are several features of this state which resolve diagnostic confusion.

(1) Eyelids are usually held firmly shut, resist opening, and when released snap shut. The slow passive closure of the lids of the comatose patient is rarely successfully reproduced.

(2) The corneal reflex evoked by a wisp of cotton wool is rarely successfully suppressed. Similarly tickling the eyelashes usually evokes eyelid twitching.

(3) Patients with psychogenic unresponsiveness do not have roving or disconjugate eye movements.

(4) Ice-water calorics evoke nystagmus, the normal response, rather than tonic deviation. This physical sign is unequivocal and diagnostic.

MANAGEMENT OF THE UNCONSCIOUS PATIENT

Evaluation of the evolution and patterns of neurological deficit should have enabled you to make a sophisticated guess at the site and nature of the lesion. However, common to all the categories are a number of basic considerations which in rough order of priority are as follows.

(1) Assure oxygenation. Measure blood gases, or minute volume (more than 4 1/min usually indicates adequate ventilation). Clear blood and vomit from the pharynx by suction.

    (i) If ventilation still seems inadequate intubate and ventilate—otherwise turn your patient into the semi-recumbent coma position.

    (ii) If there is a history of neck pain or trauma do not extend the neck to intubate. Obtain a lateral neck x-ray without moving the patient. Rarely an emergency tracheostomy may be necessary.

   (iii) Cardiac arrhythmias which may be provoked by intubation may be prevented by atropine 0.6 mg i.v. beforehand.

   (iv) Remember that inhalation of gastric contents is a frequent problem in patients who have lost the reflexes protecting their airways (see p. 101).

(2) Maintain circulation. If there is a vasomotor paresis from brainstem involvement, or if there has been inadequate fluid intake due to any prior illness, the effective circulating volume may be low. Infuse fluid in the usual way with CVP control (see p. 382). If you assess the circulating volume to be adequate, it may be necessary to infuse dopamine (see p. 340).

(3) Hypoglycaemia should be checked using BM stix, supplemented if you obtain a low reading by a formal blood glucose. This should be done whilst (1) and (2) are going on.

(4) Fits. Anything other than brief minor motor episodes should be controlled (see p. 224).

(5) If there is evidence of mass lesion (focal neurological signs and/or signs of raised intracranial pressure) start treatment for raised intracranial pressure with a bolus of mannitol and controlled hyperventilation (see p. 220). Obtain a CT scan; if no mass lesion is identified you may then proceed to a lumbar puncture.

(6) If there is evidence of metabolic disorder send blood for:

    (i)   electrolytes and urea;
    (ii)   osmolality;
    (iii) blood gases;
    (iv) calcium;
    (v)   glucose.

Save blood for toxic screen, liver function tests, coagulation studies, thyroid and adrenal function, blood culture and initial viral titre. If examining a traveller recently arrived from the tropics consider cerebral malaria, yellow fever, typhoid and typhus. Obtain a CT scan and in the absence of focal swelling do a lumbar puncture.

(7) Check the rectal temperature. Extremes of temperature should be corrected (see p. 289).

(8) If there is a history of alcoholism, or if there is opthalmoplegia, or if intravenous dextrose is to be infused, give thiamine 100 mg i.v. beforehand to prevent or treat Wernicke's encephalopathy.

(9) If you suspect a narcotic overdose give naloxone 0.4 mg every 5 min until the patient arouses (see p. 258). If there is evidence of narcotic addiction (look for needle marks), dilute 0.4 mg in 10 ml of diluent and inject slowly to avoid precipitating an acute withdrawal crisis.

(10) If coma is interrupted by agitation, small (5 mg), preferably intravenous, doses of diazepam should suffice.

(11) General care of the unconscious patient includes the following.

   (i) Attention to pressure points (a pillow between the legs, 2-hourly turning, perhaps a ripple mattress). Obviously bed linen must be frequently changed if it becomes soaked with urine or stained with faeces.

   (ii) In the absence of spontaneous blinking avoid exposure keratitis by methylcellulose eye drops, and, if necessary, securing the eyelids with adhesive tape.

   (iii) Urinary incontinence can frequently be managed satisfactorily with a sheath urinal for a man, but for women an indwelling silastic catheter inserted with strict attention to asepsis is the most satisfactory solution.

REFERENCES

1   Bates D. (1985) Predicting recovery from medical coma. *Br. J. Hosp. Med.* May p. 276.

2   Bates D. (1985) Management of the comatose patient. *Hospital Update* June, p. 425.

3   Cartlidge NEF. (1979) Clinical aspects of coma—the assessment of acute brain failure. *Trends in Neurosci.* **2:** 126.

4   Leader (1981) Outcome of non-traumatic coma. *Br. Med. J.* **283:** 3.

5   Plum E., Posner J.B. (1982) *The Diagnosis of Stupor and Coma.* Philadelphia: Davis.

Part E: Flow diagram of coma management

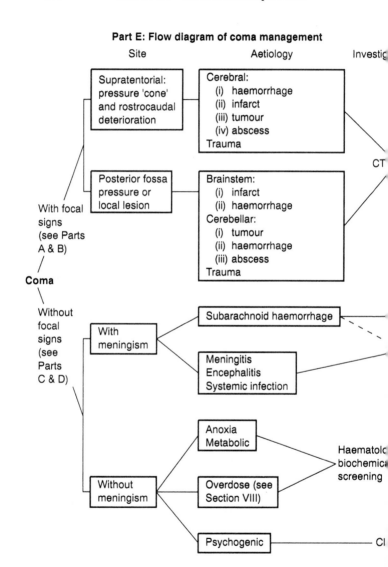

Severe chest pain[1]

DIAGNOSIS

Consider the following.

(1) The heart.
   Angina
   Myocardial infarction (see p. 11)
   Cardiac arrhythmias (see p. 26)
   Pericarditis—the pain is often affected by posture, and is usually worse lying down. It is also promptly relieved by non-steroidal anti-inflammatory agents.

(2) The lungs.
   Pneumonia (see p. 104) and other causes of pleurisy.
   Pulmonary embolus (see p. 52).
   Pneumothorax (see p. 85).
   Carcinoma of the lung.

(3) The oesophagus.
   Oesophagitis, with or without hiatus hernia.
   Oesophageal spasm.
   Oesophageal achalasia.
   Ruptured oesophagus—this gives rise to mediastinal emphysema, thus you may feel crepitus at the root of the neck.
   Oesophageal carcinoma.

(4) The aorta.
   Dissecting aneurysm (see p. 63).

(5) The mediastinum.
   Mediastinitis
   Mediastinal pneumothorax, which can give pain very like that of a myocardial infarct, and is best diagnosed by hearing a pericardial crunch, feeling air at the root of the neck and observing air in the pericardium on X-ray.

(6) The nerves.
   Cervical spondylitis or other causes of root compression.
   Herpes zoster—you will be vindicated should a characteristic rash appear.

(7) The abdomen.
   Acute cholecystitis.

Acute exacerbation or perforation of a peptic ulcer.
Pancreatitis (see p. 124).

(8) Thoracic wall.

An almost endless list of conditions involving muscles, bones and nerves—of which perhaps the commonest is an unexplained sharp pain over the precordium, lasting a few moments, called 'precordial catch'.

MANAGEMENT

The possibilities can usually be reduced to two or three by a careful history and examination. However, it is wise always to ask for:

(1) An ECG.
(2) A chest x-ray.
(3) Cardiac enzyme estimation.

If in doubt, observe the patient in hospital, bearing in mind that a normal ECG does not exclude a myocardial infarction.

REFERENCE

1 Lichstein E. *et al.* (1973) Evaluation of acute chest pain. *Med. Clin. North. Am.* **57:** 1481.

Severe headaches

The commonest cause of severe headache is migraine. Usually there is a preceding history of episodic throbbing headaches, associated with nausea and photophobia. Classically, visual symptoms such as teichopsia may precede or accompany the headache. Neck stiffness from concomitant muscle spasms, photophobia and transient focal signs (see p. 211) may mimic meningitis or subarachnoid haemorrhage, which must, in cases of doubt, be excluded by obtaining a CT scan or examination of the CSF as appropriate.

Other, more serious cases of headache which constitute emergencies are as follows.

(1) Meningitis.[7,9]

   (i)   This has four cardinal signs: headache, stiff neck, photophobia and fever. However, they may all be absent. A lumbar puncture should be considered if two of the four are present. It may also present as drowsiness, confusion, convulsions, focal neurological signs or coma.

   (ii) In the immunologically uncompromised host, three organisms account for most cases of bacterial meningitis:

      (a) *Neisseria meningitidis* (a Gram-negative coccus causing meningococcal meningitis, usually affecting young adults and invariably sensitive to penicillin).

      (b) *Haemophilus influenzae* (a Gram-negative rod usually found in the under fives, and usually sensitive to chloramphenicol).

      (c) *Streptococcus pneumoniae* (a Gram-positive coccus causing pneumococcal meningitis, the prominent organism in the elderly and, except in rare, geographically discrete instances, sensitive to penicillin).

  (iii) The organism may be identified by direct staining of CSF. However, where no organisms can be seen, for example in partially treated meningitis, distinguishing antigens may rapidly be identified after counterimmune electrophoresis.[6]

  (iv) Until positive identification is secure, give drugs as indicated below.

(a) To children above 8 years and to adults give benzyl penicillin 1.2–2.4 g i.v. in divided doses at 4-hourly intervals, on the presumption that they will be harbouring the meningococcus or pneumococcus.

(b) In cases of penicillin allergy, chloramphenicol, 50–100 mgm/kg body weight i.v. 6-hourly or cefotaxime 3 g 8-hourly (children 60–75 mg/kg 8-hourly) can be used. Both these antibiotics have a satisfactory action against all three above organisms. Some authorities recommend cefotaxime as first-line therapy.

(v) When the organism is identified, proceed as follows.

(a) Meningococcal meningitis:[7] benzyl penicillin is the drug of choice, given as above. If i.v. therapy becomes technically difficult and the organism is sensitive to sulphonamides, these may be given orally instead. Prophylaxis, either as rifampicin 10 mg/kg every 12 h for four doses, or, if the organism is sulphonamide-sensitive, sulphadimidine 500 mg 6-hourly for eight doses, should be offered to intimate contacts of your patient.[7]

(b) Pneumococcal meningitis: again, give benzyl penicillin as above.

(c) *Haemophilus influenzae*: chloramphenicol is now the drug of choice. Previously, ampicillin 300 mg/kg per day i.v. in divided doses given 6-hourly was advocated. This has now been precluded by the rapid rise in incidence of ampicillin resistance. Cefuroxime is an effective alternative to chloramphenicol. Rifampicin 20 mg/kg/day for 4 days should be given to any close contacts under the age of 4 years.

(d) Triple therapy (with penicillin, sulphonamide and chloramphenicol) and intrathecal antibiotics is unnecessary in treating meningitis caused by these organisms.

(e) Steroids. There may be a place for steroids in:
the meningitis of young children and infants;
critically ill adults with either pneumococcal or haemophilus infections.
In adults give 12 mg 12-hourly for 3 days.[3]

(iv) Differentiation from other causes of meningitis rests on examination and culture of the CSF.

(vii) Tuberculous meningitis.[5] This may present with a few weeks' history of increasing headaches, malaise and drowsiness, or have a more acute course of seizures, focal signs and progressive obtundation. Evidence of tuberculous infection elsewhere may be lacking, but the tuberculin skin test is usually positive. All cases of suspected meningitis should have CSF examined and cultured for TB organisms since, although the CSF cell response is typically lymphocytic, occasionally poly-morphs may predominate. Detection of tuberculostearic acid in the CSF is a rapid, sensitive and specific test for TB meningitis, which you should use if it is available to you.[2] Recommended therapy is isoniazid 10–15 mg/kg/d (plus pyridoxine 50 mg/day) with rifampicin 600 mg/day and either ethambutol 25 mg/kg/day or pyrazinamide (0.5 g t.i.d.).

(viii) Cryptococcal meningitis. This is of increasing importance being a major problem in immunocompromised patients, particularly those with T cell deficiencies, as in AIDS. The history is similar to that for tuberculous meningitis and likewise may be acute or more insidious. Diagnosis is made by india-ink microscopy of the CSF and examination for cryptococcal antigens. (See p. 352 for therapy.)

(ix) Amoebic meningitis. This is usually identified only when apparently pyogenic meningitis fails to respond to con-ventional therapy since the amoeba in CSF resembles white cells. Recommended therapy is amphotericin B 20 mg/day or, if the organism is a *Hartmanella* species, sulphadiazine 100 mg/kg/day given as 6-hourly doses.

(x) Unusual organisms may cause meningitis in immunolog-ically compromised people (see p. 310).

(2) Subarachnoid haemorrhage (see p. 208).
(3) Giant cell arteritis.

(i) This condition commonly causes headache by involve-ment of the medium-sized arteries of the scalp or dura, and is virtually unheard of below the age of 55 years.

(ii) In about half the cases, involvement of the central retinal artery causes blindness which usually occurs between 1 and 3 months after the onset of the headaches. However, transient or permanent amblyopia may be the presenting symptom.

(iii) In the typical case, the superficial arteries are tender, swollen and often pulseless. The ESR is usually above 60 mm/h. Occasionally, superficial arteries are not clinically involved and the ESR is normal. Where the history is suggestive, a length of temporal artery when examined serially may show the characteristic histology. High doses of steroids, e.g. 60 mg of prednisoline per day, should be given immediately the diagnosis is suspected.

(iv) Hypertensive encephalopathy (see p. 48).

(4) Herpes simplex encephalitis (HSE).[4,10]

(i) Here the headache is accompanied by 3–4 days of increasing irritability, altered level of consciousness, with behavioural and speech disturbances, and sometimes focal neurological signs, such as hemiparesis or seizures. There may be associated neck stiffness and, in the later stages, coma.

(ii) These symptoms are of course common to many causes of viral encephalitis, but focal lesions are more common with HSE. Also in HSE, percussion of the skull may demonstrate lateralised tenderness.

(iii) The CSF shows lymphocytosis, raised protein count and characteristically increased red cells.

(iv) Typically, temporal lobe involvement may be demonstrated by focal signs and symptoms and EEG abnormalities, radionuclide scan and CT scan changes.

(v) All the above may suggest the diagnosis to you. The diagnosis may be confirmed by:

(a) electron microscopy detection of virions in herpes simplex vesicles, which are, however, only rarely found in conjunction with HSE.

(b) brain biopsy, which is not now commonly undertaken, or retrospectively by a **rising** antibody titre to the herpes virus.

(vi) It is, however, unusual to be able to make a positive diagnosis, and treatment as outlined below should be given to any patient with encephalitis with or without focal clinical features, on the presumption that they have herpes simplex encephalitis.

(vii) Treatment, with i.v. acyclovir 10 mg/kg 8-hourly for 10 days has reduced the mortality to 19% at 6 months.

(viii) It is, of course, important to exclude other treatable non-viral diseases which mimic HSE. These include:

(a) Bacterial and fungal infections of the meninges, which you should identify on CSF findings.

(b) Space occupying lesions, such as brain abscess, and subdurals, the presence of which will be shown up on the CT scan.

(5) Subdural haematoma (see p. 204).

(6) Pituitary apoplexy (see p. 178).

REFERENCES

1 Davies P. (1987) Headache-including migraine. *Hospital Update* October, p. 763.

2 French G. *et al*. (1987) Diagnosis of tuberculous meningitis by detection of tuberculostearic acid in CSF. *Lancet* **ii:** 117.

3 Leader (1987) Steroids and meningitis. *Lancet* (1989) **ii:** 1307.

4 Leader (1986) Herpes simplex encephalitis. *Lancet* (1986) **i:** 535.

5 Lehrich J.R. (1982) Tuberculous meningitis. *N. Engl. J. Med.* **306:** 91.

6 Peltola H.O. (1982) C-reactive proteins for the rapid monitoring of infections of the central nervous system. *Lancet* **i:** 980.

7 Raman G. (1988) Meningococcal septicaemia and meningitis: a rising tide. *Br. Med. J.* **296:** 1141.

8 Riskind P.N. (1986) A case of pituitary apoplexy. *N. Engl. J. Med.* **314:** 229.

9 Schwartz M.N. (1984) Bacterial meningitis: more involved than just the meninges. *N. Engl. J. Med.* **311:** 912.

10 Whitley R. (1990) Viral encephalitis. *N. Engl. J. Med.* **323:** 242.

The acutely painful joint

(1) Your main objective in dealing with an acute painful joint is to exclude infection, as the consequences of delayed treatment of an infective arthropathy are disastrous.

(2) A septic arthritis gives rise to an acutely tender, swollen, reddened, hot, immobile joint (all the classic features of inflammation—calor, dolor, rubor and laesio functio are present). There is usually only a single joint involved, although a preceding flitting arthropathy is common in gonococcal arthritis. Here skin lesions, usually small papules on the trunk or limbs, and tenosynovitis are also common: 80% have positive genitourinary cultures, and this gram-negative coccus is the commonest infecting organism in the 16–40 age group; the frequency of other organisms in non-gonococcal infective arthritis is presented in Table 7.

(3) Joint infection usually occurs via haematogenous spread. Fifty per cent of patients have an obvious source for their infection—pneumonia, skin sepsis and gonorrhoea being the most common. Eighty per cent are pyrexial, although rigors are uncommon. Chronic joint disease, prosthetic joints, intra-articular injections, contiguous osteomyelitis or a deep wound all predispose toward joint infection.

(4) Other possible causes of an acutely inflamed joint or conditions that may cause confusion are:

(i) Crystal arthropathy, either gout or pseudogout. The crystals can be found in the joint fluid.

(ii) An inflammatory monoarthritis, usually a seronegative

Table 7 Organisms in non-gonococcal infective arthritis

Organism	Frquency (%)	Gram staining characteristics
Staphylococcus aureus	68	Gram+ve coccus
Streptococcus	20	Gram+ve coccus
Haemophilus influenza	1	Gram+ve bacillus
Gram-ve bacilli (various)	10	

arthropathy in association with Reiter's disease, inflammatory bowel disease, psoriasis and occasionally with rheumatoid, SLE or rheumatic fever. Evidence for the associated disease will usually be present.

(iii) Osteomyelitis. Here the pain is over the bone, rather than the joint.

(iv) Superficial cellulitis. The features of inflammation will be present, but joint movement will be relatively preserved, and the area of skin redness not necessarily locally confined to the joint.

(v) Haemorrhagic arthritis. Although pain and loss of function are prominent, other features of inflammation are not, and a history of trauma or bleeding disorders usual.

(vi) An acute episode supervening on chronic joint disease, usually rheumatoid arthritis. However, here if only one joint is involved, infection must be excluded as the cause (see (3) above).

(5) The above considerations should help with the diagnosis; the key investigation is joint aspiration and anaysis of the synovial fluid. Aspiration should be mandatory in any swollen joint where there is the faintest possibility of infection. You should aim to aspirate to dryness, as this not only relieves pain, but is said to improve long-term function.

(6) Synovial fluid should be analysed (Table 8).

Table 8 Analysis of synovial fluid

	Bacterial infection	Non-bacterial inflammation
Total leucocyte count	50 000–200 000 cells/mm^3 >90% polymorphs	>50 000 cells/mm^3 <50% polymorphs
Sugar	Low in 50% of cases	Usually normal, occasionally low in rheumatoid
Gram stain	+ve in 70%	−ve
Culture of joint fluid	+ve in the majority	−ve
Crystal	−ve	+ve in gout (uric acid) and pseudogout (calcium pyrophosphate)
Blood	−ve	+ve in haemorrhagic effusions

(7) Fifty per cent of patients suffering from infection in a joint have a total peripheral blood white cell count over 10 000/ml and 50% have positive blood cultures, both of which should therefore be undertaken.

(8) X-rays. These usually show non-specific soft tissue swelling, and are not immediately helpful.

TREATMENT

(1) Drainage. Repeated large bore needle aspiration, draining the joint completely, should be performed, twice daily if necessary.

(2) Antibiotics. There is no need for intra-articular antibiotics. Intravenous antibiotics should be used. If the gram stain is definitive be guided by this. If it is not, give i.v. penicillin 2 megaunits 6-hourly to the sexually active 16–40-year-old and a combination of gentamicin (see p. 350) and penicillin to the rest.

(3) Joint rest. In the acute phase the joint should be immobilised in an optimal functional position with a splint. Passive movements should be started as soon as pain allows.

(4) If the joint is inaccessible (as is the hip), you should consult with your orthopaedic surgical colleagues, as operative aspiration and drainage will probably be required.

FURTHER READING

1   Fraser S. *et al.* (1987) Acute arthropathies. *Hospital Update* December, p. 1039.

2   Goldenberg D.L., Reed J.I. (1985) Bacterial arthritis. *N. Engl. J. Med.* **312:** 764.

3   Leader (1986) Bacterial arthritis. *Lancet* **ii:** 721.

The acutely breathless patient

Consider the following causes.

(1) Left ventricular failure (see p. 43).
(2) Pulmonary embolus (see p. 52).
(3) Mitral stenosis (see p. 45).
(4) Cardiac tamponade (see p. 65).
(5) Asthma (see p. 80). and chronic obstructive airways disease (see p. 72).
(6) Acute respiratory tract infections (see p. 104).
(7) Pneumothorax (see p. 85).
(8) Large pleural effusion (see p. 95).
(9) Acute upper airways obstruction (see p. 92).
(10) Massive pulmonary collapse (see p. 90).
(11) Myasthenia (see p. 233).
(12) Acute infective polyneuritis (see p. 229).
(13) Overdose of salicylates, dinitrophenol or sulphanilamide (see p. 260).
(14) Overbreathing ostensibly due to anxiety (often called 'hysterical' overventilation).

Overbreathing due to anxiety

(1) This usually occurs in young women. The overbreathing may be far from obvious to the casual observer.

(2) The history is nearly always classical; first they felt breathless, then they had tingling, first around the mouth, then in the arm and legs; then they had cramps of the hands which took up the main d'accoucheur position. If sufficiently prolonged the patient may lose consciousness.

(3) You must aim to establish the sequence of events. In this condition anxiety precedes breathlessness, whereas in the other causes of breathlessness, the converse is usually the case.

(4) Emergency treatment is to persuade the patient to breathe in and out of a paper bag. This allows them to rebreathe their CO_2, lower the pH, reverse the alkalosis and relieve the tetany. This relieves most of the tension and is accompanied by massive verbal reassurance and, if necessary, sedation with 50 mg of chlorpromazine or 10 mg diazepam.

(5) Do not leave it at that—try to establish the precipitating cause. The anxiety may be due to a somatic or psychiatric condition for which the patient may need help.

(6) Do not forget that anxious overbreathing patients may also have taken an overdose of salicylates. Always test the blood for salicylates. In other states such as diabetic ketosis, the uraemic syndrome and encephalitis, the patient is obviously breathing abnormally deeply, but this is rarely attended by the distress which accompanies the above condition.

Social problems

Some people who arrive at casualty departments turn out to be unable to provide for themselves and are often referred to the medical team. They include:

(1) The frail elderly patient who does not require admission on strictly medical grounds.
(2) The patient who comes to casualty with a trivial illness, but is of no fixed abode.
(3) The mother who, as a result of contracting a minor illness, is unable to cope at home because of poor circumstances.
(4) The psychiatric patient who needs in-patient treatment, but will not come in.

The basic requirements enabling an individual to fend for himself are:

(1) Food.
(2) Money.
(3) Shelter and clothes.
(4) Companionship—in its widest sense.
(5) Mental stability (to the extent that they will neither harm themselves nor other people) and the ability to manage (1)–(4).

Help to provide for these requirements may be forthcoming from the following.

(1) Your hospital social worker, who should always be contacted first if possible.
(2) If you do not have one, or the problem arises at night and the social worker is unavailable, your local authority Social Services Department should provide a 24-hour social work service. Ring their duty officer for advice on:

   (i) Psychiatric problems. It is clearly wise to avail yourself of any local psychiatric help first, but this may not always be forthcoming. In any case you may need a social worker to help you to commit a patient against his will to hospital under the appropriate section of the Mental Health Act.

    (ii)   Problems with children. Your hospital may provide facilities for admitting young children with their mother—if not, it may be necessary that they be taken into care via the Social Services Department.

    (iii) The elderly. If the advice of a geriatrician is not easily available, social work advice regarding domiciliary services and/or residential accommodation is essential.

(3) Many areas have hostels run by the Department of Social Security (DSS), Social Services or voluntary organisations, e.g. The Salvation Army, for people of no fixed abode. Your casualty department will have the telephone number of these hostels, which, however, are under no obligation to take people. The DSS should provide for each area an emergency office which is open in the evenings for emergency payments or provision of hostel vouchers.

(4) The patient's general practitioner (if she has one) will be able to provide valuable background information and should be contacted, if available.

(5) The various voluntary organisations, for example, Samaritans, who provide a 24-hour supportive service for those in acute distress, such as potential suicides, or other similar organisations—Alcoholics Anonymous, Depressives Anonymous, Gingerbread (mainly daytime).

(6) The police, who

    (i)   can take children into emergency protection;

    (ii)   have powers to compulsorily detain someone who is mentally ill and who is a danger to themselves or others;

    (iii) are a source of information as to the whereabouts of local hostels.

(7) If these individuals or organisations cannot immediately help, the person should be admitted to hospital pro tem.

Central venous pressure and pulmonary artery occlusion catheter (Swan–Ganz)

Central venous pressure[3]

CVP measurements play an important role in many medical emergencies. This is now a standard technique in which careful attention to detail is necessary for reliable results to be obtained.

TECHNIQUE

(1) Your objective is to introduce an intravenous catheter into the superior vena cava. So introduce an intravenous catheter into a vein which will give you ready access to the superior vena cava. This is preferably done percutaneously. The veins most often used are the external or internal jugular or subclavian.

The position of the catheter **must** be checked after insertion by x-ray. If it is in the superior vena cava the level should rise and fall a few millimetres with expiration and inspiration. If it does not:

    (i)   it is not in a vein;
    (ii)   you are not far enough up the vein;
    (iii) the tip is angled against the vein wall—withdraw slightly;
    (iv) the catheter is partially blocked—flush out with 5 ml of sodium citrate;
    (v)   the catheter tip is in the right ventricle—the level is suspiciously high and pulsatile.

(2) The catheter is connected by a three-way stopcock to a water manometer. The scale should be zeroed against a fixed reference point on the patient who should, therefore, always be in the same position when the measurements are taken. The following values all apply to the horizontal patient lying supine.

Reference point	Normal values
5 cm dorsal from angle of Louis	1 to 8 cm
The angle of Louis	−4 to +3 cm

The reference point of 10 cm above the surface on which the patient is lying is not acceptable.

INTERPRETATION

(1) The measurement obtained reflects at least four variables:

  (i) intrathoracic pressure;
  (ii) efficiency of the right heart;
  (iii) venous tone; and
  (iv) volume of venous blood.

It may appear surprising, therefore, that useful results can be obtained at all. There variables are examined in more detail below.

- The gentle oscillation associated with respiration which was noted above, reflects change in the intrathoracic pressure.
- The efficiency of the right heart should not be compromised unless the circulation is being overloaded or there is myocardial disease. However, it is vital to remember that the CVP measures right atrial pressure and often fails to reflect left atrial pressure, particularly in the presence of myocardial disease. In these circumstances a patient may develop severe left ventricular failure without altering the CVP, so a pulmonary artery pressure line (with facilities for measuring pulmonary wedge pressure) should be set up wherever this is available (see p. 387).
- The fact that venous tone cannot be measured in the clinical situation neither refutes its existence nor dimishes its importance. The capacitance of the circulation is controlled by venous tone, which is therefore a primary influence upon CVP as a measure of the volume of venous blood. Venous tone is increased, for instance, by both catecholamine infusion and haemorrhagic shock. In these clinical circumstances, a relatively high CVP may be more a reflection of raised venous tone than adequate blood volume.
- In normal circumstances the venous system is readily distensible; venous tone may relax to the extent that a substantial increase of blood volume may produce no change in CVP. For these reasons a single recording of CVP is unlikely to be helpful in assessing and monitoring the replacement of blood volume. A series of readings is more likely to be informative, particularly if they are taken in response to rapid but small increments in blood volume. Specifically, if 200 ml of fluid is infused over 2 min, we recognise three patterns of response (see Fig. 25):

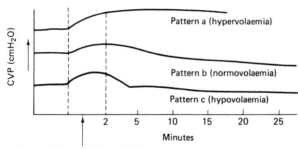

Fig. 25 Central venous pressure patterns of response to 200 ml of fluid infused over 2 min.

(a) A persistent rise of more than 3 cmH$_2$0 can be taken to exclude hypovolaemia and probably implies hypervolaemia (pattern a);

(b) A rise of 2–3 cm during the infusion with return to the base line at 15–20 min is characteristic of normovolaemia (pattern b);

(c) A rise of 2–3 cm during the infusion with return to the base line within 5 min is highly suggestive of hypovolaemia (pattern c).

(2) An initial reading of the CVP which is well within the normal range should not put you off performing this diagnostic/ therapeutic test because, as mentioned above, a high venous tone may raise the CVP and mask hypovolaemia.

(3) If hypovolaemia is suspected on clinical grounds careful expansion of the circulating volume with the CVP maintained a few cm above normal (but less than 10 cm above the angle of Louis, otherwise pulmonary oedema may be precipitated) should be tried. For details of which fluids to infuse see p. 338. An inital infusion in the setting of hypovolaemia may actually cause a slow fall of central venous pressure by inducing relaxation of the veins and allow infusion of more fluid. This gradual fall in CVP may also be observed in response to both vasodilators and steroids, or if an infusion of pressor amines is stopped.

(4) Where hypovolaemia has been confirmed:

(i)   Infuse fluid rapidly until the CVP rises into the upper half of the normal range. If this level is maintained for several hours the patient will become warmer and pinker, and will start to look better. A satisfactory urine output may also be restored (but be on your guard for acute renal failure) (see p. 153).

(ii) It is now reasonable to run the infusion at a normal rate and allow the CVP to fall. Should the CVP drop below normal, full fluid repletion has not taken place and an infusion rate sufficient to keep the CVP in the mid-normal range is required.

(iv) The deleterious effects of hypovolaemia are due to poor tissue perfusion. Although a low cardiac output is usually the primary cause of poor perfusion, the subsequent hypoxia produces locally and centrally mediated responses in the peripheral vasculature which aggravate the situation (see p. 335). Typically there is (a) arteriolar constriction producing a further reduction in tissue flow, and (b) venular dilatation which pools blood in the periphery reducing venous return and therefore cardiac output. Clearly the longer a patient remains hypovolaemic, the more firmly this vicious circle becomes established. For this reason the consequences of prolonged hypovolaemia can only be reversed by maintaining the CVP within or above the upper range of normal for several hours. Large volumes of up to 15–20 l may be required and can only be given safely with a reliable CVP line.

(v)   Any excess of water and electrolytes may be excreted after normal homeostasis has been restored without harmful effects.

OTHER USES

(1) In conditions where the problem concerns myocardial efficiency rather than hypovolaemia (e.g. myocardial infarction) a rise in CVP may give warning of impending heart failure. Remember that in these circumstances the CVP may not reflect left ventricular function, and that in any case a CVP line is no more than a jugular venous pulse with a college education.

(2) A sudden fall in the central venous pressure in a patient with

suspected gastrointestinal bleeding may herald further blood loss before this becomes clinically apparent (see p. 113).

(3) Prolonged intravenous feeding is only possible through a central venous pressure line, but you should wherever possible use enteral feeding.

(4) Blood sampling may be withdrawn through a central venous pressure line providing 20 ml is withdrawn first (and of course rejected) to clear the dead space.

COMPLICATIONS[1,2]

Although CVP measurements are of enormous help in situations of hypovolaemia and to a lesser extent myocardial infarction, venous catheters may be associated with complications and they should not therefore be used unless a definite therapeutic advantage is expected. The following complications have all been recorded.

(1) Thrombophlebitis. This is almost inevitable if the catheter is left in for more than 10 days and is probably due to mechanical irritation. The inflammation is rapidly settled by short-wave therapy but a blocked vein is inevitable and occasionally oedema of the upper arm results.

(2) Infection at the site of introduction. This is minimised by scrupulous aseptic technique. It is also a good idea to separate the sites of entry of the catheter through the skin and into the vein as far as possible.

(3) Infection of the catheter tip is less easily avoided and may give rise to septicaemia. At any rate, it is a wise precaution to culture the catheter tip after it has been removed.

(4) Erosion of the vein. If this is not recognised early it may cause widespread infusion of fluid into subcutaneous tissues, which is painful for the patient and may be dangerous if secondary infection occurs. If suspected, the catheter should be withdrawn.

(5) Arterial bleeding sufficient to cause tracheal obstruction is a potential complication of all jugular and subclavian puncture techniques.

(6) Pneumothorax is a specific complication of subclavian vein puncture.

(7) Catheter embolus into the right heart is known to occur if the

catheter is inadvertently broken at the site of entry to the skin. Surgical advice should be sought.

REFERENCES

1 Dunbar D. (1981) Aberrant location of central venous catheters. *Lancet* **i:** 711.
2 Kaye C. (1988) Complications of central venous cannulation. *Br. Med. J.* **297:** 572.
3 Leader (1974) Jugular venous pressure. *Br. Med. J.* **iv:** 367.

The pulmonary artery flotation (Swan–Ganz) catheter[1,3]

PULMONARY WEDGE PRESSURE

(1) Knowledge of the left and right atrial pressures is essential:[4]

    (i)   for the informed management of complicated acute right or left heart failure;

    (ii) to help the assessment of hypovolaemia, and thence the amount of fluid replacement required, in any critically ill patient; this is particularly useful if there is heart disease, when the usual relationship between the right and left atrial pressure may not obtain (see p. 383).

    (iii) To distinguish between non-cardiac and cardiac pulmonary oedema (see p. 44).

(2) It is also wise to have an arterial cannula for continuous monitoring of pressure and for blood gas analysis. Finally, cardiac output measurement, available if you use a catheter with a thermo dilution facility, provides all the information necessary to manage the most complex haemodynamic problems.

THE SWAN–GANZ CATHETER

Right atrial pressure is measured with a CVP line (see p. 384), while left atrial pressure is most conveniently measured using a flow-directed pulmonary artery catheter (Swan–Ganz catheter). This can be put in at the bedside without x-ray control. The left atrial pressure at which pulmonary oedema will appear is dependent on the serum albumin as an approximate index of the COP (see p. 337). A simple formula expresses the inter-relationship of serum albumin and the development of pulmonary oedema (see p. 43).

The catheter

The catheter has two lumens, one of which controls a balloon immediately behind the catheter tip, while the other opens as a single end-hole. The balloon has a dual function; during insertion it is blown up (with air or CO_2—make sure you know the correct amount) as soon as the catheter tip is in the right atrium. (The junction of the superior vena cava and the right atrium is at 15–20 cm from the usual insertion point—the internal jugular vein.) Thereafter the balloon acts as a sail, directing the catheter tip in the direction of maximal flow, i.e. through the tricuspid and pulmonary valves. Once the tip is in a small pulmonary artery, inflation of the balloon will occlude the artery proximally, leaving the end-hole exposed to the pulmonary capillary pressure (pulmonary wedge pressure), which is assumed to be identical with left atrial pressure.

Swan–Ganz catheters are usually available in two sizes:

7F with a 1.5 ml balloon
5F with a 0.8 ml balloon

We have found the larger size easier to manipulate and less likely to clot.

For cardiac output measurement, using the thermodilution technique, catheters are available with an additional injection lumen in the right atrium and two thermistors beyond, and so you can also use most catheters to measure CVP.

Catheter insertions

The catheter is usually inserted percutaneously into a large central vessel, either the internal jugular or subclavian. 7F catheters require a guide-wire technique; we use Desselet insertion sheaths. Remember to use a sheath one size larger than the catheter to allow for the deflated balloon. 5F catheters can be passed through large cannulae, e.g. a 12G. medicut, but a guide-wire technique is probably safer.

(1) Advance the catheter into the vein—say 10 cm—and connect to the transducer (see Measurement below).
(2) Blow up the balloon when the tip is in a central vein, preferably just at the junction of the vein and right atrium.
(3) Advance slowly allowing the catheter tip to be guided by flow. Except in conditions of very low flow, it is usually easy to cross the valves. If there is trouble crossing the pulmonary valve it is worth trying the balloon both deflated and inflated to get across. Sometimes loops form in the right atrium which

make manipulation difficult. Withdraw the catheter with the balloon blown up in order to straighten it out.

(4) Try to find a position which gives a good pulmonary artery tracing with the balloon deflated (Fig. 26b) and a good wedge pressure with it inflated (Fig. 26c). The right ventricular pressure tracing (Fig. 26a) is shown for comparison.

(5) X-ray the chest.

Measurement

The exact set-up will vary with the equipment available. Most equipment designed for continuous monitoring is pre-calibrated such that a given pressure change produces a set deflection on the scale. It therefore only remains to zero the transducer to atmospheric pressure. Some equipment may require both zero and calibration adjustment in which case it is necessary to adjust the calibration using a mercury column.

(1) The catheter is connected via a manometer line, a three-way tap and an Intraflo continuous flushing device to the transducer. The Intraflo is also connected to a pressure bag containing N saline and 500 units heparin.

(2) As the transducer is set up, exclude all air bubbles from the system.

(3) To zero the transducer:

    (i)   Close the tap between catheter and transducer (if this is not done, blood will flow back up the catheter into the transducer dome).

    (ii)   Open the tap on the side arm of the transducer to air.

    (iii) Adjust the tracing on the monitor to zero.

    (iv) Close the transducer side arm and open the transducer to the catheter; zero the transducer after it has warmed up—this will take about 30 min. Remember that the wave form used for catheter positioning does not have to be quantitatively accurate; we ordinarily put the catheter in first and then zero (and calibrate if necessary) afterwards.

    (v)   You should of course take expert advice if you are not familiar with these practicalities.

(4) Recordings are made:

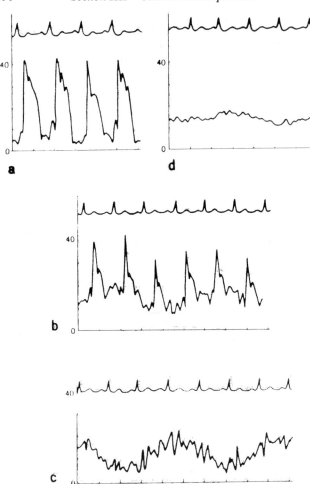

Fig. 26 Pressure tracings from the right heart. (**a**) Right ventricle.
(**b**) Pulmonary artery. (**c**) Pulmonary artery wedge pressure. (**d**) Damped
wedge pressure tracing. The pressure scale is in mmHg. The paper speed
is 25 mm/s with 10 mm spaces shown. The baseline variation in the
tracings is due to the effect of respiration. An ECG recording is also
displayed.

(i)   with the patient flat;
(ii) with the transducer at the level of the angle of Louis or mid chest (see CVP, p. 381)—this is most important;
(iii) of phasic and then mean pulmonary wedge pressure. The phasic nature of the recording is due to the pressure swings related to respiration, and it is the mean pulmonary wedge pressure which you should act on. (Many monitors produce a digital display of systolic, diastolic and mean pressures.)

(5) Before acting on a single or serial recording, it is essential to check their validity. Check:

(i)   Mechanical factors, such as the level of the transducer and the zero level.
(ii) (a) that there is recognizable wave form (see p. 390).
      (b) that there is respiratory variation of the wave form;
      (c) that the pulmonary artery trace returns on deflation of the balloon;
      (d) the pulmonary capillary wedge pressure should be less than the systolic pulmonary artery pressure, but similar to the diastolic PA pressure (see below).

If you have any reason to disbelieve the calibration of a preset machine, it is easy to attach a manometer line to the transducer side arm and produce a vertical column of water (13.5 cmH$_2$O = mmHg). Important decisions may be made on the basis of differences of less than 4 mmHg in the wedge pressure, that is 20% of the upper limit of normal. It is easy to make errors of this order in recording.

Problems

(1) 'Over-wedging'. Sometimes the catheter tip is lodged in a small pulmonary artery whose diameter is less than that of the balloon. As the balloon is blown up a wedge tracing appears and starts climbing continuously. If this happens, deflate the balloon, pull it back and then fill it slowly again, stopping as soon as the wedge appears. Make sure the trace rises and falls with respiration.
(2) Failure to wedge. Try repositioning the catheter. Alternatively, pulmonary artery diastolic pressure usually approximates to wedge pressure.

(3) Damped trace (Fig. 26d) and blocked catheters. This is the major problem with continuous monitoring.

  (i)   Check that there is no air in the system and that the transducer is not open both to air and to the patient.
  (ii) Try flushing the catheter using the fast flush mechanism on the Intraflo.
  (iii) Try a hand flush. Use a 1 ml syringe—being of narrow bore this generates the highest pressures. Make sure you flush only the catheter and not the transducer. Be careful not to introduce any air.

The catheter is more likely to block while the balloon is inflated. For this reason flush the catheter after each reading. If the trace does become damped it is important to try to clear it as soon as possible otherwise the catheter will become blocked.

(4) Positive end expiratory pressure (PEEP). Remember PEEP will add to the intrathoracic pressure and that PA and wedge recordings will be accordingly higher.

Complications[2]

These are infrequent.

(1) As in the insertion of any central line, damage to the lung or large arteries may occur. It is wise to do a chest x-ray after inserting the catheter.
(2) Arrhythmias related to the passage of the catheter may occur, and will require a standard therapeutic approach (see p. 26).
(3) The line may be a source of infection. It should be inserted with scrupulous aseptic technique, and removed as soon as possible.
(4) Pulmonary infarction is a hazard, particularly if there is persistent wedging of the catheter.
(5) Air embolism is said to be a hazard, which can be overcome by filling the balloon with CO_2.

REFERENCES

1   George R.J.D., Banks R.A. (1983) Bedside measurement of capillary wedge pressure. *Br. J. of Hosp. Med.* March, p. 287.

2   Leader (1983) Complications of pulmonary artery balloon flotation catheters. *Lancet* **1:** 37.
3   Shaver J.A. (1983) Hemodynamic monitoring in the critically ill. *N. Engl. J. Med.* **308:** 277.
4   Young D. (1990) Indications for pulmonary artery flow directed catheters. *Br. J. Hosp. Med.* **44:** 413.

Index

Doctors Stott and Robinson want this book to be as useful and informative as possible. If therefore you have any specific comments about the recommendations or advice contained in the book, please send your suggestions to the address below. Please indicate whether you wish your name to be made known to the authors.

Butterworth Heinemann Ltd
Linacre House, Jordan Hill, Oxford OX2 8DP